Clinical Approaches to Hospital Medicine

Kevin Conrad
Editor

Clinical Approaches to Hospital Medicine

Advances, Updates and Controversies

Second Edition

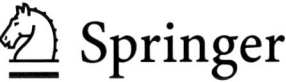

Editor
Kevin Conrad
Ochsner Health
New Orleans, LA, USA

ISBN 978-3-030-95163-4   ISBN 978-3-030-95164-1   (eBook)
https://doi.org/10.1007/978-3-030-95164-1

© The Editor(s) (if applicable) and The Author(s), under exclusive license to Springer Nature Switzerland AG 2022
This work is subject to copyright. All rights are solely and exclusively licensed by the Publisher, whether the whole or part of the material is concerned, specifically the rights of translation, reprinting, reuse of illustrations, recitation, broadcasting, reproduction on microfilms or in any other physical way, and transmission or information storage and retrieval, electronic adaptation, computer software, or by similar or dissimilar methodology now known or hereafter developed.
The use of general descriptive names, registered names, trademarks, service marks, etc. in this publication does not imply, even in the absence of a specific statement, that such names are exempt from the relevant protective laws and regulations and therefore free for general use.
The publisher, the authors and the editors are safe to assume that the advice and information in this book are believed to be true and accurate at the date of publication. Neither the publisher nor the authors or the editors give a warranty, expressed or implied, with respect to the material contained herein or for any errors or omissions that may have been made. The publisher remains neutral with regard to jurisdictional claims in published maps and institutional affiliations.

This Springer imprint is published by the registered company Springer Nature Switzerland AG
The registered company address is: Gewerbestrasse 11, 6330 Cham, Switzerland

*To the courage, commitment, and dedication
to duty of our frontline workers now
and always.*

Preface

Welcome to the second edition of *Clinical Approaches to Hospital Medicine: Advances, Updates and Controversies*.

As this text is completed, my colleagues and I are recovering from the devasting impact of Hurricane Ida. The rapidly intensifying storm made land fall as category 4 hurricane near New Orleans. Here, in southern Louisiana, we are ground zero for the effects of climate change and severe weather events. It is no longer an abstract concept. Climate change directly affects the practice of medicine in this region on a daily basis. After landfall of hurricane Ida, several regional hospitals and nursing homes were closed due to damage, and patients were urgently transferred to functioning locations. The impact on areas south of New Orleans was devastating and its recovering, including its healthcare infrastructure, will take years. Many of our most vulnerable patients were particularly impacted. Oxygen tanks ran out, dialysis centers lacked clean water, and nursing homes struggled to meet the basic needs of their residents. The fragile network that supports these patients was suddenly gone. As expected, our emergency rooms and hospital services were stretched beyond their capacity.

At the same time, in this region, the COVID-19 pandemic, at the time of this publication, is in its fourth and largest surge. I cannot imagine how either emergency alone could have been dealt with without the flexibility and adaptability of hospitalists. In our program, as with others, providers took extra shifts, missed family events, slept in the hospital, and traveled to whatever hospital they were needed. It is the nature of hospital medicine to fill the void in care and that is exactly what has happened over the past 2 years, but it has been a long 2 years. What once was an occasional event now seems to be routine.

If there was any doubt, hospital medicine has demonstrated its essential value to healthcare administration and the community. In a time of need, hospitalists stood up and delivered. This will not be the last pandemic or severe climate event. Possibly it is the beginning of a new way of functioning. One thing is certain, our current practices are not sustainable. Hospital medicine will accordingly need to plan for a new future. Into each program, emergency plans must be further refined, resiliency must be planned for, and sustainability must be built into the expected emergencies that are certain to come. After nearly 2 years of upheaval, we must contemplate that this is the new normal.

Our dedication has been tested, and in the short run we are surviving. The long-term implications are much less certain. Will these practice circumstances appeal to the new a bread of doctors or serve as a deterrent? I have been through several hurricanes in my career. The first one was exciting, the next few not so much. The same can be expected for all of the recent stressors. How will this impact us?

As with the first edition, the overall purpose of this text is not so much to be a reference book, but an in-depth review of timely topics. Feedback from the first edition provided some guidance in chapter selection. We have strived to include topics that are not only clinical but sit at the intersection of medicine and society. The consensus from the readers is that medicine can no longer function isolated from changes in society. Indeed healthcare providers must use their scientific background, communication skills, and perceived moral currency to be a force of change. The issues are just too large and urgent to ignore . For this reason, several chapters deal with societal issues.

In our region, and as in many, the single most common admission to the hospital service over the past 1.5 years has been COVID-19. Never has one disease so dominated our practice for such an extended time. We rapidly had to become experts in its management as well all of the nuances that has come with treating this highly infectious disease. Correct allocation of resources, infection control, and urgent palliative care all became emphasized in our daily practice. Treatment decisions had to be made with insufficient data and modified, sometimes based on daily feedback. The management of COVID-19 continues to evolve. In reviewing the chapter on COVID-19, I was struck by how our initial approach has changed. For those reasons, the COVID-19 chapter offers a snapshot of what COVID-19 strategies are currently employed and is not intended as reference. I expect that those strategies will continue to evolve and be far different form the treatment modalities presented in this text.

Since the first edition, rapid cultural change has impacted society and the practice of medicine. Gender, racial, and fair career advancement in the practice of medicine have all come to the forefront. Several chapters from a variety of viewpoints take aim at those issues.

In my last edition, I stressed it was important that we define what we do, do it well, and communicate our value to the healthcare community. Due to circumstances, I think this has been accomplished, faster than I could have imagined. Now it is our opportunity to utilize that accomplishment to establish a thriving specialty – one that is sustainable and has a vigorous academic output. In the past and at present, we have filled the gaps in care. We must expand beyond that. Now that our practice is viewed as essential, we have the ability to define our future. Let's take advantage of that.

I hope you enjoy this edition, and I welcome any feedback.

New Orleans, LA, USA Kevin Conrad

Acknowledgments

This book would not be possible without the contributions of the medical staff at Ochsner Health in New Orleans, Louisiana, and the University of Queensland Medical school in Australia. Their international educational collaboration over the past 10 years has served as a catalyst for the development of this project. Each institution has brought a unique perspective to the practice of medicine and has guided the overall theme of this text. I am appreciative of the chapter authors who have found the time in a very disruptive year to contribute their expertise.

I extend specific gratitude to my managing editors, Mounika Kandalam and Dileep Mandali, and chief managing editor Margaret Malone. I relied on their expertise, insight, and dedication to a difficult project. I believe the collaborative approach fostered by them has served the goal of providing an expansive and inclusive overview of hospital medicine and of social topics influencing the practice of medicine.

Contents

1 **Clinical Approaches to the COVID-19 Pandemic** 1
   Kristen M. Rogers, Marianne Maumus, Margaret Malone,
   Neiki Amiri-Rasavian, Safa Gul, Nupur Savalia, Brett Pearce,
   Angela J. Conway, and Sinead Brenner

2 **Management of Inflammatory Bowel Disease** 23
   Gregory Gaspard, Samir Hussaini, Dileep Mandali,
   and Ethan Lieberamn

3 **Updates in Nephrology for the Hospitalist** 41
   Juan Carlos Q. Velez, Santoshi M. Kandalam, Margaret Malone,
   Thomas Vu, Lukas Kuhnel, Dustin Chalmers, Jaye Frances Espinas,
   and Brett Pearce

4 **Heart Failure Management for the Inpatient Provider** 59
   Tripti Gupta, Vishak Venkataraman, and Sunny Dengle

5 **Advances in the Evaluation and Treatment of Sepsis and Shock** 71
   Kevin Conrad and Emily Kelsoe

6 **Current Trends in Stroke Management** 85
   Mohammad Moussavi and Kiana Moussavi

7 **Co-management of Orthopedic Patients** 99
   Allison Leonard, James Mautner, and Andrew Bennie

8 **Pediatric Hospital Medicine** 119
   Alexandra Wright and Margaret Malone

9 **Management of Psychiatric Disorders in the Hospital** 131
   Shilpa Amara and Brett Pearce

10 **Opioids: History, Pathophysiology, and Stewardship
   for Hospitalists** 151
   Marianne Maumus, Daniel Zumsteg, and Dileep Mandali

| 11 | Overview, Updates, and New Topics in Perioperative Care 179
Lakshmi N. Prasad Ravipati and Marisa Doran |
|---|---|
| 12 | Virtual Hospital Medicine 195
Charit Fares and Margaret Malone |
| 13 | Palliative Care for Hospitalists 201
Susan Nelson and Megha Koduri |
| 14 | Barriers to Advance Care Planning (ACP) in the Hospital:
A Review and Case Study. 213
Christian Goodwin and Kevin Conrad |
| 15 | Value-Based Care in the Hospital 225
Jason B. Hill, Santoshi M. Kandalam, and Sneha Panganamamula |
| 16 | Wellness in Physicians in the Era of the COVID-19 Pandemic 243
Kevin Conrad and Rula Saeed |
| 17 | LGBTQ Healthcare Issues. 255
Leise Knoepp and Olivia Mirabella |
| 18 | Racial Disparities in Healthcare 265
Veronica Gillispie and Ryan Abrigo |
| 19 | Gender and Racial Disparities in Career Advancement
in the United States. 275
Anna Garbuzov, Jessica Koller-Gorham, and Tamika Webb-Detiege |
| 20 | Research in Medicine 293
Tonchanok Intaprasert, Audrey Lim, and Rob Eley |
| 21 | Sustainability and Healthcare: Expanding the Scope
of "Do No Harm" Models of Success. 311
Kevin Conrad and Margaret Conrad |
| 22 | The Evolution of International Health: Lessons to Be Learned. 321
Rajasekaran Warrier, Haripriya Madabushi, Santoshi M. Kandalam,
Ahmed Noreddin, and Carl Kim |
| 23 | Update in Hospital Medicine: Trends in Compensation,
COVID-19, Workplace Environment and Malpractice. 339
Kevin Conrad |

Index. 349

Contributors

Ryan Abrigo The University of Queensland School of Medicine, Ochsner Clinical School, New Orleans, LA, USA

Shilpa Amara Ochsner Health, New Orleans, LA, USA

Neiki Amiri-Rasavian The University of Queensland Faculty of Medicine, Ochsner Clinical School, New Orleans, LA, USA

Andrew Bennie The University of Queensland Faculty of Medicine, Ochsner Clinical School, New Orleans, LA, USA

Dustin Chalmers University of Queensland School of Medicine - Ochsner Clinical School, New Orleans, LA, USA

Kevin Conrad Ochsner Health, New Orleans, LA, USA

Margaret Conrad Louisiana State University School of Medicine, New Orleans, LA, USA

Angela J. Conway The University of Queensland Faculty of Medicine, Ochsner Clinical School, New Orleans, LA, USA

Sunny Dengle University of Queensland School of Medicine, Ochsner Clinical School, New Orleans, LA, USA

Marisa Doran University of Queensland-Ochsner Clinical School, New Orleans, LA, USA

Rob Eley Emergency Department, Princess Alexandra Hospital, and Southside Clinical Unit, Faculty of Medicine, University of Queensland, Brisbane, QLD, Australia

Jaye Frances Espinas University of Queensland School of Medicine - Ochsner Clinical School, New Orleans, LA, USA

Charit Fares Hospital Medicine, Ochsner Health, New Orleans, LA, USA

Anna Garbuzov University of Queensland-Ochsner Clinical School, New Orleans, LA, USA

Gregory Gaspard Ochsner Health, New Orleans, LA, USA

Veronica Gillispie Women's Health, Ochsner Medical Center, New Orleans, LA, USA

Christian Goodwin University of North Carolina Medical School at Chapel Hill, Chapel Hill, NC, USA

Jessica Koller-Gorham Department of Surgery, Ochsner Health, New Orleans, LA, USA

Safa Gul The University of Queensland Faculty of Medicine, Ochsner Clinical School, New Orleans, LA, USA

Tripti Gupta Ocshner Health, New Orleans, LA, USA

Jason B. Hill Ochsner Medical Center - North Shore, Ochsner, New Orleans, LA, USA

Samir Hussaini University of Queensland- Ochsner Clinical School of Medicine, New Orleans, LA, USA

Tonchanok Intaprasert University of Queensland, Faculty of Medicine, Herston, QLD, Australia

Santoshi M. Kandalam University of Queensland, Faculty of Medicine, QLD, Australia

Emily Kelsoe The University of Queensland School of Medicine, Ochsner Clinical School, New Orleans, LA, USA

Carl Kim The University of Queensland-Ochsner Clinical School, New Orleans, LA, USA

Leise Knoepp Ochsner Health, New Orleans, LA, USA

Megha Koduri The University of Queensland School of Medicine, Ochsner Clinical School, New Orleans, LA, USA

Lukas Kuhnel University of Queensland School of Medicine - Ochsner Clinical School, New Orleans, LA, USA

Allison Leonard Hospital Medicine, Ochsner Health, New Orleans, LA, USA

Ethan Lieberamn University of Queensland- Ochsner Clinical School of Medicine, New Orleans, LA, USA

Audrey Lim University of Queensland, Faculty of Medicine, Herston, QLD, Australia

Contributors   xv

Haripriya Madabushi   Jawaharlal Nehru Medical College, Belgaum, India

Margaret Malone   The University of Queensland-Ochsner Clinical School, New Orleans, LA, USA

Dileep Mandali   The University of Queensland-Ochsner Clinical School, New Orleans, LA, USA

Marianne Maumus   Hospital Medicine, Ochsner Health, New Orleans, LA, USA

James Mautner   Orthopedics, Ochsner Health, New Orleans, LA, USA

Olivia Mirabella   University of Queensland School of Medicine, Ochsner Clinical School, New Orleans, LA, USA

Kiana Moussavi   The University of Queensland School of Medicine, Ochsner Clinical School, New Orleans, LA, USA

Mohammad Moussavi   Neurovascular Surgery, Northwell Health, Staten Island, NY, USA

Susan Nelson   Ochsner Health, New Orleans, LA, USA

Ahmed Noreddin   The University of Queensland-Ochsner Clinical School, New Orleans, LA, USA

Sneha Panganamamula   New York University, New York, NY, USA

Brett Pearce   The University of Queensland-Ochsner Clinical School, New Orleans, LA, USA

Lakshmi N. Prasad Ravipati   Perioperative Care Center, Ochsner Health, New Orleans, LA, USA

Kristen M. Rogers   Hospital Medicine, Ochsner Health, New Orleans, LA, USA

Rula Saeed   University of Queensland School of Medicine, Ochsner Clinical School, New Orleans, LA, USA

Nupur Savalia   The University of Queensland Faculty of Medicine, Ochsner Clinical School, New Orleans, LA, USA

Juan Carlos Q. Velez   Ochsner Clinical School / The University of Queensland, Brisbane, QLD, Australia

Department of Nephrology, Ochsner Health, New Orleans, LA, USA

Vishak Venkataraman   University of Queensland School of Medicine, Ochsner Clinical School, New Orleans, LA, USA

Thomas Vu   University of Queensland School of Medicine - Ochsner Clinical School, New Orleans, LA, USA

Rajasekaran Warrier The University of Queensland-Ochsner Clinical School, New Orleans, LA, USA

Tamika Webb-Detiege Department of Rheumatology, Ochsner Health, New Orleans, LA, USA

Alexandra Wright, MD Ochsner Hospital for Children, New Orleans, LA, USA

Daniel Zumsteg The University of Queensland School of Medicine, Ochsner Clinical School, New Orleans, LA, USA

Chapter 1
Clinical Approaches to the COVID-19 Pandemic

Kristen M. Rogers, Marianne Maumus, Margaret Malone, Neiki Amiri-Rasavian, Safa Gul, Nupur Savalia, Brett Pearce, Angela J. Conway, and Sinead Brenner

Introduction

In late 2019, reports emerged of a small cluster of cases of an acute respiratory illness in Wuhan, Hubei province, China. By February 2020, 20,471 cases in China had been reported, and the illness had been found in 26 other countries [1]. Coronavirus disease 2019 (COVID-19), caused by severe acute respiratory syndrome coronavirus 2 (SARS-CoV-2), would go on to be the worst pandemic in at least a century. As of this writing, there have been almost 208 million cases worldwide, with 4.3 million deaths [2]; by the time of publication, the numbers will almost certainly be higher.

The United States has seen the highest total case rate of COVID-19 in the world, at 112,451 cases per one million population [2]. As this continues to be a new and evolving situation, the authors understand that much of the following information and guidance may change. However, this chapter is an overview of our current knowledge of the characteristics, presentation, management, and special considerations of COVID-19 with an emphasis on inpatient care.

K. M. Rogers (✉) · M. Maumus
Hospital Medicine, Ochsner Health, New Orleans, LA, USA
e-mail: kristen.rogers@ochsner.org

M. Malone · B. Pearce
The University of Queensland-Ochsner Clinical School, New Orleans, LA, USA

N. Amiri-Rasavian · S. Gul · N. Savalia · A. J. Conway · S. Brenner
The University of Queensland Faculty of Medicine, Ochsner Clinical School, New Orleans, LA, USA

© The Author(s), under exclusive license to Springer Nature Switzerland AG 2022
K. Conrad (ed.), *Clinical Approaches to Hospital Medicine*, https://doi.org/10.1007/978-3-030-95164-1_1

Epidemiology

As of August 2021, over 200 million confirmed cases of COVID-19 have been reported, with cases on every continent [3]. It is believed that these counts underestimate the overall burden of COVID-19 as only a fraction of acute infections are diagnosed or reported [4]. Seroprevalence surveys suggest the rate of prior exposure exceeds the incidence of reported cases by approximately tenfold or greater [4]. Among adult populations in the United States, underrepresented racial and ethnic groups appear to have higher rates of infection [5]. Preexisting conditions disproportionately impact racial and ethnic minorities, and poorer patients are more likely to be exposed to the virus due to employment in essential industries and limited ability to telecommute or work from home [47]. Children, who make up 12–14% of all cases, are also seen to be affected more greatly in underrepresented racial and ethnic groups [6]. According to the American Academy of Pediatrics, children account for about 20% of newly identified cases each week; the majority of transmission occurs from household exposure [6].

The primary means of transmission of SARS-CoV-2 is via the direct person-to-person transmission of respiratory particles via large droplets and very fine aerosol particles [4]. Respiratory transmission appears to occur mainly through close-range contact of around six feet or less; the particles are produced by coughing, sneezing, or talking and are then inhaled by the uninfected person. Aerosol particles are small enough that they can remain suspended in the air for minutes to hours, and transmission of the virus from air farther than six feet from an infectious source is thought to be rare but can occur under specific circumstances, such as inadequate ventilation, prolonged exposure, or increased exhalation of particles (from coughing, exercise, singing) [4, 50]. Asymptomatic and presymptomatic transmission has been well documented [48]. Direct contact from contaminated hands which then touch the mucous membranes of the eye, nose, or mouth is another route of transmission. Fomite transmission from contaminated surfaces is not thought to contribute significantly to new infections though the virus can remain viable on surfaces for extended durations [4, 49]. Furthermore, although SARS-CoV-2 has been detected in non-respiratory specimens such as stool, other routes of transmission, such as fecal-oral or blood-borne, do not appear to be significant [4, 50].

Another factor to consider regarding transmission is the period of infectiousness and viral shedding. The incubation period is estimated to be between 4 and 7 days in most cases, with a range up to 14 days. The serial interval – the time between symptom development in one person and symptom development in a person they infect – appears to be between 3 and 8 days [51]. Viral shedding can be present 1–3 days prior to onset of symptoms and may persist for weeks after recovery, though longer durations are consistent with shedding of viral debris rather than live virus capable of transmission [52]. Transmission is unlikely to occur 10 days after symptom onset in individuals without underlying immunocompromise and who have had either asymptomatic infection or mild-to-moderate illness. For patients who have experienced severe or critical illness or who are immunocompromised, transmission of virus may occur for up to 20 days after symptom onset [53].

Virology

SARS-CoV-2 is a member of the coronavirus family. Coronaviruses are enveloped positive-stranded RNA viruses. SARS-CoV-2 is from the same subgenus as the severe acute respiratory syndrome (SARS-CoV-1) virus but a different clade [7]. The RNA sequence is similar to two bat coronaviruses, and bats are likely the primary source of this zoonotic disease; however, the means by which SARS-CoV-2 was initially transmitted to humans is still unknown [8]. SARS-CoV-2 and SARS-COV-1 use the same host receptor, angiotensin-converting enzyme 2 (ACE2). The viruses bind to ACE2 through the receptor-binding domain of its spike protein [9].

Since the start of the pandemic, SARS-CoV-2 has evolved. While some mutations have no impact on viral function, other variants have gained worldwide attention for their rapid emergence and greater risk of transmission. The new variants are named according to the Greek alphabet. The alpha variant (B.1.1.7 lineage) was first identified in the United Kingdom (UK) in late 2020. The alpha variant had more than a dozen mutations, including several specifically within the spike protein. Among these were the receptor-binding domain of the spike protein (N501Y) and a mutation which abuts the furin-cleavage site, an area thought to be involved in cell entry of SARS- CoV-2 [10]. The alpha variant is approximately 50% more transmissible than the original form of the virus [10]. There is also an increased severity seen in the alpha strain when examining hospitalization and case fatality rates [10].

The beta variant (B.1.351 lineage) was first identified in South Africa in late 2020. Data from South Africa showed that the variant rapidly became the dominant strain, showing the possibility of increased transmissibility. This pattern was then seen in other countries, including the United States [11]. This mutation is in another region of the spike protein (E484K) [11].

The gamma variant (P.1 lineage) was identified in Japan in travelers from Brazil. Studies showed that this variant accounted for 42% of specimens in the Amazonas states of Brazil [12]. There are several mutations, including a few in the spike protein receptor-binding domain (N501Y, E484K, and K417T) [12]. Both the beta variant and the gamma variant have been shown to have significant impact on neutralization by some monoclonal antibody therapies [13].

The delta variant (B.1.617.2 lineage) was first identified in India in December 2020 and has become the most prevalent variant in India as well as in the United States and UK [14]. Even more transmissible than the alpha variant, studies showed that such a large proportion of new SARS-CoV-2 infections were caused by delta that the alpha variant decreased. Furthermore, reports state that delta is associated with higher risk of hospitalization than alpha [15].

Presentation

Children

Overall, COVID-19 appears to be milder in children than adults, but that does not exclude children from having severe cases [16]. A systematic review showed that symptoms in children may be unrecognized prior to diagnosis. However, in a case surveillance of 5188 children aged 0–9 years who tested COVID-19 positive, over 60% had either fever, cough, or shortness of breath, while 10% had myalgia, 15% had headaches, and 14% had diarrhea [17]. Other symptoms included rhinorrhea, sore throat, nausea, vomiting, and abdominal pain. Only 1% had loss of smell or taste. Children aged 10–19 years had similar symptoms; however, up to 10% had loss of smell or taste and up to 42% had headache [17]. A meta-analysis of 9335 children showed that fever was the most significant symptom, but other symptoms (excluding earlier list) included Kawasaki-like symptoms, conjunctivitis, and pharyngeal erythema [18]. Multisystem inflammatory syndrome in children (MIS-C) has been reported in pediatric cases of COVID-19. This condition presents similarly to Kawasaki disease and/or toxic shock syndrome. Symptoms include persistent fever, hypotension, myocarditis, and rash; the diagnosis is supported by increased inflammation on laboratory findings [19]. MIS-C is more thoroughly discussed in the Chap. 8.

Adults

For adult patients, fever, cough, myalgia, and headaches are the most commonly reported symptoms (20). Diarrhea, fatigue, anorexia, sore throat, and loss of smell/taste are also common. Symptomatic infections may range from mild to critical, with dyspnea, hypoxemia, pneumonia, acute respiratory distress syndrome, dysrhythmia, cardiomyopathy, acute renal failure, neurologic complications, thromboses, and more [54]. Table 1.1 classifies presentation from mild to critical based on symptoms.

Admission Criteria

One of the hallmarks of managing patients with COVID-19 is determining whether inpatient or outpatient care is appropriate and understanding disease severity to provide treatment accordingly.

In terms of disease severity, mild disease consisting of fever, malaise, cough, or upper respiratory symptoms, without evidence of respiratory failure, typically does not require hospitalization [20, 25]. Presence of lower respiratory symptoms such as

Table 1.1 Classification of COVID-19 symptoms, adapted from NIH [25]

Classification	Signs/symptoms	Site of care
Mild	Any of the various symptoms of COVID-19 (including fever, malaise, cough, sore throat, diarrhea) without hypoxemia, dyspnea, or abnormal chest imaging	Outpatient
Moderate	Evidence of lower respiratory disease (chest imaging, dyspnea, cough) but with $SpO_2 \geq 94\%$ on room air	Evaluate in emergency department Consider admission or observation on a case-by-case basis
Severe	Evidence of severe respiratory illness with any of these findings: SpO_2 <94% on room air Respiratory rate >30 breaths/min PaO_2/FiO_2 <300 mmHg Lung infiltrates >50%	Admit to hospital
Critical	Respiratory failure, septic shock, and/or multiple organ dysfunction	Admit to hospital

dyspnea raises concern for at least moderate severity disease [20]. General indications for emergency department evaluation and hospital admission include one or more of the following features: severe dyspnea, peripheral oxygen saturation on ambient air of ≤94%, or significantly altered mental status or other symptoms of hypoperfusion or hypoxia (e.g., falls, hypotension, cyanosis, anuria, chest pain) [20]. In addition to clinical considerations, there are social factors that might support earlier hospitalization such as patients in settings with more limited outpatient resources [20]. Patients may have infiltrates on chest imaging and still be considered to have moderate disease, but hypoxemia (oxygen saturation ≤94% on ambient air) and the need for supplemental oxygenation or ventilatory support indicate severe disease. In the United States, the National Institute of Health (NIH) suggests hospitalization for patients with any of the following: an oxygen saturation of <94% on room air, respiratory rate of >30 breaths/minute, PaO_2/FiO_2 <300 mmHg, or lung infiltrates >50% [20].

COVID-19 Management

General Therapy Guidelines

There are several important aspects to consider regarding therapy for COVID-19 including but not limited to severity of disease, possible or confirmed coinfection, comorbidities, and ongoing investigations into the efficacy of novel treatments. It is also important to understand the pathophysiology of COVID-19. The earlier stage of the disease course is primarily driven by replication of SARS-CoV-2 [20]. The later stage is driven by an exaggerated immune/inflammatory response to the virus that leads to extensive tissue damage. Based on this, it is understood that antiviral therapies have the greatest benefit early in the disease course, while immunosuppressive/anti-inflammatory therapies are more efficacious in the later stages of infection.

For both ambulatory and hospitalized patients who do not require supplemental oxygen, the NIH strongly recommends [AIIa] against use of dexamethasone or other glucocorticoids [25]. Remdesivir is approved for use in hospitalized patients only, not in the ambulatory population. In hospitalized patients with mild to moderate disease, there is not sufficient data to support or refute routine use of remdesivir, but it may be considered in patients who are classified as high risk of deterioration or disease progression [25]. In hospitalized patients with severe or critical disease, it is recommended to use one of the following options: remdesivir, dexamethasone plus remdesivir, or dexamethasone [25].

Hydroxychloroquine and chloroquine received an initial emergency use authorization (EUA) from the United States Food and Drug Administration (FDA) for treatment of patients with COVID-19. In June 2020, the FDA revoked its emergency use authorization (EUA) for these agents, given lack of clear benefit and potential toxic side effects [21]. It is recommended that hydroxychloroquine or chloroquine not be used to treat COVID-19 patients.

Dexamethasone and Other Corticosteroids

Dexamethasone or other systemic glucocorticoids should be used in COVID-19 patients with severe illness who require supplemental oxygenation or mechanical ventilation to maintain SpO2 ≥94%. Patients should be closely monitored for adverse effects such as opportunistic infection and hyperglycemia. Prophylactic treatment with ivermectin should be considered for patients at high risk of *Strongyloides*, most notably those from endemic tropical or subtropical regions. Typical therapy with dexamethasone is 6 mg IV or oral daily. Duration of therapy with corticosteroids should not exceed 10 days [25]. NIH does not recommend either for or against the use of inhaled corticosteroids (e.g., budesonide) in the management of COVID-19 [25].

Remdesivir

Remdesivir is an antiviral therapy that inhibits viral replication and has in vitro activity against SARS-CoV-2. It is the only drug approved by the FDA for treatment of COVID-19 in hospitalized adults and children 12 years or older. The recommended adult dose is 200 mg intravenously (IV) on day 1 followed by 100 mg IV daily for 5 days total or until the patient is stable for discharge, whichever is sooner. Remdesivir is not recommended in patients with an estimated glomerular filtration rate (eGFR) <30 mL/min per 1.73 m^2 because of potential for renal accumulation and toxicity unless the benefit outweighs the risk. Liver enzymes should be checked before and during remdesivir administration; alanine aminotransferase elevations >10 times the upper limit of normal should prompt consideration of remdesivir discontinuation. The optimal role of remdesivir remains uncertain, and some guideline panels (including the World Health Organization) suggest not using it in hospitalized patients because there is no clear evidence that it improves patient-important outcomes for hospitalized patients. In a meta-analysis of four trials that included over 7000 patients with all severities of COVID-19, remdesivir did not reduce mortality (OR 0.9, 95% CI 0.7–1.12) or need for mechanical ventilation (OR 0.90, 95% CI 0.76–1.03) compared with standard of care or placebo [35, 41].

Antibody Therapy

Convalescent plasma obtained from individuals who have recovered from COVID-19 may provide passive antibody-based immunity [23, 24]. Convalescent plasma has potential clinical benefit when given early in the course of disease and may have notable value for individuals with antibody production deficiencies [23, 24]. However, there is a lack of evidence for use of convalescent plasma in patients with severe or critical disease [23, 24]. In the United States, EUA has been granted for high-titer convalescent plasma among hospitalized patients with COVID-19 who are early in the course of disease or have impaired humoral immunity [23, 24]. Nonetheless, treatment of hospitalized patients with convalescent plasma is not recommended outside of clinical trials [23, 24].

Anti-SARS-CoV-2 monoclonal antibodies including bamlanivimab, sotrovimab, and casirivimab-imdevimab have each received EUAs from the FDA for treatment of nonhospitalized high-risk patients age >12 years with mild-to-moderate COVID-19. The NIH recommends use of a monoclonal antibody infusion to treat nonhospitalized patients with mild or moderate COVID-19 who are at high risk of progression and for postexposure prophylaxis in high-risk individuals [25]. SARS-CoV-2 variants (alpha, beta, gamma, delta) have shown marked differences in susceptibility to the authorized monoclonal antibodies, and choice of agent should be tailored to the prevalent SARS-CoV-2 variant at the time of therapy [25].

Other Therapies

Baricitinib (a Janus kinase inhibitor) and tocilizumab (an interleukin-6 inhibitor) are immunomodulators which have shown some mortality benefit in severe and critical COVID-19, and either may be used as adjunctive therapy for hospitalized severely ill patients. NIH recommends against the use of baricitinib in combination with tocilizumab due to the elevated risk of opportunistic infection [25]. Baricitinib is an oral medication which is dose-dependent on renal eGFR. Duration of therapy is up to 14 days or until the patient is ready for hospital discharge, whichever is sooner. Tocilizumab is dosed as a single IV dose 8 mg/kg of actual body weight, and a second dose may be considered if no clinical improvement is observed in the first 8 hours after therapy. NIH recommends against the use of JAK inhibitors other than baricitinib and tofacitinib (e.g., ruxolitinib) and against the use of IL-6 monoclonal antibodies (siltuximab).

Hospitalized patients with COVID-19 should receive routine prophylactic dose anticoagulation for prevention of venous thromboembolism (VTE), unless contraindicated. Patients on full-dose anticoagulation for chronic medical conditions or acute indications should continue therapy. Clinical trials (ATTACC) are ongoing to investigate the role of higher-than-prophylactic dose anticoagulation and antiplatelet agents in hospitalized patients with COVID-19. NIH recommends against the use of anticoagulants or antiplatelets for COVID-19 in nonhospitalized patients or in patients who are discharged from the hospital [25–27].

Since the onset of the pandemic, numerous therapies have been proposed and investigated for the management of COVID-19 but have failed to show efficacy in clinical trials while demonstrating potential for harm. Additionally, several medications have been proposed as having a potential role in the severity of COVID-19 and are routinely discontinued upon diagnosis.

NIH does not recommend either for or against SARS-CoV-2-specific immunoglobulins, GM-CSF inhibitors (granulocyte-macrophage colony-stimulating factor inhibitors), vitamin C, vitamin D, zinc, or fluvoxamine (SSRI). NIH recommends against the use of the following specifically for the treatment of COVID-19: chloroquine/hydroxychloroquine, zinc dosed above dietary recommendations, azithromycin, ivermectin, colchicine, interferons, nonspecific intravenous immunoglobulin (IVIG, non-SARS-CoV-2 specific), Bruton's tyrosine kinase inhibitors (e.g., ibrutinib), lopinavir/ritonavir and other HIV protease inhibitors, IL-6 monoclonal antibodies (siltuximab), interleukin-1 inhibitors (canakinumab, anakinra), low-titer convalescent plasma, statins, ACE inhibitors or angiotensin receptor blockers, famotidine, or nitazoxanide [25]. NIH recommends against the routine discontinuation of a patient's inhaled corticosteroids, statins, NSAIDs, acid-suppressive therapy (PPI, H2RA), ACE inhibitors, or ARBs specifically for COVID-19 unless otherwise warranted by clinical condition.

Treatment of Coinfections

The clinical features of seasonal influenza and COVID-19 overlap, and coinfection with both is possible. The NIH recommends empiric therapy for influenza for patients hospitalized with suspected or documented COVID-19 in locations where influenza virus is prevalent [25]. Antiviral therapy for influenza should be discontinued if molecular testing for influenza is negative from upper respiratory tract specimens in non-intubated patients and from both upper and lower respiratory tract specimens in intubated patients [25].

For patients with documented COVID-19, empiric therapy for bacterial pneumonia is not recommended because bacterial superinfection does not appear to be a prominent feature of infection [25]. Empiric treatment for bacterial pneumonia may be reasonable in patients with documented COVID-19 if there is clinical suspicion for concomitant bacterial infection. If empiric antibiotic therapy is initiated, a microbial diagnosis should be made (e.g., sputum Gram stain and culture or urinary antigen testing), and the need to continue antibiotic therapy should be reevaluated regularly.

Management of Complications

Complications of COVID-19 are varied and may include secondary bacterial pneumonia, pulmonary embolism, or myocardial inflammation. For patients who have experienced cardiopulmonary symptoms during their disease course, a computed tomography (CT) scan of the chest can be performed at 12 weeks if radiographic imaging shows persistent abnormalities [25]. This timeline is variable considering that patients may have other underlying factors for disease, for example, malignancy or interstitial lung disease. Cardiac testing should include an electrocardiogram (ECG), and if needed, extended Holter monitoring. Transthoracic echocardiograms (TTE) are not routinely performed unless there is a suspicion for myocarditis. Management for cardiopulmonary symptoms includes optimization of any current medications, breathing exercises including incentive spirometry and awake self-proning, and consideration of steroids, particularly in cases of organizing pneumonia [21].

Acute respiratory distress syndrome (ARDS) is another significant complication of COVID-19. ARDS presents in approximately 42% of patients with COVID-19 pneumonia, with a majority of these patients requiring intensive care [22]. Management for ARDS due to COVID-19 focuses on ventilation, with particular success with prone positioning, which allows homogenous aeration of the lungs [22]. Success with prone ventilation is seen when it is initiated early in the disease course and for >12 hours per day [22]. The Society for Critical Care Medicine recommends therapy with supplemental oxygen to maintain SpO_2 92–96%, which can be administered via nasal cannula, face mask, high-flow nasal cannula, or noninvasive positive pressure ventilation (NIPPV) with the use of appropriate safety measures and personal protective equipment (PPE). Intubation and mechanical ventilation may be considered if clinical worsening occurs [56].

Severe acute kidney injuries (AKI) have been found in 20–31% of COVID-19 patients, particularly in those who require mechanical ventilation [24]. Standard management for AKI should be initiated in these patients, for example, avoidance of nephrotoxic agents, optimization of volume, and consideration of renal replacement therapy [28]. One study found that patients who develop AKI from COVID have a low recovery rate when compared to non-COVID AKIs, with a third of patients not recovering to their baseline kidney function [29].

Diabetic ketoacidosis has been observed in some patients without a prior diagnosis of diabetes, either during infection with COVID-19 or weeks to months after the resolution of symptoms [24]. Testing for type 1 diabetes autoantibodies should be obtained for patients without type 2 diabetes risk factors. Patients can also present with incidental thyrotoxicosis due to COVID-induced thyroiditis [24]. These patients can be treated with corticosteroids but should also be evaluated for new-onset Graves' disease.

COVID-19 is associated with coagulopathy and thrombotic events, and investigations are ongoing to determine if these events occur at higher-than-expected rates [30]. One study showed that COVID-19 has similar rates of thrombosis as hospitalized patients with identical levels of critical illness [31]. Initial elevated D-dimer levels as well as elevated inflammatory markers are associated with bleeding complications, thrombosis, and death [31]. On August 4, 2021, the New England Journal of Medicine published results of the ATTACC trial, which provided evidence that full-dose anticoagulation in severely ill (but not critically ill) hospitalized patients may reduce the progression to organ support, such as mechanical ventilation, and improved patient's chances of leaving the hospital. At this time, NIH and other guideline bodies continue to recommend routine prophylactic dose anticoagulation for prevention of venous thromboembolism (VTE) in hospitalized COVID-19 patients, unless contraindicated. NIH recommends against the use of anticoagulants or antiplatelets for COVID-19 in nonhospitalized patients or in patients who are discharged from the hospital [25].

Discharge from the Hospital

Similar to most other health conditions, the guidelines for discharging a patient with COVID-19 vary on a case-by-case basis at the discretion of the medical provider and team.

Requirement for infection control should not prevent discharge if the patient can appropriately self-isolate at home. Patients older than 65 years, those with underlying medical comorbidities, and those being discharged to a nursing facility have been associated with an increased risk of readmission following hospitalization [25]. Patients with COVID-19 should receive outpatient follow-up via telehealth or an in-person visit following discharge from the hospital. Vaccination should be considered prior to hospital discharge for all patients, including those hospitalized with COVID-19. Contraindications to vaccination prior to hospital discharge include receipt of antibody therapy (convalescent plasma or monoclonal antibodies sotrovimab and casirivimab-imdevimab). For those who have received passive antibody therapy, vaccination can be administered after 90 days.

Vaccination

Vaccination is the most effective way to prevent SARS-CoV-2 infection and COVID-19 disease and complications [46]. Two mRNA vaccines (Pfizer-BioNTech BNT162b2 and Moderna mRNA-1273) are available. BNT162b2 is a two-dose series FDA approved for individuals aged 16 years and older. The FDA has issued an EUA for BNT162b2 for individuals 12 years and older, for the two-dose Moderna mRNA-1273 series in individuals 18 years and older, and for a single-dose human adenovirus vector vaccine (Johnson & Johnson/Janssen) Ad25.COV2.S for those 18 years and older.

In large placebo-controlled trials, the two-dose mRNA vaccines have shown >90% effectiveness for preventing symptomatic COVID-19 and >95% effectiveness at preventing severe COVID-19 after completion of the two-dose series. The single-dose Ad25.COV2.S was 66% effective in preventing moderate to critical COVID-19.

CDC has recommended a third dose vaccine booster for individuals who have received either of the mRNA vaccines for several populations. For immunocompromised people (active cancer treatment, organ or stem cell transplant recipient, immunodeficiency conditions, or treatment with immunosuppressants), CDC recommends a third dose of the same mRNA vaccine product at least 28 days after the second dose of either BNT162b2 or mRNA-1273 [25]. For people who have received either of the mRNA vaccines who are over 65 years, people age 18 or older who reside in long-term care, have underlying medical conditions, or who work in high-risk settings, CDC has recommended a booster dose of the same mRNA vaccine (BNT162b2 or mRNA-1273) 6 months or more after the initial series. For individuals who received the single-dose Ad25.COV2.S, CDC recommends booster doses after two months for those 18 years and older [55].

Special Considerations

Psychiatric Complications of COVID-19

The COVID-19 pandemic has been linked with the presentation of psychiatric sequela both patients affected by COVID-19 as well as health-care workers caring for those affected. This section aims to serve as a concise presentation of some of the data regarding possible cognitive and psychiatric side effects, both acute and chronic, associated with the COVID-19 pandemic, as well as to highlight the need for more research in this area.

While currently limited by the sparse number of studies directed at the psychiatric sequelae of the ongoing COVID-19 pandemic, retrospective and cross-sectional studies as well as analysis of past coronavirus pandemics suggest that individuals with COVID-19, as well as health-care workers, are at an increased risk of experiencing psychiatric symptoms [32, 33].

Little information is available regarding long-term psychiatric complications among patients affected by COVID-19. However, analysis of previous coronavirus pandemics, specifically Middle East respiratory syndrome (MERS) and severe acute respiratory syndrome (SARS), suggests that a significant number of patients affected by COVID-19 will develop psychiatric disorders or symptoms during the course of their disease [34]. Among patients hospitalized with MERS or SARS, there was a greater than 5% chance of experiencing any of the following: aggression, altered consciousness, auditory hallucinations, confusion, and memory impairment. Additionally, it may be possible that the existence of a preexisting psychiatric illness may lead to the development of novel comorbid psychiatric disorders or symptoms [35]. Furthermore, there may be an association between the severity of COVID-19 infection and the development of psychiatric symptoms. A meta-analysis of critically ill patients being treated for various illnesses revealed that 1 year after treatment, 20–40% reported the manifestation of clinically significant symptoms, including anxiety, post-traumatic stress disorder (PTSD), and symptoms of depression [36].

While there may not be an abundance of data demonstrating the long-term psychiatric effects of COVID-19, there have been multiple studies demonstrating some of the acute neurologic and psychiatric complications. Especially in the acute phase of COVID-19, there appears to be an association between infection and the development of neuropsychiatric symptoms. In a study with 144 infected patients, it was found that anxiety was present in 35% of participants while depressive symptoms were present in 28% [37]. Additionally, a retrospective analysis involving 214 patients hospitalized with COVID-19 demonstrated central nervous system manifestations in 25% [38].

Health-care workers exposed to COVID-19 may also experience psychiatric symptoms. A cross-sectional study consisting of over 1200 physicians, nurses, and other frontline health-care personnel operating from hospitals in China showed the following prevalence of symptoms: anxiety 45%, depression 50%, insomnia 34%, and traumatic stress 71% [32]. Additionally, a review of 59 studies regarding viral outbreaks (including past SARS and current COVID pandemics) was undertaken in order to identify protective factors and risk factors for the development of psychiatric symptoms. The strongest identified risk factor for the development of psychiatric symptoms was found to be the degree of contact with affected patients. Other risk factors included prior history of a psychiatric disorder and a perceived lack of organizational support [39]. On the other hand, the strongest protective factor was access to adequate personal protective equipment (PPE). Other protective factors included adequate time off from work and supportive peers [39]. This highlights the importance of organizational structure in employee mental health.

The COVID-19 pandemic appears to be responsible for a number of psychiatric complications in multiple populations. Therefore, it is important to determine effective ways of mitigating or treating the psychiatric sequelae of this pandemic. As a general paradigm, "stepped care" may be an effective way to distribute care in a cost-efficient manner. This principle relies on using the fewest possible resources to the greatest effect and is accomplished by delivering the least resource-heavy option first before "stepping up" to more intensive treatment. For example, individuals experiencing a mild degree of symptoms may benefit from self-help (whether clinician-guided or pure self-help), cognitive behavioral therapy (CBT), group therapies, or the option of seeing a mental health professional if the individual has additional concerns.

For individuals with moderate or severe psychiatric symptoms, more intensive treatments such as interpersonal therapy and counseling are available based on the discretion of either the general practitioner or a mental health professional.

Antenatal Care and Pregnancy Issues

Changes to Regular Prenatal Care

Patients should be assessed based on their pregnancy risk factors, including comorbidities, and the necessity of in-person visits [40]. Modifications to the regular prenatal care schedule involve reducing the number of in-person visits, laboratory tests, and ultrasounds or scheduling appointments in groups that would occur during the same visit or on the same day. Patients could opt to perform their genetic screening using cell-free DNA blood screening instead of the combined screening method to reduce lab and office visits. Additionally, those with telehealth capabilities and home blood pressure cuffs can take their blood pressure measurements at home and see their clinician through telehealth to reduce in-person visits.

Unvaccinated women can also safely receive the COVID-19 vaccine before or during pregnancy, especially if they are at higher risk of exposure to the virus or at a higher risk of having severe disease. If vaccination is performed while pregnant, it may be administered with other routine vaccinations without requiring a time separation [40].

Implications for Pregnant and COVID-19-Positive Patients

Women should not alter reproductive decisions based on COVID-19 concerns as congenital infection is unlikely. In utero and intrapartum transmission or ascending infection is uncommon. Similarly, the risk of first- or second-trimester miscarriages does not appear to be increased [40].

There are mixed data regarding the rate of stillbirth. Data from 12 countries, including the United States and UK, reported similar rates of intrauterine fetal death rates in those with confirmed or suspected infection and national population-based data. However, another study in the United States showed the stillbirth rate in pregnant patients hospitalized with COVID-19 was approximately 3%, compared to 0.4–0.5% among the overall population [40]. This increase is generally attributed to severe and critical maternal illness, disruptions in prenatal care, or a higher incidence of home birth. Transient elevations in lupus anticoagulant levels have also been found in patients with COVID-19. Because the rate of stillbirth is generally quite low, the increase may simply be because of sensitivity to random variation [40].

Classification of disease severity follows the NIH categories for nonpregnant women. Pregnant women are more likely to be asymptomatic than nonpregnant women of reproductive age. For those that are symptomatic, common symptoms are comparable to nonpregnant women and include cough, headache, myalgias, fevers, sore throat, and shortness of breath [41]. As some of these symptoms overlap with common pregnancy complaints, it is important to consider COVID-19 in afebrile symptomatic patients. Similarly, laboratory and chest imaging reveal similar results in pregnant and nonpregnant patients. Elevated C-reactive protein, lymphopenia, and leukocytosis are the three most common findings from blood work, with ground-glass opacities in the lungs found on CT [41].

Pregnancy does not increase the risk of acquiring COVID-19 infection but appears to worsen the clinical course of infection. While over 90% of infected pregnant women will recover from infection without requiring hospitalization, patients may deteriorate rapidly. Symptomatic pregnant patients are at increased risk of severe disease and death, while women greater than 35 years of age or with obesity or preexisting medical conditions are at the highest risk of adverse outcomes. CDC reports found pregnant women are at increased risk of ICU admission, invasive ventilation, ECMO requirement, and death compared to nonpregnant women [40]. Complications from infection are comparable to nonpregnant women. Therefore, pregnant hospitalized patients with severe or critical disease should be cared for by a multispecialty team at a facility with obstetric services and an adult ICU.

Patients should be admitted to the hospital if they develop a comorbid condition that requires admission, fever >39C resistant to acetaminophen, or symptoms of moderate, severe, or critical disease [42].

Respiratory support for patients with severe disease should be focused on maternal oxygenation saturation remaining at or above 95% or maternal PaO_2 greater than 70 mmHg to maintain a favorable diffusion gradient across the placenta. Prone positioning, often used in the ICU for patients with severe disease, may be used in pregnant patients in the latter half of pregnancy as long as padding is placed above and below the uterus to avoid aortocaval compression [40].

The preferred treatment for fevers and pain is acetaminophen although NSAIDs may be used at the lowest effective dose and require monitoring for fetal complications, such as oligohydramnios or premature closure of the ductus arteriosus. In patients who meet the criteria for use of glucocorticoids for treatment of COVID-19 and to induce fetal lung maturity, the usual doses of dexamethasone (4 doses of 6 mg intravenously, 12 hours apart) may be used [40].

Primary antiviral treatment should start with remdesivir, which may be used without restriction in COVID-positive pregnant patients. Baricitinib, a JAK inhibitor often used with remdesivir in hospitalized patients, along with tocilizumab and sarilumab, IL-6 antagonists used with dexamethasone inpatient, should only be used after shared decision-making has occurred with the patient. They are not recommended for primary treatment as there is a concern for placental transfer, and their use should be considered after comparing the maternal benefit to fetal risks, such as increased rate of preterm birth [43]. Ribavirin should be completely avoided as it is a known teratogen [40].

Prophylactic anticoagulation is recommended for pregnant women hospitalized with severe disease. For those unlikely to deliver within a few days, prophylactic or intermediate dose LMWH can be used. Unfractionated heparin is preferred for patients who may imminently deliver because of its ease of reversal compared to LMWH or for those with contraindications to LMWH. If all pharmacologic anticoagulation is contraindicated, intermittent pneumatic compression should be used [40].

Outpatient follow-up for pregnant patients should be scheduled within a few days of discharge. Fetuses should be monitored for suboptimal growth, which is a theoretical risk of placental insufficiency because of vascular malperfusion, which can occur secondary to infection. Patients with confirmed COVID-19 infection in the first or second trimester should have a detailed morphology scan at 18–23 weeks of gestation. There should also be at least one ultrasound with amniotic fluid volume in the third trimester, occurring at least 14 days after symptoms resolve or 21 days from prior fetal biometry ultrasound [40].

Labor and Delivery

Hospitals and registered birthing centers are still safer alternatives for delivery than home births. Similar to processes for nonpregnant patients, guidelines involve screening patients for symptoms, patient and visitor mask use, and proper use of PPE by health-care personnel [40].

COVID-19 infection is not an indication to alter the delivery plan in patients who are asymptomatic or without severe disease, and there is no association with adverse perinatal outcomes in these patients. Methods of induction can include outpatient mechanical cervical ripening with a balloon catheter to prevent facility exposure or inpatient use of two methods to decrease the time from induction to birth [40].

For patients with severe or critical infection, delivery modifications are determined on a case-by-case basis. These infections are associated with an increased risk of preterm labor, preterm rupture of membranes, abnormal fetal heart rate patterns, and cesarean section, which may all result from fever and hypoxemia [40, 44]. Many physiologic changes of pregnancy can affect pulmonary function, including increased oxygen consumption, decreased functional residual capacity, and excessive uterine distention which may occur with multi-fetal gestations or polyhydramnios. While induction of labor may be performed safely, it is often not ideal for patients intubated in the OR or ICU; therefore, a C-section is recommended for these patients [40].

Patients under 32 weeks gestational age (GA) should not deliver, and maternal supportive care and fetal monitoring should progress as long as the patient remains stable or improving. For non-intubated patients without severe disease, delivery is indicated after 32 weeks to prevent respiratory deterioration. For those with severe disease who are intubated, delivery may be considered after 32 weeks if their clinical status is stable, worsening, or if they have refractory hypoxemic respiratory failure [40].

The labor course and fetal monitoring can progress as normal in patients that are not severely ill. There is no benefit for oxygen supplementation in non-hypoxemic mothers as there has been no proven benefit for the fetus [42]. Expectant mothers hospitalized with normal oxygenation levels can undergo once- or twice-daily fetal nonstress tests (NSTs) [40]. However, if a patient has pneumonia with suspected or confirmed COVID-19 infection or is unstable, continuous electronic fetal monitoring is recommended [40, 44]. This may be deferred if the parents would not opt for an emergency C-section if non-reassuring fetal heart tones develop [40]. The differential for patients with intrapartum fever should include COVID-19 infection and the usual diagnoses like chorioamnionitis and epidural fever [44].

Pharmacological treatment during labor and delivery can continue unmodified for COVID-positive patients. Neuraxial anesthesia is not contraindicated and is recommended to reduce cardiopulmonary stress from maternal pain and anxiety, which can reduce the risk of viral particle spread and is useful if delivery progresses to an emergency C-section. It is not recommended to use nitrous oxide systems in suspected or confirmed COVID-19 patients as there is uncertainty regarding these systems' ability to adequately filter viral particles [44].

If magnesium sulfate is administered, patients who are not intubated but suffering from respiratory compromise should be monitored for respiratory paralysis, a sign of magnesium toxicity. Maternal-fetal medicine and pulmonary critical care specialists should be consulted if magnesium is administered to intubated patients as the first sign of toxicity could be cardiac arrhythmias. Magnesium should also be renally dosed if the patient has a suspected COVID-induced kidney injury [44].

The second stage of labor may involve more viral particle spread, and personnel should increase their PPE to include airborne precautions. There are no recommended modifications to delayed cord clamping, cord blood banking, or skin-to-skin protocols. However, infected mothers should continue to wear face masks and practice hand hygiene with infants.

Management of the third stage of labor is unchanged although some clinicians prefer to avoid tranexamic acid use for the management of postpartum hemorrhage in COVID-19-positive or COVID-19-suspected patients because of the underlying hypercoagulable state [45].

Postpartum Care

In the immediate postpartum period, there is no need to room the mother and infant separately although COVID-positive mothers should use proper hand hygiene, wear masks, and safely distance from the child where possible. Separation should only be considered if the mother is too ill to care for the child as for most families, continued separation after discharge is highly unlikely. These precautions can be discontinued when the mother is greater than 10 days from positive test result if asymptomatic or from the first symptom or over 24 hours since last fever [44].

COVID-19 status does not alter postpartum analgesia options. As in pregnancy, acetaminophen remains the preferred antipyretic agent although there are no restrictions to NSAID use if clinically indicated [44].

Asymptomatic or mildly symptomatic mothers do not require anticoagulation. COVID-19-positive mothers with severe disease should have venous thromboembolism prophylaxis using low molecular weight heparin or unfractionated heparin. Both are compatible with breastfeeding and may be discontinued before discharge [44].

Infants of mothers with confirmed or suspected COVID infection should be tested twice using reverse transcriptase PCR at 24 hours and 48 hours of age as viral fragments transmitted during delivery and the postnatal environment can cause an initial false-positive result.

The risk of viral transmission through breast milk is very low, and so breastfeeding should still be encouraged because of the benefits to mother and infant. However, if the infant is formula-fed and the mother is COVID-positive, another caregiver should feed the child [44].

Patients without COVID-19 should be discharged as early as possible to reduce the risk of acquiring infection, while those with COVID-19 should be discharged based on clinical assessment. All patients should receive the COVID-19 vaccine, including breastfeeding mothers, as antibodies from the vaccine are transmitted to the infant with no adverse effects [44].

Conclusion

SARS-CoV-2 is a highly contagious virus that can affect almost any system in the body. New developments in understanding its transmissibility, management, and sequelae are unfolding almost daily. However, no medical publication in 2021 would be complete without a snapshot of the current status of this pandemic. The virus continues to mutate to more contagious, and therefore more dangerous, strains. The best path forward through this pandemic is vaccination against SARS-CoV-2 for all those who are eligible.

References

1. Patel A, Jernigan D. Initial public health response and interim clinical guidance for the 2019 novel coronavirus outbreak - United States. MMWR Morb Mortal Wkly Rep. 2020;2020:140–6. https://doi.org/10.15585/mmwr.mm6905e1.
2. COVID-19 Coronavirus Pandemic. Worldometer. 2021. https://www.worldometers.info/coronavirus/. Accessed 15 Aug 2021.
3. WHO. Weekly epidemiological update on COVID-19 World Health Organization. 2021. https://www.who.int/publications/m/item/weekly-epidemiological-update-on-covid-19%2D%2D-27-july-2021. Accessed 15 Aug 2021.
4. CDC. Commercial laboratory seroprevalence survey data. Centers for Disease Control and Prevention. 2021. https://www.cdc.gov/coronavirus/2019-nCoV/index.html. Accessed 15 Aug 2021.

5. CDC. Health equity considerations and racial and ethnic minority groups. Centers for Disease Control and Prevention. 2021. https://www.cdc.gov/coronavirus/2019-ncov/community/health-equity/race-ethnicity.html. Accessed 15 Aug 2021.
6. AAP. Children and COVID-19: state-level data report. American Academy of Pediatrics. 2021. https://www.aap.org/en/pages/2019-novel-coronavirus-covid-19-infections/children-and-covid-19-state-level-data-report/. Accessed 15 Aug 2021.
7. The species Severe acute respiratory syndrome-related coronavirus: classifying 2019-nCoV and naming it SARS-CoV-2. Nat Microbiol. 2020;5(4):536–44. https://doi.org/10.1038/s41564-020-0695-z.
8. Perlman S. Another decade, another coronavirus. N Engl J Med. 2020;382(8):760–2. https://doi.org/10.1056/NEJMe2001126.
9. Zhou P, Yang XL, Wang XG, Hu B, Zhang L, Zhang W, Si HR, Zhu Y, Li B, Huang CL, Chen HD, Chen J, Luo Y, Guo H, Jiang RD, Liu MQ, Chen Y, Shen XR, Wang X, Zheng XS, Zhao K, Chen QJ, Deng F, Liu LL, Yan B, Zhan FX, Wang YY, Xiao GF, Shi ZL. A pneumonia outbreak associated with a new coronavirus of probable bat origin. Nature. 2020;579(7798):270–3. https://doi.org/10.1038/s41586-020-2012-7.
10. Davies NG, Abbott S, Barnard RC, Jarvis CI, Kucharski AJ, Munday JD, Pearson CAB, Russell TW, Tully DC, Washburne AD, Wenseleers T, Gimma A, Waites W, Wong KLM, van Zandvoort K, Silverman JD, Diaz-Ordaz K, Keogh R, Eggo RM, Funk S, Jit M, Atkins KE, Edmunds WJ. Estimated transmissibility and impact of SARS-CoV-2 lineage B.1.1.7 in England. Science. 2021;372(6538) https://doi.org/10.1126/science.abg3055.
11. Tegally H, Wilkinson E, Giovanetti M, Iranzadeh A, Fonseca V, Giandhari J, Doolabh D, Pillay S, San EJ, Msomi N, Mlisana K, von Gottberg A, Walaza S, Allam M, Ismail A, Mohale T, Glass AJ, Engelbrecht S, Van Zyl G, Preiser W, Petruccione F, Sigal A, Hardie D, Marais G, Hsiao NY, Korsman S, Davies MA, Tyers L, Mudau I, York D, Maslo C, Goedhals D, Abrahams S, Laguda-Akingba O, Alisoltani-Dehkordi A, Godzik A, Wibmer CK, Sewell BT, Lourenço J, Alcantara LCJ, Kosakovsky Pond SL, Weaver S, Martin D, Lessells RJ, Bhiman JN, Williamson C, de Oliveira T. Detection of a SARS-CoV-2 variant of concern in South Africa. Nature. 2021;592(7854):438–43. https://doi.org/10.1038/s41586-021-03402-9.
12. Faria NR, Mellan TA, Whittaker C, Claro IM, Candido DDS, Mishra S, Crispim MAE, Sales FCS, Hawryluk I, McCrone JT, Hulswit RJG, Franco LAM, Ramundo MS, de Jesus JG, Andrade PS, Coletti TM, Ferreira GM, Silva CAM, Manuli ER, Pereira RHM, Peixoto PS, Kraemer MUG, Gaburo N Jr, Camilo CDC, Hoeltgebaum H, Souza WM, Rocha EC, de Souza LM, de Pinho MC, Araujo LJT, Malta FSV, de Lima AB, Silva JDP, Zauli DAG, Ferreira ACS, Schnekenberg RP, Laydon DJ, Walker PGT, Schlüter HM, Dos Santos ALP, Vidal MS, Del Caro VS, Filho RMF, Dos Santos HM, Aguiar RS, Proença-Modena JL, Nelson B, Hay JA, Monod M, Miscouridou X, Coupland H, Sonabend R, Vollmer M, Gandy A, Prete CA Jr, Nascimento VH, Suchard MA, Bowden TA, Pond SLK, Wu CH, Ratmann O, Ferguson NM, Dye C, Loman NJ, Lemey P, Rambaut A, Fraiji NA, Carvalho M, Pybus OG, Flaxman S, Bhatt S, Sabino EC. Genomics and epidemiology of the P.1 SARS-CoV-2 lineage in Manaus, Brazil. Science. 2021;372(6544):815–21. https://doi.org/10.1126/science.abh2644.
13. Administration UFaD. Fact sheet for health care providers emergency use authorization (EUA) of bamlanivimab and etesevimab. 2021.
14. Public Health England. (2021). SARS-CoV-2 variants of concern and variants under investigation in England: Technical briefing 19, p.21, https://assets.publishing.service.gov.uk/government/uploads/system/uploads/attachment_data/file/1005517/Technical_Briefing_19.pdf.
15. Sheikh A, McMenamin J, Taylor B, Robertson C. SARS-CoV-2 Delta VOC in Scotland: demographics, risk of hospital admission, and vaccine effectiveness. Lancet. 2021;397(10293):2461–2. https://doi.org/10.1016/s0140-6736(21)01358-1.
16. Mehta NS, Mytton OT, Mullins EWS, Fowler TA, Falconer CL, Murphy OB, Langenberg C, Jayatunga WJP, Eddy DH, Nguyen-Van-Tam JS. SARS-CoV-2 (COVID-19): what do we know about children? A systematic review. Clin Infect Dis. 2020;71(9):2469–79. https://doi.org/10.1093/cid/ciaa556.

17. Stokes EK, Zambrano LD, Anderson KN, Marder EP, Raz KM, El Burai FS, Tie Y, Fullerton KE. Coronavirus disease 2019 case surveillance - United States, January 22–May 30, 2020. MMWR Morb Mortal Wkly Rep. 2020;69(24):759–65. https://doi.org/10.15585/mmwr.mm6924e2.
18. Irfan O, Muttalib F, Tang K, Jiang L, Lassi ZS, Bhutta Z. Clinical characteristics, treatment and outcomes of paediatric COVID-19: a systematic review and meta-analysis. Arch Dis Child. 2021;106(5):440–8. https://doi.org/10.1136/archdischild-2020-321385.
19. Feldstein LR, Tenforde MW, Friedman KG, Newhams M, Rose EB, Dapul H, Soma VL, Maddux AB, Mourani PM, Bowens C, Maamari M, Hall MW, Riggs BJ, Giuliano JS Jr, Singh AR, Li S, Kong M, Schuster JE, McLaughlin GE, Schwartz SP, Walker TC, Loftis LL, Hobbs CV, Halasa NB, Doymaz S, Babbitt CJ, Hume JR, Gertz SJ, Irby K, Clouser KN, Cvijanovich NZ, Bradford TT, Smith LS, Heidemann SM, Zackai SP, Wellnitz K, Nofziger RA, Horwitz SM, Carroll RW, Rowan CM, Tarquinio KM, Mack EH, Fitzgerald JC, Coates BM, Jackson AM, Young CC, Son MBF, Patel MM, Newburger JW, Randolph AG. Characteristics and outcomes of US children and adolescents with multisystem inflammatory syndrome in children (MIS-C) compared with severe acute COVID-19. JAMA. 2021;325(11):1074–87. https://doi.org/10.1001/jama.2021.2091.
20. Huang C, Huang L, Wang Y, Li X, Ren L, Gu X, Kang L, Guo L, Liu M, Zhou X, Luo J, Huang Z, Tu S, Zhao Y, Chen L, Xu D, Li Y, Li C, Peng L, Li Y, Xie W, Cui D, Shang L, Fan G, Xu J, Wang G, Wang Y, Zhong J, Wang C, Wang J, Zhang D, Cao B. 6-month consequences of COVID-19 in patients discharged from hospital: a cohort study. Lancet. 2021;397(10270):220–32. https://doi.org/10.1016/s0140-6736(20)32656-8.
21. Myall KJ, Mukherjee B, Castanheira AM, Lam JL, Benedetti G, Mak SM, Preston R, Thillai M, Dewar A, Molyneaux PL, West AG. Persistent post-COVID-19 interstitial lung disease. An observational study of corticosteroid treatment. Ann Am Thorac Soc. 2021;18(5):799–806. https://doi.org/10.1513/AnnalsATS.202008-1002OC.
22. Gibson PG, Qin L, Puah SH. COVID-19 acute respiratory distress syndrome (ARDS): clinical features and differences from typical pre-COVID-19 ARDS. Med J Aust. 2020;213(2):54–56. e51. https://doi.org/10.5694/mja2.50674.
23. Welker C, Huang J, Gil IJN, Ramakrishna H. 2021 acute respiratory distress syndrome update, with coronavirus disease 2019 focus. J Cardiothorac Vasc Anesth. 2021. https://doi.org/10.1053/j.jvca.2021.02.053.
24. Nalbandian A, Sehgal K, Gupta A, Madhavan MV, McGroder C, Stevens JS, Cook JR, Nordvig AS, Shalev D, Sehrawat TS, Ahluwalia N, Bikdeli B, Dietz D, Der-Nigoghossian C, Liyanage-Don N, Rosner GF, Bernstein EJ, Mohan S, Beckley AA, Seres DS, Choueiri TK, Uriel N, Ausiello JC, Accili D, Freedberg DE, Baldwin M, Schwartz A, Brodie D, Garcia CK, Elkind MSV, Connors JM, Bilezikian JP, Landry DW, Wan EY. Post-acute COVID-19 syndrome. Nat Med. 2021;27(4):601–15. https://doi.org/10.1038/s41591-021-01283-z.
25. NIH. Coronavirus disease 2019 (COVID-19) treatment guidelines. Bethesda: National Institutes of Health; 2021.
26. Cuker A, Tseng EK, Nieuwlaat R, Angchaisuksiri P, Blair C, Dane K, Davila J, DeSancho MT, Diuguid D, Griffin DO, Kahn SR, Klok FA, Lee AI, Neumann I, Pai A, Pai M, Righini M, Sanfilippo KM, Siegal D, Skara M, Touri K, Akl EA, Bou Akl I, Boulos M, Brignardello-Petersen R, Charide R, Chan M, Dearness K, Darzi AJ, Kolb P, Colunga-Lozano LE, Mansour R, Morgano GP, Morsi RZ, Noori A, Piggott T, Qiu Y, Roldan Y, Schünemann F, Stevens A, Solo K, Ventresca M, Wiercioch W, Mustafa RA, Schünemann HJ. American Society of Hematology 2021 guidelines on the use of anticoagulation for thromboprophylaxis in patients with COVID-19. Blood Adv. 2021;5(3):872–88. https://doi.org/10.1182/bloodadvances.2020003763.
27. Roberts LN, Whyte MB, Georgiou L, Giron G, Czuprynska J, Rea C, Vadher B, Patel RK, Gee E, Arya R. Postdischarge venous thromboembolism following hospital admission with COVID-19. Blood. 2020;136(11):1347–50. https://doi.org/10.1182/blood.2020008086.

28. Hassanein M, Thomas G, Taliercio J. Management of acute kidney injury in COVID-19. Cleve Clin J Med. 2020. https://doi.org/10.3949/ccjm.87a.ccc034.
29. Chan L, Chaudhary K, Saha A, Chauhan K, Vaid A, Zhao S, Paranjpe I, Somani S, Richter F, Miotto R, Lala A, Kia A, Timsina P, Li L, Freeman R, Chen R, Narula J, Just AC, Horowitz C, Fayad Z, Cordon-Cardo C, Schadt E, Levin MA, Reich DL, Fuster V, Murphy B, He JC, Charney AW, Böttinger EP, Glicksberg BS, Coca SG, Nadkarni GN, Center obotMSCI. AKI in hospitalized patients with COVID-19. J Am Soc Nephrol. 2021;32(1):151–60. https://doi.org/10.1681/asn.2020050615.
30. Kreuziger L, Lee A, Garcia D, Cushman M, DeSancho M, Connors JM. COVID-19 and VTE/Anticoagulation: Frequently Asked Questions. American Society of Hematology. https://www.hematology.org/covid-19/covid-19-and-vte-anticoagulation. 2021.
31. Al-Samkari H, Karp Leaf RS, Dzik WH, Carlson JCT, Fogerty AE, Waheed A, Goodarzi K, Bendapudi PK, Bornikova L, Gupta S, Leaf DE, Kuter DJ, Rosovsky RP. COVID-19 and coagulation: bleeding and thrombotic manifestations of SARS-CoV-2 infection. Blood. 2020;136(4):489–500. https://doi.org/10.1182/blood.2020006520.
32. Lai J, Ma S, Wang Y, Cai Z, Hu J, Wei N, Wu J, Du H, Chen T, Li R, Tan H, Kang L, Yao L, Huang M, Wang H, Wang G, Liu Z, Hu S. Factors associated with mental health outcomes among health care workers exposed to coronavirus disease 2019. JAMA Netw Open. 2020;3(3):e203976. https://doi.org/10.1001/jamanetworkopen.2020.3976.
33. Xiang YT, Jin Y, Cheung T. Joint international collaboration to combat mental health challenges during the coronavirus disease 2019 pandemic. JAMA Psychiat. 2020;77(10):989–90. https://doi.org/10.1001/jamapsychiatry.2020.1057.
34. Galea S, Merchant RM, Lurie N. The mental health consequences of COVID-19 and physical distancing: the need for prevention and early intervention. JAMA Intern Med. 2020;180(6):817–8. https://doi.org/10.1001/jamainternmed.2020.1562.
35. Rogers JP, Chesney E, Oliver D, Pollak TA, McGuire P, Fusar-Poli P, Zandi MS, Lewis G, David AS. Psychiatric and neuropsychiatric presentations associated with severe coronavirus infections: a systematic review and meta-analysis with comparison to the COVID-19 pandemic. Lancet Psychiatry. 2020;7(7):611–27. https://doi.org/10.1016/s2215-0366(20)30203-0.
36. Hatch R, Young D, Barber V, Griffiths J, Harrison DA, Watkinson P. Anxiety, depression and post traumatic stress disorder after critical illness: a UK-wide prospective cohort study. Crit Care. 2018;22(1):310. https://doi.org/10.1186/s13054-018-2223-6.
37. Varatharaj A, Thomas N, Ellul MA, Davies NWS, Pollak TA, Tenorio EL, Sultan M, Easton A, Breen G, Zandi M, Coles JP, Manji H, Al-Shahi Salman R, Menon DK, Nicholson TR, Benjamin LA, Carson A, Smith C, Turner MR, Solomon T, Kneen R, Pett SL, Galea I, Thomas RH, Michael BD. Neurological and neuropsychiatric complications of COVID-19 in 153 patients: a UK-wide surveillance study. Lancet Psychiatry. 2020;7(10):875–82. https://doi.org/10.1016/s2215-0366(20)30287-x.
38. Mao L, Jin H, Wang M, Hu Y, Chen S, He Q, Chang J, Hong C, Zhou Y, Wang D, Miao X, Li Y, Hu B. Neurologic manifestations of hospitalized patients with coronavirus disease 2019 in Wuhan, China. JAMA Neurol. 2020;77(6):683–90. https://doi.org/10.1001/jamaneurol.2020.1127.
39. Kisely S, Warren N, McMahon L, Dalais C, Henry I, Siskind D. Occurrence, prevention, and management of the psychological effects of emerging virus outbreaks on healthcare workers: rapid review and meta-analysis. BMJ. 2020;369:m1642. https://doi.org/10.1136/bmj.m1642.
40. Berghella V, Hughes B. COVID-19: Pregnancy issues and antenatal care. UpToDate. 2021.
41. Allotey J, Stallings E, Bonet M, Yap M, Chatterjee S, Kew T, Debenham L, Llavall AC, Dixit A, Zhou D, Balaji R, Lee SI, Qiu X, Yuan M, Coomar D, Sheikh J, Lawson H, Ansari K, van Wely M, van Leeuwen E, Kostova E, Kunst H, Khalil A, Tiberi S, Brizuela V, Broutet N, Kara E, Kim CR, Thorson A, Oladapo OT, Mofenson L, Zamora J, Thangaratinam S. Clinical manifestations, risk factors, and maternal and perinatal outcomes of coronavirus disease 2019 in pregnancy: living systematic review and meta-analysis. BMJ. 2020;370:m3320. https://doi.org/10.1136/bmj.m3320.

42. Halscott T, Vaught J, Miller E. Management considerations for pregnant patients with COVID-19. 2020.
43. Hoeltzenbein M, Beck E, Rajwanshi R, Gøtestam Skorpen C, Berber E, Schaefer C, Østensen M. Tocilizumab use in pregnancy: analysis of a global safety database including data from clinical trials and post-marketing data. Semin Arthritis Rheum. 2016;46(2):238–45. https://doi.org/10.1016/j.semarthrit.2016.05.004.
44. Berghella V, Hughes B. COVID-19: labor, birth, and postpartum issues. UpToDate. 2021.
45. Ogawa H, Asakura H. Consideration of tranexamic acid administration to COVID-19 patients. Physiol Rev. 2020;100(4):1595–6. https://doi.org/10.1152/physrev.00023.2020.
46. Prevention CfDCa. Vaccine effectiveness. CDC. 2021. https://www.cdc.gov/vaccines/covid-19/effectiveness-research/protocols.html. Accessed 16 Aug 2021.
47. Yancy CW. COVID-19 and African Americans. JAMA. 2020;323(19):1891–2. https://doi.org/10.1001/jama.2020.6548.
48. Lee S, Kim T, Lee E, et al. Clinical course and molecular viral shedding among asymptomatic and symptomatic patients with SARS-CoV-2 infection in a community treatment center in the Republic of Korea. JAMA Intern Med. 2020;180(11):1447–52. https://doi.org/10.1001/jamainternmed.2020.3862.
49. Van Doremalen N, et al. Aerosol and surface stability of SARS-CoV-2 as compared with SARS-CoV-1. N Engl J Med. 2020;382:1564–7. https://doi.org/10.1056/NEJMc2004973.
50. CDC. Scientific brief: SARS-CoV-2 transmission. 2021. https://www.cdc.gov/coronavirus/2019-ncov/science/science-briefs/sars-cov-2-transmission.html. Accessed 23 Oct 2021.
51. Wiersinga WJ, Rhodes A, Cheng AC, Peacock SJ, Prescott HC. Pathophysiology, transmission, diagnosis, and treatment of coronavirus disease 2019 (COVID-19): a review. JAMA. 2020;324(8):782–93. https://doi.org/10.1001/jama.2020.12839.
52. Perera R, Tso E, Tsang O, et al. SARS-CoV-2 virus culture and subgenomic RNA for respiratory specimens from patients with mild coronavirus disease. Emerg Infect Dis. 2020;26(11):2701–4. https://doi.org/10.3201/eid2611.203219.
53. CDC. Interim infection prevention and control recommendations for healthcare personnel during the coronavirus disease 2019 (COVID-19) pandemic. 2021. https://www.cdc.gov/coronavirus/2019-ncov/hcp/infection-control-recommendations.html. Updated September 10, 2021. Accessed 23 Oct 2021.
54. Wang D, Hu B, Hu C, et al. Clinical characteristics of 138 hospitalized patients with 2019 novel coronavirus–infected pneumonia in Wuhan, China. JAMA. 2020;323(11):1061–9. https://doi.org/10.1001/jama.2020.1585.
55. CDC. CDC expands eligibility for COVID-19 booster shots. 2021. Published October 21, 2021. https://www.cdc.gov/media/releases/2021/p1021-covid-booster.html. Accessed 23 Oct 2021.
56. Alhazzani W, et al. Surviving sepsis campaign guidelines on the management of adults with coronavirus disease 2019 (COVID-19) in the ICU: first update. Crit Care Med. 2021;49(3):e219–34. https://doi.org/10.1097/CCM.0000000000004899.

Chapter 2
Management of Inflammatory Bowel Disease

Gregory Gaspard, Samir Hussaini, Dileep Mandali, and Ethan Lieberamn

Introduction

Inflammatory bowel disease (IBD) describes chronic, relapsing inflammatory disorders of the gastrointestinal (GI) tract, likely due to an abnormal immune response to enteric flora. The two most common types are Crohn's disease (CD) and ulcerative colitis (UC), each with its own distinct characteristics. CD may affect the entire GI tract, from mouth to anus, but classically affects the ileum or the distal part of the small intestine, whereas UC classically affects the rectum and extends in a continuous fashion, proximally through the colon; it spares the small intestine and everything above.

Treatment and management of IBD are aimed at bringing the disease into a state of remission and sustaining that state for as long as possible. IBD typically presents in an inpatient setting during an acute flare or due to a complication of the disease process. A flare is described as the reappearance of symptoms due to active disease-related inflammation, and the most common symptoms at presentation include:

- Increased frequency and urgency of bowel movements (BMs)
- Bloody BMs
- Abdominal pain
- Nausea, vomiting, and diarrhea
- Reduced appetite

G. Gaspard (✉)
Ochsner Health, New Orleans, LA, USA
e-mail: Gregory.gaspard@ochsner.org

S. Hussaini · E. Lieberamn
Ochsner Health, New Orleans, LA, USA

University of Queensland- Ochsner Clinical School of Medicine, New Orleans, LA, USA

D. Mandali
The University of Queensland-Ochsner Clinical School, New Orleans, LA, USA

© The Author(s), under exclusive license to Springer Nature Switzerland AG 2022
K. Conrad (ed.), *Clinical Approaches to Hospital Medicine*,
https://doi.org/10.1007/978-3-030-95164-1_2

Several factors can cause a flare or worsen existing symptoms. These include:

- Inefficacy of IBD medications due to medication resistance, inadequate dosing, antidrug antibodies, and/or nonadherence to treatment
- Infection
- Stress
- Dietary factors
- Smoking
- Antibiotics
- Nonsteroid anti-inflammatory drugs (NSAIDs)

An exacerbation of symptoms warrants an evaluation of the cause of ongoing issues. The nature and process of evaluation for both CD and UC are discussed later in the chapter.

Factors Causing IBD Flares

A large percentage of Americans use NSAIDs to relieve headaches, fever, musculoskeletal issues, and other common body discomforts. People with IBD are cautioned against the use of NSAIDs due to its induced GI toxicity through several mechanisms: increased mucosal permeability, intracellular adenosine triphosphate (ATP) depletion, and formation of drug-enterocyte adducts [1]. However, the most discussed mechanism of NSAID-induced GI toxicity is the effect on prostaglandin synthesis. Prostaglandins are pivotal in maintaining the microcirculation and modulation of the gastroenteric immune system. Experimental models have shown that inhibition of COX1, COX2, and their prostaglandins (E2, F2A, and D2) resulted in the development of intestinal ulcers, exacerbation of dextran sulfate sodium-induced colitis, and frequent flares of IBD [1].

Smoking is implicated in both the development of CD and in subsequent flares. Those who regularly smoke tend to have increased severity of disease, reduced response to medical treatment, and an increased risk of disease complications. The pathogenesis of CD through smoking is thought to be due to generation of reactive oxygen species and their effects on the immune system by intensifying vasodilation in chronically inflamed GI microvasculature [2]. Paradoxically, smoking is considered a protective factor for UC. This is potentially due to nicotine and/or its byproduct, cotinine, having an immunomodulatory effect that leads to decreased production of pro-inflammatory cytokines through the activation of nicotinic receptors $\alpha 7$ in macrophages and dendritic cells. However, this benefit was only observed in mild to moderate UC, whereas smoking has shown to increase the activity of disease in severe UC [2].

Recent studies show that chronic stress, depression, and even adverse life events may increase the likelihood of IBD flares. The damaging effects of stress on the gut involve a comprehensive integrated interaction among the neuronal, endocrine, and immune systems. Stress contributes to the development of IBD via dysbiosis, alterations in intestinal permeability and mobility, and release of inflammatory factors by activating the brain-gut axis, hypothalamic pituitary-adrenal axis (HPA axis), autonomic nervous system (ANS), and enteric nervous system (ENS) [3]. In the HPA axis, the main culprit is corticotropin-releasing factor, which increases inflammation by activating mast cell degranulation and increasing tumor necrosis factor-alpha (TNF-α) and protease production, thereby damaging the intestinal barrier. Stress also activates the sympathetic part of the ANS, leading to increased production of catecholamines and inhibition of the vagus nerve, which is responsible for intestinal inflammation attenuation by activating cholinergic enteric neurons that have inhibitory effects on macrophages in the muscularis externa [3, 4]. Catecholamines induce increased intestinal inflammation through increased activation of inflammatory nuclear factor kB. Stress also induces dysbiosis by abundance reduction in *Lactobacillus*, leading to opportunistic infections, notably *Shigella flexneri* and *Campylobacteri jejuni*. This also alters the functionality of proteins constituting the gut flora; specifically, this inhibits nucleotide-binding oligomerization domain-like receptors (NOD-like receptors) and pyrin domain containing (NLRP)-6 inflammasome, leading to inflammation of the intestine [3]. Increased intestinal permeability through inflammation further causes immune dysregulation by allowing microbiota to cross the gut-epithelial barrier and activating the innate immune system.

Dietary causes of IBD flares have several plausible mechanisms including alterations in gut microbiome, dietary antigen presentation, and mucosal immune system and epithelial barrier function. Two theories attempt to highlight the etiology of diet-induced IBD. The "cold chain hypothesis" suggests that prolonged refrigeration of food promotes growth of psychotropic pathogens such as *Yersinia* and *Listeria*, which have been identified in patients with CD [5]. The "hygiene hypothesis," on the other hand, suggests that reduced exposure to various enteric organisms in early childhood due to hygienic practices results in an ineffective and aberrant immune response, triggering IBD later in life. A high fermentable oligosaccharides, disaccharides, monosaccharides, and polyols (FODMAP) diet has been associated with increased gastrointestinal symptoms since these substances are poorly absorbed, draw water, and ferment in intestines causing abdominal bloating and distension, crampy pain, flatulence, and diarrhea [5].

Crohn's Disease

Presentation of Crohn's Disease Flares

CD can affect the entire GI tract. It generally involves full-thickness or transmural inflammation with deep fissuring ulcers. Granulomatous lymphoid aggregates can be seen. Based on the location of active disease, patients may also present with symptoms of enteritis related to small bowel inflammation, colitis related to large bowel inflammation, bowel obstruction due to fibrotic or inflammatory structuring disease, and complications such as fistulas and abscesses [6].

"Enteritis" is defined as inflammation of the small intestine, whereas "colitis" is defined as inflammation of the colon. In CD, enteritis is more common with approximately 80% of patients presenting with small bowel involvement. One-third of patients with CD have isolated ileitis. About 50% of patients present with involvement of both the ileum and colon (ileocolitis). About 20% of patients have disease limited to the colon, with half of them sparing the rectum. About a third have perianal disease [7].

The cardinal symptoms of CD include abdominal pain, diarrhea (typically non-bloody), weight loss, and fatigue. A patient may present specifically with right lower quadrant (RLQ) pain due to involvement of ileum; however, CD can often lead to localized pain in other areas of the abdomen due to formation of fibrotic strictures leading to small bowel obstruction or less commonly colonic obstruction [7]. Intermittent diarrhea can result from excessive fluid secretion and lack of fluid absorption by inflamed bowel, bile salt malabsorption due to ileitis, and enteroenteric or enterocolic fistulas leading to bypass of segments of bowel. Additionally, patients with predominant colitis may have grossly bloody bowel movements [7].

The transmural nature of inflammation in CD can create sinus tracts, which are responsible for fistula and abscess formation. Fistulas are connections between two epithelial-lined organs, and in CD, they may connect one segment of bowel to another (enteroenteric), bowel to bladder (enterovesical), bowel to vagina (enterovaginal), and/or bowel to skin (enterocutaneous). Each type of fistula presents with a specific presentation as seen in Table 2.1.

Some sinus tracts may simply cause abscess formation, e.g., a sinus tract extending to the retroperitoneum causing a psoas abscess and presenting with fever and localized abdominal pain and tenderness. Some may even present with phlegmon, an acute suppurative inflammation that occurs subcutaneously and can spread within the connective tissue as it is unbound and lacks a capsule.

Table 2.1 Fistulas in inflammatory bowel disease

Fistula type	Presentation
Enteroenteric	Palpable mass, diarrhea, or asymptomatic
Enterovesical	Pneumaturia (passage of gas in urine); recurrent UTIs with multiple organisms
Enterovaginal	Passage of fecal matter or gas through the vagina
Enterocutaneous	Drainage of fecal matter through the surface of skin or subcutaneous abscess

Severity of Crohn's Disease

Crohn's Disease Activity Index (CDAI) is the gold standard for defining CD clinical activity and assessing clinical response and remission. CDAI takes into consideration signs, symptoms, and history during a 7-day period; its criteria include number of liquid stools, abdominal pain, general well-being, extraintestinal/physical complaints (i.e., arthritis/arthralgia, mucocutaneous lesions such as erythema nodosum and aphthous ulcers, uveitis/iritis, anal disease such as fistulas and fissures, and fever over 37.8 C), antidiarrheal drugs, abdominal mass, hematocrit, and body weight [9]. A CDAI score <150 indicates remission of CD, while a score >450 indicates severe CD. CDAI was developed to assess disease activity at any given point, but since CD is a chronic, progressive disorder, evaluating long-term disease severity is also important. This requires exploring three main domains relevant to evaluating disease severity: (1) disease impact on the patient, (2) disease burden, and (3) disease course. Clinical symptoms, quality of life, and disability are some of the factors considered to assess CD's impact on the patient [8]. To assess disease burden, a combination of lab testing, imaging, and endoscopic evaluation is typically required.

Disease Impact on the Patient

Harvey-Bradshaw Index (HBI) is a modified CDAI assessment that only requires 1 day of patient diary entries rather than 7 day and omits hematocrit level, antidiarrheal medication use, and body weight. Both allowed for the development of disease activity thresholds but correlate poorly with mucosal inflammation [9]. As a result, the van Hees Index was derived to combine clinical and laboratory data contributing most to the activity index, and Perianal Disease Activity Index is derived to more adequately quantify symptoms specific to perianal fistulizing disease. The Manitoba IBD index and Inflammatory Bowel Disease Questionnaire were commonly used to assess the impact of CD on a patient's quality of life, and in recent years, the Crohn's Disease Patient-Reported Outcomes Signs and Symptoms (CD-PRO/SS) was developed to best assess CD's impact on a patient's quality of life and to assess primary outcome measures in pivotal clinical trials per recommendation by the US Food and Drug Administration and the International Society for Pharmacoeconomics and Outcomes Research [8, 10].

Disease Burden

The degree of mucosal inflammation, location, and complications are important measures of disease severity. Biomarkers (i.e., CRP, fecal calprotectin, fecal lactoferrin) can be used to assess disease activity, but they are nonspecific and should not be used exclusively. CRP levels can be normal in up to one-third of CD patients with active disease [8].

Endoscopy, usually ileocolonoscopy, continues to be the gold standard to assess disease activity. Crohn's Disease Endoscopic Index of Severity and the Simple Endoscopic Score for Crohn's Disease have been developed to assess severity. CT and MRI are also useful in assessing disease activity, complications, and distribution and are important tools to aid in the assessment of patients with Crohn's disease. Additionally, ultrasound can differentiate active from inactive disease with a specificity of 85% and sensitivity of 71%, respectively, when assessed against endoscopy or surgery [11] and can be a useful assessment tool in locations where expertise in this technique is available.

Disease Course

Disabling CD can be defined as having one of the following: steroid dependence, need for more than two steroid courses, disabling chronic symptoms for a cumulative time of 12+ months, and need for immunosuppressive therapy or surgery. Severe disease can be defined as having one or more of the following: any colonic resection, complex perianal disease, two or more small bowel resections, or permanent stoma reconstruction. "Aggressive" CD can be defined as penetrating disease, complications or flares of the disease requiring hospitalization, EIMs involving two or more systems, disease refractory to currently available treatments, and need for surgery. "Complicated" disease can be defined as presence of bowel damage, presence of EIMs, and/or the need for surgery [9].

Evaluation of Crohn's Disease

There are no laboratory tests that definitively rule out or rule in CD, but serum and stool testing can assist with reaching a diagnosis. An initial evaluation of a patient presenting with symptoms thought to be related to CD should start with stool studies, including tests for parasitic and bacterial pathogens such as *C. difficile*, to rule out other causes of diarrhea and gastrointestinal symptoms. Patients with severe and longer duration of CD may have thrombocytosis and anemia from chronic inflammation, iron deficiency, and cobalamin (vitamin B12) deficiency, and these findings can be evident on serum studies [12]. Inflammatory markers such as C-reactive protein (CRP) and/or erythrocyte sedimentation rate (ESR) may be elevated, but normal levels do not rule out CD. Fecal calprotectin or fecal lactoferrin may be used to evaluate the degree of gastrointestinal tract inflammation [9].

CD is diagnosed using a combination of clinical features, endoscopic findings, and radiologic findings. In cases of colonic or ileal involvement, endoscopic findings classically indicate skip lesions next to areas of normal-appearing mucosa and with varying degrees of transmural inflammation [9]. In some cases, such as isolated jejunal involvement, affected area(s) may not be easily visualized. As a result, capsule endoscopy may be performed to visualize and assess the small bowel mucosa

[13]. It is a highly sensitive test for finding abnormal mucosa, but it has low specificity for a diagnosis of CD and has the risk of the capsule being impacted or retained in structuring CD; this risk is around 13% in known CD cases [14]. To reduce the risk, patency capsule, specifically designed to disintegrate in 2–3 days, is placed, and small bowel imaging is obtained 24 hours after placement to determine if it has passed through the small bowel. If it is successful in passing through, then regular capsule endoscopy is performed without significant risk of capsule retention [13].

Both magnetic resonance enterography (MRE) and computed tomography enterography (CTE) also allow for visualization of the bowel wall, mucosa, and extraluminal complications. CTE allows for accurate assessment of disease activity and is economical compared to MRE, but it has high radiation exposure and requires iodinated contrast. MRE, on the other hand, is expensive, but it lacks radiation and is an accurate tool for assessment of disease distribution and assessment with its ability to often capture perianal fistulation [15].

Management for Crohn's Disease

When a patient is hospitalized with an increase in or new-onset gastrointestinal symptoms concerning for either a Crohn's disease flare or a possible new diagnosis of Crohn's disease, it is imperative to not immediately assume that the symptoms are solely related to disease-related inflammation and not another cause. Initial evaluation should include an evaluation of labs and stool studies as noted above to assess for signs of inflammation and disease severity. Arguably, the most important step in the evaluation is to assess for infection. Stool testing for *C. difficile* is important for all patients presenting with diarrheal symptoms, especially those with IBD or suspected IBD. Stool testing for other infections should be done in the appropriate clinical situation (i.e., acute diarrhea, especially with fevers). If the patient is immunosuppressed, consider additional testing including serum testing for cytomegalovirus (CMV) and Epstein-Barr virus (EBV). In febrile patients, a chest x-ray, urinalysis with microscopic analysis, and blood cultures should also be obtained.

In addition to the evaluation noted above, cross-sectional imaging – usually with a contrast enhanced CT or MRE – is usually helpful if there is any concern for possible structural complications such as bowel obstruction from stricturing disease or penetrating disease with a possible abscess or phlegmon as well as to evaluate for other possible causes of the patient's symptoms. If a perianal abscess or fistula is suspected, MRI of the pelvis can be a helpful adjunct to a careful physical examination.

Endoscopic evaluation is often needed to complete the evaluation of a patient with gastrointestinal symptoms suspected to be related to Crohn's disease. For any patient with an unclear diagnosis or with suspected new-onset Crohn's disease, endoscopic evaluation is an absolutely necessary part of making the diagnosis. In a patient with known Crohn's disease with a known disease distribution presenting with typical symptoms and having undergone a recent ileocolonoscopy for disease evaluation, this may not be needed, but if there is any question about disease activity or possible CMV colitis or enteritis, colonoscopy with biopsy should be performed. If imaging suggests disease activity in a location that might not be able to be assessed through routine colonoscopy, then other endoscopic techniques such as upper endoscopy or enteroscopy (routine or balloon assisted) can be considered.

Once the underlying cause of the patient's issues is identified, then treatment can be initiated. Appropriate treatment of luminal inflammatory CD depends on the severity of disease, location and extent of inflammation, and the disease phenotype. Severity of disease is classified into mild, moderate, and severe disease. The medical management for mild to moderate disease differs from the medical management of moderate to severe disease. The medical management of inflammatory CD typically involves induction and maintenance therapy. The goal of induction therapy is to acutely control the inflammation and achieve symptomatic remission in a period of less than 3 months. The goal of maintenance therapy is to gain long-term control of the inflammation for the period following 3 months, preventing symptoms (diarrhea and abdominal pain) and consequences (fistulas and strictures). Maintenance therapy is typically done in an outpatient setting by a gastroenterologist. Induction therapy used for acute exacerbations of inflammatory CD can involve corticosteroids, biologics, and antibiotics in addition to diet modification.

For patients with mild to moderate disease that is limited to the proximal colon or ileum, treatment with 9 mg of enteric-release budesonide daily for 4 weeks is an effective induction therapy. If the patient responds to the treatment, tapering budesonide by 3 mg every 2–4 weeks for 8–12 weeks can begin [16]. If the disease involves the distal colon or is diffusely spread throughout the colon, it is recommended to begin an induction of 40 mg of prednisone daily for 1 week. A taper of 5–10 mg per week over the next 1–2 months can begin if the patient responds to initial treatment. The use of 5-aminosalicylates is not recommended in the treatment of inflammatory CD in patients hospitalized with active Crohn's disease [17, 18].

Management of patients with moderate to severe inflammatory CD is more complicated as there are several factors that need to be considered in determining the best treatment. A gastroenterologist should be consulted as treatment is often individualized. Similar to the management of mild to moderate inflammatory CD, steroids can be used in hospitalized patients with acute flares. Typically, intravenous methylprednisolone is used to mitigate exacerbations. In addition, induction for moderate to severe inflammatory CD may involve the use of TNF inhibitors such as infliximab. Infliximab, a monoclonal antibody against TNF-alpha, can be used as an induction treatment and has been shown to be effective at obtaining remission quickly in patients with severe disease [19]. Prior to treatment, the patient should undergo testing for hepatitis B (HBsAg, HBsAb, HBcAb) and tuberculosis as reactivation of latent disease has been reported with infliximab. Infliximab is given intravenously in dosages of 5 mg/kg at zero, two, and six weeks for induction therapy [20]. There is evidence to demonstrate that combination therapy (infliximab plus immunomodulator) is more effective than monotherapy, but immunomodulators are not indicated for induction of remission, so this treatment strategy is more suited for maintenance therapy than for induction therapy [21].

Current therapies for moderate to severe CD include methotrexate, TNF inhibitors, thiopurines, IL 12/23 inhibitors, and integrin inhibitors. Difficulties in tolerating these medications and increased rates of treatment failure in the case of TNF inhibitors due to the development of antidrug antibodies, for instance, have prompted increased interest in novel CD therapies [22]. Such novel therapies include small molecule therapies, like Janus kinase (JAK) inhibitors that have advantages over biologics like TNF inhibitors such as less variability in pharmacokinetics, convenient oral route of administrations, and minimal risk of immunogenicity. Despite a greater risk of drug-drug interactions compared to biologics, the unique benefits of small molecule therapies make them a promising alternative to the management of CD [22]. Currently, JAK inhibitors are not FDA approved for induction or maintenance of CD.

Management of Intra-abdominal Abscesses (IAA) Due to Crohn's Disease

Intra-abdominal abscesses secondary to CD are treated using antibiotics or a combination of antibiotics and drainage. Antibiotics used to target intra-abdominal abscesses should cover enteric pathogens, such as gram-negative aerobic and facultative bacteria, gram-positive streptococci, and obligate anaerobic bacilli. Rueken et al. compiled a microbiological spectrum of those with IAA from perforating Crohn's disease, finding E. coli as the most frequent isolated pathogen (45 patients), then Streptococcus spp (28 patients), then Enterococci (27 patients), then Candida (12 patients), and finally anaerobic bacteria (11 patients) [23]. Appropriate antibiotic monotherapy would include any of the following: cefoxitin, ertapenem, moxifloxacin, or tigecycline [24]. Combination therapy with metronidazole plus either cefazolin, cefuroxime, ceftriaxone, cefotaxime, levofloxacin, or ciprofloxacin can also be used [24]. There has been no clear indication on whether parenteral or oral antibiotics are superior in resolution of abscess [24]. Some IAA have resolved with antibiotic use only. Two previous studies found that 37% of patients treated with antibiotics alone had IAA recurrence with these reoccurrences occurring within 12–47.5 months of follow-up [25, 26]. More recently, Graham et al. found 31% of patients treated with solely antibiotics had recurrence of IAA; however, their follow-up period was only 6 months [27]. There are no clear indications for what patient qualifies for treatment of IAA solely with antibiotics, but it has been suggested that abscesses larger than 3 cm in size are not likely to resolve with antibiotic therapy alone [24].

Percutaneous vs. Surgical Drainage

If antibiotics do not resolve an intra-abdominal abscess, or if recurrent intra-abdominal abscesses develop, abscesses should be drained percutaneously or surgically. Gutierrez et al. conducted a retrospective cohort study comparing percutaneous and surgical abscess drainage, which showed no significant time difference for time to resolution of abscess. It did however show about one-third of percutaneous drainage patients underwent surgical drainage for abscess within 1 year [28]. Clancy et al. conducted a recent meta-analysis searching for comparisons between percutaneous and surgical drainage for spontaneous Crohn's disease-related intra-abdominal abscesses and found that 29.3% of surgical drainage can be avoided by percutaneous drainage [29] although an increased likelihood of abscess reformation with percutaneous drainage (OR of 6.54, 95% CI: 1.78–24.0, $p = 0.005$) was also noted [29].

Management of Structural Issues Secondary to Crohn's Disease (CD)

Over time, chronic inflammation in CD can lead to fibrostenotic disease that can ultimately result in mechanical bowel obstruction. According to the European Crohn's and Colitis Organisation (ECCO) guidelines, stricturing CD is defined as persistent, localized narrowing whereby functional effects may be evident by pre-stenotic dilation with accompanying obstructive symptoms [30]. Strictures can be inflammatory, fibrotic, or mixed, and they appear in roughly 50% of patients with CD after 20 years of disease [31]. Up to 80% of patients with ileal or ileocecal disease require surgery within 10 years from onset of diagnosis for stricturing disease [32, 33]. Traditionally, the use of steroid therapy and procedures like bowel resections were utilized to treat stricturing CD. In the case of resection, they carried with them the high risk of malabsorptive disorders and short bowel syndrome.

Many factors contribute to the consideration of using medical therapy vs. surgical therapy for stricturing CD. Patients with the following characteristics have demonstrated better outcomes from medical therapy initially rather than surgical treatment: previous resection or short bowel syndrome, current smoker, naiveté toward anti-TNF drugs, severe nutritional deficiency, and acute history of obstructive symptoms. Mechanical features like multifocal strictures, long strictures (>40 cm), limited dilatation of upstream tract (<35 mm), and absence of complex fistulizing disease also support the use of medical therapy initially. Conversely, patients without these characteristics or morphologic features should be considered for surgical intervention [31].

Procedures involving conservative endoscopic approaches and surgical strictureplasty have been utilized more recently and were developed as bowel-sparing techniques providing excellent short-term and moderate long-term efficacy. Endoscopic balloon dilatation can be performed during regular colonoscopies. This technique is best reserved for short (<2–3 cm), noncomplicated strictures (minimal inflammation, no fistula, single stenosis). The procedural success rate of endoscopic balloon dilatation is 71–100%, whereby success is defined as the ability to pass a scope through the stricture. Symptomatic recurrence can occur, requiring repeat dilatation or surgery in 30–41% of patients after 15–36 months [34, 35]. Risks of bowel perforation during endoscopic balloon dilatation are low at 1.1% compared to a risk of postoperative complications at 8.8%. Bowel-sparing surgical options like strictureplasty are a viable option when medical therapies and endoscopic balloon dilatations fail or are unable to be performed due to multiple small bowel strictures. Strictureplasty works to maintain absorptive function of the bowel by increasing its luminal diameter rather than resecting large portions. Strictureplasty has been proven to be a safe and effective alternative to bowel resection. The overall short-term complication rate ranged from 5% to 20% with no mortalities and a long-term recurrence rate of 25–70% [36]. It is important for hospitalists to get gastroenterologists and general surgeons onboard early in the decision-making process to optimize care in patients with complicated CD.

Ulcerative Colitis

Ulcerative Colitis Flares

Ulcerative colitis is characterized by recurrent inflammation limited to the mucosal and submucosal layers of the colon. It begins in the rectum and extends proximally toward the cecum in a continuous fashion with the extent of distribution varying [6]. On imaging, plain films showing a loss of haustra ("lead pipe" sign) is classic for UC. Otherwise, cross sectional imaging may show inflammatory changes of the colon. On colonoscopy, continuous inflammation in a circumferential pattern generally starting in the rectum can be seen, and the classic findings include ulcerations, friability, granularity, erythema, and the loss of a normal vascular pattern. Histological findings of distortion of crypt architecture with crypt shortening, basal plasmacytosis, Paneth cell metaplasia, and mucin depletion are suggestive of UC [37].

Patients with UC typically present with frequent diarrhea that may be bloody and in small volumes. They may also have colicky abdominal pain (often in the left lower quadrant), urgency, tenesmus, and fecal incontinence due to rectal inflammation [37]. Severity can range from mild (four or less bowel movements per day with or without blood) to severe (10+ bowel movements daily with severe cramps and bleeding). Patients may also have fatigue, weight loss, fever, and symptoms of anemia secondary to iron deficiency from blood loss or chronic inflammation. Progression of these symptoms can be gradual, occurring over several weeks [38].

Up to 15% of patients can present with acute severe UC [37]. Massive hemorrhage can be present in up to 3% of these patients during the course of their disease and may warrant urgent colectomy [37]. Urgency and tenesmus are typically seen in proctitis, whereas bloody diarrhea and abdominal pain are more prominent in pancolitis. Physical examination may reveal signs of abdominal tenderness, signs of anemia, blood on digital rectal exam, and tympany on percussion of the abdomen which may indicate colonic dilatation and requires prompt imaging [37]. Patients with fulminant colitis (10+ stools per day with bleeding, abdominal pain/distension, and toxic presentation such as fever and anorexia) are at risk for toxic megacolon (colonic diameter of equal/greater than 6 cm or cecal diameter greater than 9 cm and the presence of systemic toxic symptoms). Toxic megacolon commonly leads to perforation that has a high mortality rate.

Severity of Ulcerative Colitis

When describing the severity of ulcerative colitis, the Truelove and Witt's criteria has been the most prevalently used. The Truelove and Witt's criteria published in 1955 differentiates between mild and severe disease [39]. Mild colitis according to this criterion will have fewer than four bowel movements a day, normal vitals, a hemoglobin of greater than 11 g/dL, and an ESR less than 22 mm/hr. Severe disease according to this criterion will have six or more bowel movements a day, with fever, tachycardia, anemia, or elevated ESR. These criteria do not take account endoscopic information [39]. The most commonly used criteria that take account of endoscopic information are the Mayo score and Ulcerative Colitis Endoscopic Index of Severity. These three criteria have been incorporated by the American College of Gastroenterology to make their own disease activity index that combines clinical and endoscopic data [39].

Evaluation of Ulcerative Colitis

While laboratory tests are not used to diagnose UC, they are useful to describe the severity of disease, evaluate nutritional status of the patient, and evaluate for any infectious etiology of the patient's symptoms. Complete blood count (CBC), comprehensive metabolic panel (CMP), ESR, C-reactive protein, and albumin are helpful to assess for disease severity. A fecal calprotectin can also be helpful to assess for bowel inflammation. Evaluation of prealbumin, vitamin D, vitamin B12, and iron studies (iron, total iron binding capacity, and ferritin) is helpful to evaluate the patient's nutritional status as well as evaluating patients with anemia. It is very important to evaluate for possible infections. Stool cultures for Salmonella, Shigella, Campylobacter, and Yersinia, stool testing for Escherichia coli O157:H7, giardia stool antigen, C. difficile toxin, and stool microscopy for ova and parasites are helpful in the appropriate clinical setting. In febrile patients, an evaluation for other sources of fever should be completed with urinalysis and urine culture, blood cultures, and a chest radiograph. In patients who are immunosuppressed or in patients with fevers, testing for cytomegalovirus infection and Epstein-Barr virus infection should be done.

Imaging with computed tomography of the abdomen or an abdominal x-ray can be helpful to evaluate for bowel obstruction, colonic dilatation, or perforation. CT scans or MRIs can be used to identify intra-abdominal abscesses or pelvic abscesses, fistulizing disease, or stricturing disease although these are much less common in UC than in CD due to the nature of the disease [40].

Once hospitalized, the care of all patients with severe ulcerative colitis should involve a gastroenterologist, and in most cases, colonoscopy to assess disease severity and to get allow for biopsy looking for CMV or EBV infection will be helpful. If not done within the past 6 months or if risk factors exist, evaluation for hepatitis B and tuberculosis should be performed at the time of admission in the event that TNF inhibitors are needed as to avoid delaying care.

Management of Ulcerative Colitis

Systemic Glucocorticoids

As outlined in Fig. 2.1, systemic glucocorticoids are first-line treatment for inpatient management of acute severe ulcerative colitis (ASUC). According to the American Gastroenterological Association (AGA) guidelines, treatments with 60 mg of IV methylprednisolone (IVMP) or 300 mg IV of hydrocortisone (IVHC) daily is recommended [41]. Doses can be divided. ASUC patients usually respond within 3–5 days of initiation of IV steroids. Systemic glucocorticoids treatment exceeding 7 days for ASUC without clinical improvement is not recommended as the potential for significant improvement past the 7-day mark is minimal. Additionally, longer treatment with glucocorticoids increases the risk for adverse effects such as infection, venous thromboembolism, fractures, poor wound healing, mood changes, irritability, psychosis, weight gain, and increased appetite [42]. While the AGA does not specify whether to use methylprednisolone or

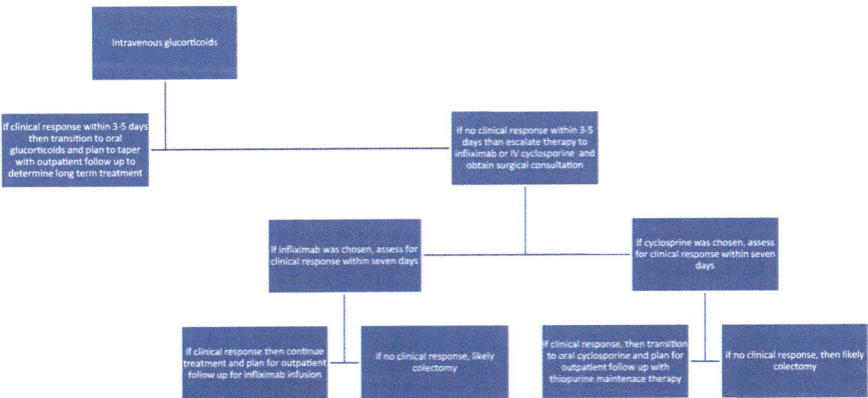

Fig. 2.1 Algorithm for inpatient management of moderate to severe ulcerative colitis flares

hydrocortisone, some research suggests that IVMP use in ASUC may lead to increased need to step up treatment to cyclosporine or biologics compared to IVHC [43]. IVHC has however been seen to have higher rates of hypokalemia and need for potassium supplement compared to IVMP.

Cyclosporine

One of the two established therapies for corticosteroid-resistant ASUC is intravenous cyclosporine, a calcineurin inhibitor. The recommended dose of cyclosporine is 2–4 mg/kg/day given as an intermittent intravenous dose with a serum level goal between 250 and 400 ng/mL [41]. A randomized double-blind study between 2 mg/kg and 4 mg/kg of cyclosporine showed no difference in clinical efficacy for ASUC [44]. Response to cyclosporine in ASUC patients is reported to occur at a median of 4–5 days [43]. Contraindications to cyclosporine include hypocholesteremia, due to its increased risk of precipitating seizures, and decreased renal function as cyclosporine is cleared renally [45].

Infliximab

The other established therapy for corticosteroid resistant is infliximab, an antitumor necrosis factor (TNF) monoclonal antibody [41]. Infliximab is the first agent mentioned that can be used in both acute management and being used as a maintenance treatment. Administration of infliximab is 5 mg/kg at weeks 0, 2, and 6 followed by maintenance dosing of 5 mg/kg every 8 weeks [41]. Expected timing to clinical response for ASUC should be noted by 7 days [43]. Infliximab is contraindicated in those with congestive heart failure, demyelinating diseases, any active infections, latent TB, and hepatitis B [46]. It is also contraindicated in patients with prior antibodies to infliximab or with prior infusion reactions to infliximab.

Infliximab vs. Cyclosporine

Currently, the AGA makes no direct recommendation on preference of treatment between infliximab and cyclosporine [41]. The most recent trial of 135 patients comparing these two drugs found no statistically significant difference in quality of life and 12-month colectomy rate around 40% [47]. Cost-utility analysis demonstrated a significantly higher cost of infliximab due to acquisition costs, but cyclosporine treatment is estimated to have longer hospital stay by a factor of 1.527 times longer (95% CI 1.278–1.817, $p < 0.001$) [47]. This study was done in the United Kingdom under the National Health Service health-care system, so cost analysis may differ when applied to the United States health-care system.

Novel Treatments for ASUC

There are two promising novel treatments for ASUC, vedolizumab and tofacitinib. Vedolizumab is a monoclonal antibody that is an integrin antagonist targeting T lymphocytes. For corticosteroid refractory ASUC, once a calcineurin inhibitor has been used for rescue therapy, the patient can then be bridged to vedolizumab. Ollech et al. conducted a retrospective observational study showing a 7% colectomy rate at 3 months for patients treated with vedolizumab after rescue therapy with cyclosporine [48]. A year later, 33% of this patient cohort had a colectomy and 45% had a colectomy after 2 years [48, 49].

Tofacitinib is a small-molecule Janus kinase inhibitor that has demonstrated efficacy in the inpatient management of corticosteroid-resistant ASUC. Berinstein et al. conducted a retrospective observational study evaluating colectomy rates in patients treated with tofacitinib compared to intravenous corticosteroids [50]. They found that tofacitinib was protective against colectomy at the 90 day mark compared to intravenous corticosteroids with a hazard ratio 0.28, 95% confidence interval of 0,10–0.81, and $p = 0.018$ [12]. It was also noted that 10 mg three times daily dosing of tofacitinib was significantly protective, while 10 mg twice daily was not [50]. This is an exciting prospect as this drug has a rapid-onset action, rapid clearance, and lower costs compared to infliximab [50].

References

1. Klein A, Eliakim R. Non steroidal anti-inflammatory drugs and inflammatory bowel disease. Pharmaceuticals (Basel). 2010;3(4):1084–92. https://doi.org/10.3390/ph3041084.
2. Berkowitz L, Schultz BM, Salazar GA, Pardo-Roa C, Sebastián VP, Álvarez-Lobos MM, Bueno SM. Impact of cigarette smoking on the gastrointestinal tract inflammation: opposing effects in Crohn's disease and ulcerative colitis. Front Immunol. 2018;9(74). https://doi.org/10.3389/fimmu.2018.00074.
3. Sun Y, Li L, Xie R, Wang B, Jiang K, Cao H. Stress triggers flare of inflammatory bowel disease in children and adults. Front Pediatr. 2019;7:432. https://doi.org/10.3389/fped.2019.00432.
4. Stakenborg N, Boeckxstaens GE. Bioelectronics in the brain–gut axis: focus on inflammatory bowel disease (IBD). Int Immunol. 2021;33(6):337–48. https://doi.org/10.1093/intimm/dxab014.
5. Limdi JK. Dietary practices and inflammatory bowel disease. Indian J Gastroenterol. 2018;37(4):284–92. https://doi.org/10.1007/s12664-018-0890-5.
6. Lee JM, Lee KM. Endoscopic diagnosis and differentiation of inflammatory bowel disease. Clin Endosc. 2016;49(4):370–5. https://doi.org/10.5946/ce.2016.090.
7. Peppercorn MA, Kane SV. Clinical manifestations, diagnosis, and prognosis of Crohn disease in adults. UpToDate. 2021. https://www.uptodate.com/contents/clinical-manifestations-diagnosis-and-prognosis-of-crohn-disease-in-adults. Accessed 18 June 2021.
8. Peyrin-Biroulet L, Panes J, Sandborn WJ, Vermeire S, Danese S, Feagan BG, Colombel JF, Hanauer SB, Rycroft B. Defining disease severity in inflammatory bowel diseases: current and future directions. Clin Gastroenterol Hepatol. 2016;14(3):348–354 e317. https://doi.org/10.1016/j.cgh.2015.06.001.

9. Best WR. Predicting the Crohn's disease activity index from the Harvey-Bradshaw index. Inflamm Bowel Dis. 2006;12(4):304–10. https://doi.org/10.1097/01.MIB.0000215091.77492.2a.
10. Dulai PS, Jairath V, Khanna R, Ma C, McCarrier KP, Martin ML, Parker CE, Morris J, Feagan BG, Sandborn WJ. Development of the symptoms and impacts questionnaire for Crohn's disease and ulcerative colitis. Aliment Pharmacol Ther. 2020;51(11):1047–66. https://doi.org/10.1111/apt.15726.
11. Panes J, Bouzas R, Chaparro M, Garcia-Sanchez V, Gisbert JP, Martinez de Guerenu B, Mendoza JL, Paredes JM, Quiroga S, Ripolles T, Rimola J. Systematic review: the use of ultrasonography, computed tomography and magnetic resonance imaging for the diagnosis, assessment of activity and abdominal complications of Crohn's disease. Aliment Pharmacol Ther. 2011;34(2):125–45. https://doi.org/10.1111/j.1365-2036.2011.04710.x.
12. Vermeire S, Van Assche G, Rutgeerts P. Laboratory markers in IBD: useful, magic, or unnecessary toys? Gut. 2006;55(3):426–31. https://doi.org/10.1136/gut.2005.069476.
13. Feuerstein JD, Cheifetz AS. Crohn disease: epidemiology, diagnosis, and management. Mayo Clin Proc. 2017;92(7):1088–103. https://doi.org/10.1016/j.mayocp.2017.04.010.
14. Cheifetz AS, Kornbluth AA, Legnani P, Schmelkin I, Brown A, Lichtiger S, Lewis BS. The risk of retention of the capsule endoscope in patients with known or suspected Crohn's disease. Am J Gastroenterol. 2006;101(10):2218–22. https://doi.org/10.1111/j.1572-0241.2006.00761.x.
15. Dambha F, Tanner J, Carroll N. Diagnostic imaging in Crohn's disease: what is the new gold standard? Best Pract Res Clin Gastroenterol. 2014;28(3):421–36. https://doi.org/10.1016/j.bpg.2014.04.010.
16. Coward S, Kuenzig ME, Hazlewood G, Clement F, McBrien K, Holmes R, Panaccione R, Ghosh S, Seow CH, Rezaie A, Kaplan GG. Comparative effectiveness of mesalamine, sulfasalazine, corticosteroids, and budesonide for the induction of remission in Crohn's disease: a Bayesian network meta-analysis. Inflamm Bowel Dis. 2017;23(3):461–72. https://doi.org/10.1097/MIB.0000000000001023.
17. Ford AC, Kane SV, Khan KJ, Achkar JP, Talley NJ, Marshall JK, Moayyedi P. Efficacy of 5-aminosalicylates in Crohn's disease: systematic review and meta-analysis. Am J Gastroenterol. 2011;106(4):617–29. https://doi.org/10.1038/ajg.2011.71.
18. Hanauer SB, Stromberg U. Oral Pentasa in the treatment of active Crohn's disease: a meta-analysis of double-blind, placebo-controlled trials. Clin Gastroenterol Hepatol. 2004;2(5):379–88. https://doi.org/10.1016/s1542-3565(04)00122-3.
19. Kawalec P, Mikrut A, Wisniewska N, Pilc A. Tumor necrosis factor-alpha antibodies (infliximab, adalimumab and certolizumab) in Crohn's disease: systematic review and meta-analysis. Arch Med Sci. 2013;9(5):765–79. https://doi.org/10.5114/aoms.2013.38670.
20. Hanauer SB, Feagan BG, Lichtenstein GR, Mayer LF, Schreiber S, Colombel JF, Rachmilewitz D, Wolf DC, Olson A, Bao W, Rutgeerts P, Group AIS. Maintenance infliximab for Crohn's disease: the ACCENT I randomised trial. Lancet. 2002;359(9317):1541–9. https://doi.org/10.1016/S0140-6736(02)08512-4.
21. Colombel JF, Sandborn WJ, Reinisch W, Mantzaris GJ, Kornbluth A, Rachmilewitz D, Lichtiger S, D'Haens G, Diamond RH, Broussard DL, Tang KL, van der Woude CJ, Rutgeerts P, Group SS. Infliximab, azathioprine, or combination therapy for Crohn's disease. N Engl J Med. 2010;362(15):1383–95. https://doi.org/10.1056/NEJMoa0904492.
22. Boland BS, Vermeire S. Janus kinase antagonists and other novel small molecules for the treatment of Crohn's disease. Gastroenterol Clin N Am. 2017;46(3):627–44. https://doi.org/10.1016/j.gtc.2017.05.015.
23. Reuken PA, Kruis W, Maaser C, Teich N, Büning J, Preiß JC, Schmelz R, Bruns T, Fichtner-Feigl S, Stallmach A, Group TGIS. Microbial spectrum of intra-abdominal abscesses in perforating Crohn's disease: results from a prospective German registry. J Crohn's Colitis. 2018;12(6):695–701. https://doi.org/10.1093/ecco-jcc/jjy017.
24. Feagins LA, Holubar SD, Kane SV, Spechler SJ. Current strategies in the management of intra-abdominal abscesses in Crohn's disease. Clin Gastroenterol Hepatol. 2011;9(10):842–50. https://doi.org/10.1016/j.cgh.2011.04.023.

25. Lee H, Kim YH, Kim JH, Chang DK, Son HJ, Rhee PL, Kim JJ, Paik SW, Rhee JC. Nonsurgical treatment of abdominal or pelvic abscess in consecutive patients with Crohn's disease. Dig Liver Dis. 2006;38(9):659–64. https://doi.org/10.1016/j.dld.2005.12.001.
26. Garcia JC, Persky SE, Bonis PAL, Topazian M. Abscesses in Crohn's disease: outcome of medical versus surgical treatment. J Clin Gastroenterol. 2001;32(5):409–12.
27. Graham E, Rao K, Cinti S. Medical versus interventional treatment of intra-abdominal abscess in patients with Crohn disease. Infect Dis Res Treat. 2017;10:1179916117701736. https://doi.org/10.1177/1179916117701736.
28. Gutierrez A, Lee H, Sands BE. Outcome of surgical versus percutaneous drainage of abdominal and pelvic abscesses in Crohn's disease. Am J Gastroenterol. 2006;101(10):2283–9. https://doi.org/10.1111/j.1572-0241.2006.00757.x.
29. Clancy C, Boland T, Deasy J, McNamara D, Burke JP. A meta-analysis of percutaneous drainage versus surgery as the initial treatment of Crohn's disease-related intra-abdominal abscess. J Crohns Colitis. 2016;10(2):202–8. https://doi.org/10.1093/ecco-jcc/jjv198.
30. Gionchetti P, Dignass A, Danese S, Magro Dias FJ, Rogler G, Lakatos PL, Adamina M, Ardizzone S, Buskens CJ, Sebastian S, Laureti S, Sampietro GM, Vucelic B, van der Woude CJ, Barreiro-de Acosta M, Maaser C, Portela F, Vavricka SR, Gomollón F. 3rd European evidence-based consensus on the diagnosis and management of Crohn's disease 2016: part 2: surgical management and special situations. J Crohns Colitis. 2017;11(2):135–49. https://doi.org/10.1093/ecco-jcc/jjw169.
31. Rieder F. Managing intestinal fibrosis in patients with inflammatory bowel disease. Gastroenterol Hepatol. 2018;14(2):120–2.
32. Thienpont C, Van Assche G. Endoscopic and medical management of fibrostenotic Crohn's disease. Dig Dis. 2014;32 Suppl 1:35–8. https://doi.org/10.1159/000367824.
33. Molodecky NA, Soon IS, Rabi DM, Ghali WA, Ferris M, Chernoff G, Benchimol EI, Panaccione R, Ghosh S, Barkema HW, Kaplan GG. Increasing incidence and prevalence of the inflammatory bowel diseases with time, based on systematic review. Gastroenterology. 2012;142(1):46–54.e42; quiz e30. https://doi.org/10.1053/j.gastro.2011.10.001.
34. Hassan C, Zullo A, De Francesco V, Ierardi E, Giustini M, Pitidis A, Taggi F, Winn S, Morini S. Systematic review: endoscopic dilatation in Crohn's disease. Aliment Pharmacol Ther. 2007;26(11–12):1457–64. https://doi.org/10.1111/j.1365-2036.2007.03532.x.
35. Bettenworth D, Gustavsson A, Atreja A, Lopez R, Tysk C, van Assche G, Rieder F. A pooled analysis of efficacy, safety, and long-term outcome of endoscopic balloon dilation therapy for patients with stricturing Crohn's disease. Inflamm Bowel Dis. 2017;23(1):133–42. https://doi.org/10.1097/mib.0000000000000988.
36. Campbell L, Ambe R, Weaver J, Marcus SM, Cagir B. Comparison of conventional and non-conventional strictureplasties in Crohn's disease: a systematic review and meta-analysis. Dis Colon Rectum. 2012;55(6):714–26. https://doi.org/10.1097/DCR.0b013e31824f875a.
37. Ungaro R, Mehandru S, Allen PB, Peyrin-Biroulet L, Colombel JF. Ulcerative colitis. Lancet. 2017;389(10080):1756–70. https://doi.org/10.1016/S0140-6736(16)32126-2.
38. Silverberg MS, Satsangi J, Ahmad T, Arnott ID, Bernstein CN, Brant SR, Caprilli R, Colombel JF, Gasche C, Geboes K, Jewell DP, Karban A, Loftus EV Jr, Pena AS, Riddell RH, Sachar DB, Schreiber S, Steinhart AH, Targan SR, Vermeire S, Warren BF. Toward an integrated clinical, molecular and serological classification of inflammatory bowel disease: report of a Working Party of the 2005 Montreal World Congress of Gastroenterology. Can J Gastroenterol. 2005;19 Suppl A:5A–36A. https://doi.org/10.1155/2005/269076.
39. Rubin DT, Ananthakrishnan AN, Siegel CA, Sauer BG, Long MD. ACG clinical guideline: ulcerative colitis in adults. Off J Am Coll Gastroenterol | ACG. 2019;114(3):384–413. https://doi.org/10.14309/ajg.0000000000000152.
40. Feuerstein J. Hospital management of acute severe ulcerative colitis. Gastroenterol Hepatol (N Y). 2021;17(3):128–31.
41. Feuerstein JD, Isaacs KL, Schneider Y, Siddique SM, Falck-Ytter Y, Singh S, Chachu K, Day L, Lebwohl B, Muniraj T, Patel A, Peery AF, Shah R, Sultan S, Singh H, Singh S, Spechler S, Su G, Thrift AP, Weiss JM, Weizman AV, Feuerstein J, Singh S, Isaacs K, Schneider Y, Falck-

Ytter Y, Siddique SM, Allegretti J, Terdiman J, Singh S, Siddique SM. AGA clinical practice guidelines on the management of moderate to severe ulcerative colitis. Gastroenterology. 2020;158(5):1450–61. https://doi.org/10.1053/j.gastro.2020.01.006.
42. Waljee AK, Rogers MAM, Lin P, Singal AG, Stein JD, Marks RM, Ayanian JZ, Nallamothu BK. Short term use of oral corticosteroids and related harms among adults in the United States: population based cohort study. BMJ. 2017;357:j1415. https://doi.org/10.1136/bmj.j1415.
43. Vasudevan A, Gibson PR, van Langenberg DR. Time to clinical response and remission for therapeutics in inflammatory bowel diseases: what should the clinician expect, what should patients be told? World J Gastroenterol. 2017;23(35):6385–402. https://doi.org/10.3748/wjg.v23.i35.6385.
44. Van Assche G, D'haens G, Noman M, Vermeire S, Hiele M, Asnong K, Arts J, D'hoore A, Penninckx F, Rutgeerts P. Randomized, double-blind comparison of 4 mg/kg versus 2 mg/kg intravenous cyclosporine in severe ulcerative colitis. Gastroenterology. 2003;125(4):1025–31. https://doi.org/10.1016/S0016-5085(03)01214-9.
45. Rubin DT, Traboulsi C, Rai V. A practical clinical approach to the management of high-risk ulcerative colitis. Gastroenterol Hepatol (N Y). 2021;17(2):59–66.
46. Rosiou K, Selinger CP. Acute severe ulcerative colitis: management advice for internal medicine and emergency physicians. Intern Emerg Med. 2021. https://doi.org/10.1007/s11739-021-02704-0.
47. Williams JG, Alam MF, Alrubaiy L, Arnott I, Clement C, Cohen D, Gordon JN, Hawthorne AB, Hilton M, Hutchings HA, Jawhari AU, Longo M, Mansfield J, Morgan JM, Rapport F, Seagrove AC, Sebastian S, Shaw I, Travis SPL, Watkins A. Infliximab versus ciclosporin for steroid-resistant acute severe ulcerative colitis (CONSTRUCT): a mixed methods, open-label, pragmatic randomised trial. Lancet Gastroenterol Hepatol. 2016;1(1):15–24. https://doi.org/10.1016/S2468-1253(16)30003-6.
48. Ollech JE, Dwadasi S, Rai V, Peleg N, Normatov I, Israel A, Sossenheimer PH, Christensen B, Pekow J, Dalal SR, Sakuraba A, Cohen RD, Rubin DT. Efficacy and safety of induction therapy with calcineurin inhibitors followed by vedolizumab maintenance in 71 patients with severe steroid-refractory ulcerative colitis. Aliment Pharmacol Ther. 2020;51(6):637–43. https://doi.org/10.1111/apt.15616.
49. Narula N, Marshall JK, Colombel J-F, Leontiadis GI, Williams JG, Muqtadir Z, Reinisch W. Systematic review and meta-analysis: infliximab or cyclosporine as rescue therapy in patients with severe ulcerative colitis refractory to steroids. Am J Gastroenterol. 2016;111(4):477–91. https://doi.org/10.1038/ajg.2016.7.
50. Berinstein JA, Sheehan JL, Dias M, Berinstein EM, Steiner CA, Johnson LA, Regal RE, Allen JI, Cushing KC, Stidham RW, Bishu S, Kinnucan JAR, Cohen-Mekelburg SA, Waljee AK, Higgins PDR. Tofacitinib for biologic-experienced hospitalized patients with acute severe ulcerative colitis: a retrospective case-control study. Clin Gastroenterol Hepatol. https://doi.org/10.1016/j.cgh.2021.05.038.

Chapter 3
Updates in Nephrology for the Hospitalist

Juan Carlos Q. Velez, Santoshi M. Kandalam, Margaret Malone, Thomas Vu, Lukas Kuhnel, Dustin Chalmers, Jaye Frances Espinas, and Brett Pearce

Introduction

The purpose of this chapter is to give a broad overview of nephrology as it affects hospitalists while also hoping to answer a few of the burning questions hospitalists may ask their nephrology colleagues. The majority of the chapter will be focused on discussing a few new updates in the field of nephrology and how these updates could potentially change hospital care.

There is no doubt that kidney-related conditions are extremely common problems within the setting of hospital medicine, especially in the last year due to an increased incidence of kidney injury in patients who have coronavirus disease 2019 (COVID-19). Evaluation and treatment of both acute and chronic kidney disease is constantly evolving as the small but tight-knit community of hospital-nephrologists continue to collect, review, and research data. Chronic kidney disease (CKD) and end-stage renal disease (ESRD) make a significant impact on our health-care system, accounting for

---

J. C. Q. Velez (✉)
Ochsner Clinical School / The University of Queensland, Brisbane, QLD, Australia

Department of Nephrology, Ochsner Health, New Orleans, LA, USA
e-mail: juancarlos.velez@ochsner.org

S. M. Kandalam
University of Queensland, Faculty of Medicine, QLD, Australia

M. Malone · B. Pearce
The University of Queensland-Ochsner Clinical School, New Orleans, LA, USA
e-mail: v-marmalone@ochsner.org

T. Vu · L. Kuhnel · D. Chalmers · J. F. Espinas
University of Queensland School of Medicine - Ochsner Clinical School,
New Orleans, LA, USA
e-mail: v-thomvu@ochsner.org; v-lukkuhnel@ochsner.org; v-duschalmers@ochsner.org; v-jayespinas@ochsner.org

a significant portion of the Medicare budget [1]. The United States Renal Data System is a large-scale data collection system that stores and analyzes detailed data regarding CKD and ESRD, making it easier for researchers and physicians to understand the varying trends that are prevalent in different communities. The Kidney Disease Improving Global Outcome (KDIGO) is a global nonprofit that provides guidelines for management of patients with kidney disease. Though KDIGO and other resources publish detailed guidelines that account for comorbidities, hospitalists commonly report difficulties in understanding and treating nephrology-related conditions within the hospital [2]. Acid-base disorders, glomerular diseases, dialysis, and electrolyte disorders are commonly considered some of the most challenging conditions to manage by medical students as well as internal medicine fellows training in non-nephrology programs [3, 4]. This chapter does not provide a comprehensive guide to the management of kidney disease within the hospital but hopes to highlight important resources and new developments within the field of nephrology.

Hospital-Acquired Acute Kidney Injury

Acute kidney injuries have a high prevalence in hospital settings. While approximately 1% of all hospital admissions are due to an AKI, a much higher percentage of patients (5–10%) develop an AKI while hospitalized [5]. This percentage is significantly increased in critically ill patients. The CDC published a study in 2018 that estimated the incidence of AKI in the United States and found increasing rates from 2000 to 2014, irrespective of whether patients had diabetes [5]. Many studies show that the rate and severity of acute kidney injury is continuing to increase around the globe [6]. The recent pandemic has also been shown to increase rates and severities of AKI in the hospital. A study done at Ochsner Medical Center not only found a higher prevalence of AKIs in COVID patients but also increased need for renal replacement therapy and increased mortality in patients with CoV-related AKI [7].

AKIs typically present as an abrupt decline in kidney function. This can be detected as a marked decrease in urine output; an increase in serum blood urea nitrogen (BUN), creatinine, or other dialyzable substances normally excreted by the kidneys; or a decline in GFR. The two primary metrics used to define an AKI are urine output and serum creatinine concentration; together, they can help determine the severity of an AKI as well, the least severe defined as stage 1 AKI to the most severe, stage 3. The current KDIGO guidelines, published in 2012, define AKIs based on urine output and change in creatinine from a patient's baseline.

If urine output does not correlate with change in serum creatinine, it is advised to manage the patient as if they had the higher stage of AKI. Using urine output to determine stage in a hospital setting has its own challenges. It is important to ensure that a patient with renal injury has urine output measured very carefully. Guidelines also recommend being aware of fluid overloaded states, especially in patients with certain comorbidities. When urine output is low, regardless of their serum creatinine, patients should be closely monitored for signs of fluid overload [8].

Identifying the etiology for kidney injury is vital to determine management and prognosis. Recent data shows that there is a need for better education with the goals

3 Updates in Nephrology for the Hospitalist

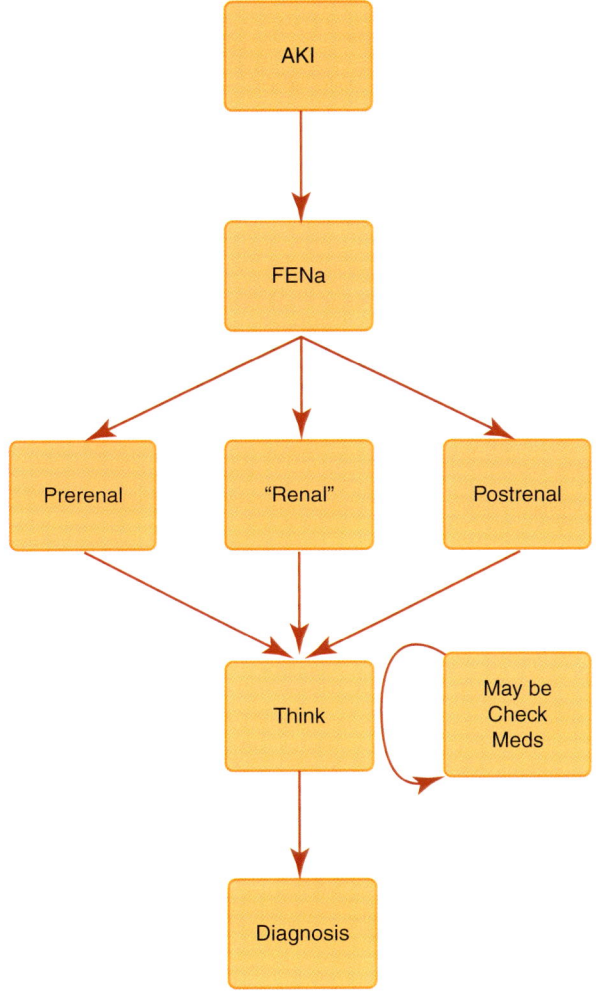

Fig. 3.1 The process of working up a suspected AKI

of recognizing and treating AKI more efficiently within the hospital [9]. Quality measures and initiatives addressing the management of AKI are in the process of being developed [10].

The process of working up a suspected AKI is commonly approached via the process shown in Fig. 3.1: Calculate the fractional excretion of sodium and urea to differentiate between prerenal and renal, think about other causes once the differentiation has been made, and check for possible nephrotoxins before arriving at a diagnosis [11]. Though this method was initially thought to make diagnosis simpler, most prerenal causes in hospital settings can be determined with good history taking and thorough chart review. Furthermore, the fractional excretion of sodium or urea have not consistently shown to correlate with histopathologic findings in systemic reviews [12]. While this method works well for learning the different etiologies of

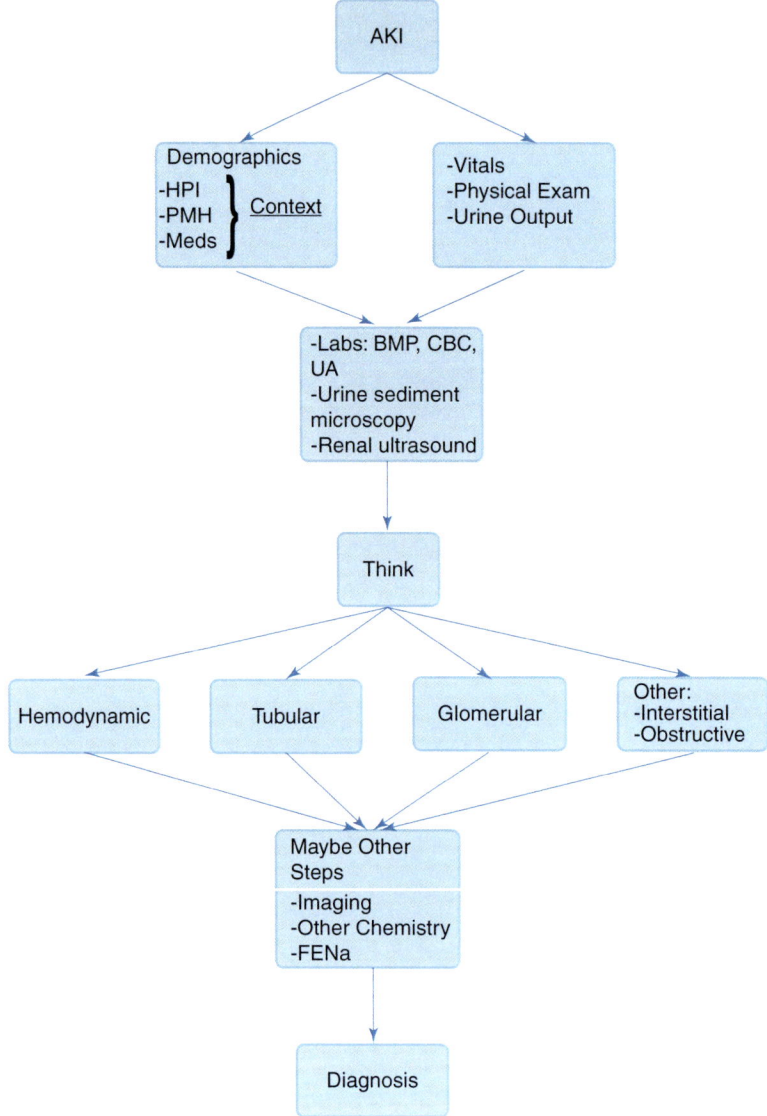

Fig. 3.2 Alternative AKI classification system

kidney damage, a more nuanced approach can better differentiate the pathophysiology involved in the hospitalized patient with AKI.

An alternative AKI classification system with four different categories (hemodynamic, tubular injury, glomerular, and other), as shown in Fig. 3.2, can be beneficial in complex patients. As with any condition, it is important to take a patient's background, demographics, past medical history, and current medications as context for their vitals and physical exam findings. Urine output, as discussed above, is also vital to determining the cause of an AKI. Labs that can differentiate between these causes include a comprehensive metabolic panel, urinalysis, complete blood count, and urine sediment microscopy. A renal ultrasound is also a useful tool in narrowing the diagnosis. Further modalities of imaging can be considered when there is ambiguity in the diagnosis [13].

The temporal association of the injury relative to surgery or use of contrast is another factor to consider in patients with AKIs. The challenge in determining the etiology is often due to multiple processes occurring simultaneously. Urine microscopy can help aid in diagnosis by differentiating between these processes. For example, ATN, the most common type of AKI, often presents with confounding conditions but is identifiable with urine microscopy [14]. Urine microscopy can also aid in making decisions about management and indicate whether further testing, for example, biopsy, is needed.

Medication management in the setting of kidney injury is important for identifying an etiology for the injury itself, modifying medications until renal function improves, and AKI prevention. Avoiding nephrotoxins and renally dosing medications is the recommendation most hospitalists initiate for patients with hospital-acquired AKI; however, renally dosing medication can be challenging. Newer clinical trials with good evidence constantly evolve our understanding of which medications are harmful for patients with renal disease. Some earlier studies have found a link between angiotensin-converting enzyme (ACE) inhibitors and AKI; however, other studies do not recommend unilaterally ceasing ACEi, ARBs, and diuretics in all patients with renal disease [15]. As in all fields of medicine, it is important to individualize treatment plans to the patient and their unique medical history.

Acute Kidney Injury and COVID-19

The newest challenge in managing AKIs is in the setting of COVID-19. The novel coronavirus has presented as a new, independent cause of AKI, warranting an investigation into novel management approaches [7]. This section will cover recent hospital inpatient AKI developments including the most recent diagnostic pathway, COVID-19-associated nephropathy, and new morphometric parameters of the kidney.

Currently, the management of CoV-AKI is traditional in nature employing the standard renal supportive treatments. Implementation of the KDIGO supportive care guideline is likely to reduce the occurrence and severity of CoV-AKI, but this has yet to be validated [16].

The pharmacotherapy for COVID-19 is still undergoing investigation, and over the course of the pandemic, multiple agents have been put forth and trialed. However, only remdesivir and dexamethasone are currently approved for the treatment of COVID-19. Remdesivir is an IV-administered antiviral prodrug that interferes with the action of viral RNA-dependent RNA polymerase. Like many antivirals, concerns have been raised about its effect on kidney function and use during CoV-AKI. Fortunately, initial trials have found that remdesivir is well tolerated in patients with AKI and CKD including those on hemodialysis [17].

Collapsing glomerulopathy is an aggressive variant of focal segmental glomerulosclerosis (FSGS). During the 1980s human immunodeficiency virus (HIV) and acquired immunodeficiency syndrome (AIDS) pandemic, collapsing glomerulopathy was recognized as a specific type of renal involvement in individuals of African ancestry. This clinical entity was subsequently became recognized as HIV-associated nephropathy (HIVAN) [18].

Similar to what was observed during the AIDS epidemic, COVID-19 has been found to affect the kidneys by leading to the development of collapsing glomerulopathy among susceptible individuals. The pathophysiology behind this phenomenon is very similar to that of HIVAN, and as such, a new classification has been proposed entitled COVID-19-associated nephropathy (COVAN). The primary risk factor for the development of COVAN is thought to be genetic. Similar to HIVAN, where the *APOL1* gene risk variants confer a 30- to 90-fold risk increase for the development of collapsing glomerulopathy in the setting of HIV, COVAN is currently suspected to develop in the same *APOL1* gene risk demographic [18]. Patients with COVAN have been found to present clinically with AKI in addition to nephrotic-range proteinuria. Treatment options for COVAN are still being explored and currently only supportive in the hospital medicine setting [18].

Electrolyte Abnormalities: Hyperkalemia and Hyponatremia

Electrolyte abnormalities are extremely common in the hospital setting. Nephrology consults are commonly placed for electrolyte abnormalities independently of underlying renal disease. Electrolyte abnormalities account for a significant amount of hospitalizations in the United States and have placed a significant burden on our health-care system [19].

Hyperkalemia is the most common electrolyte abnormality in patients with CKD and contributes significantly to mortality and morbidity of patients with CKD. Around half of all patients with hyperkalemia have CKD and/or heart failure, amounting to approximately 1.85 million people in 2014 [20]. The burden of disease on the health-care system is immense as well. Hospitalization rates are much higher and mortality rates more than double for CKD patients with hyperkalemia compared to CKD patients with normal potassium levels [20]. According to the AHRQ's data from 2015, around 40,000 admissions occur with the primary diagnosis of hyperkalemia. Furthermore, more than 10% of these patients are discharged to locations other than home, highlighting the need for better management.

There is a widely accepted regimen for patients who have acute, severe hyperkalemia [21]. However, the chronic management of this condition, especially in patients with renal disease or other comorbid conditions, is challenging. Often, comorbid conditions such as hypertension and diabetes, either directly through pathology or indirectly through the medications used to treat the conditions, create even more challenges in the management of hyperkalemia. Many times, patients who have CKD with subsequent hyperkalemia are unable to continue taking medications for coexisting conditions due to the side effect of increased levels of potassium [22]. Medications that can cause hyperkalemia include nonsteroidal anti-inflammatory drugs (NSAIDs), potassium-sparing diuretics, renin-angiotensin system blockers/inhibitors (RASi), epithelial sodium channel blockers, calcineurin inhibitors and heparin. Patients who develop or worsen their hyperkalemia while using RASi are often prescribed a subtherapeutic dose or have the medications discontinued altogether, leading to worse outcomes [23].

Hyperkalemia is defined as extracellular potassium levels above 5.5 mEq/L [24]. Patients with progressing CKD are eventually unable to excrete sufficient potassium for homeostasis; consequently, serum levels of potassium increase. Insulin deficiency can contribute as insulin is a primary driver of potassium uptake by cells.

Other common occurrences contributing to hyperkalemia include the use of angiotensin-converting enzyme inhibitors (ACEi) and potassium-sparing diuretics in patients with coexisting heart failure. A study evaluating the effect of ACEi given to hospitalized patients showed that 10–38% of these patients developed hyperkalemia. Additionally, Collin et al. found that for every 0.1 mEq/L change in potassium either above or below threshold, all-cause mortality increases [25]. As a result, heart failure medications are frequently decreased or discontinued due to concerns for worsening hyperkalemia. However, suboptimal treatment of underlying comorbidities has consequences. Multiple trials have shown that patients who decrease or discontinue RASi have worse overall outcomes than patients who continue to be treated at optimal levels [23]. Newer potassium binders have been shown to maintain potassium levels without needing to change these medications, allowing physicians better options for care of these patients.

Kayexalate, sodium polystyrene sulfonate (SPS), approved in 1958, was the standard treatment of hyperkalemia in patients for decades. It wasn't until recently that newer medications were developed. Studies initially evaluating the validity of using SPS as a treatment option for hyperkalemia found the medication to be effective for lowering potassium levels; however, subsequent studies identified confounding variables [26]. For example, one study found that sorbitol alone reduces potassium levels just as effectively as SPS [27]. Other studies have highlighted the severity of the GI side effects, such as fatal bowel necrosis, associated with SPS [28]. Moreover, the management for patients on SPS is associated with suboptimal use of renin-angiotensin-aldosterone system inhibitors (RAASi) and spironolactone [29]. Strict potassium-restricted diet was also recommended for patients on SPS. Ingesting less than 3 g of potassium in a healthy patient triggers an RAAS response, indicating the importance of the daily ingestion of potassium. Potassium is found in healthier foods such as green vegetables, which have been shown time and time again to be better for the body [30]. Newer potassium binders may allow patients predisposed to hyperkalemia to continue normal diets without the fear of developing hyperkalemia.

Zirconium cyclosilicate and patiromer, newer potassium binders, have been shown to be effective in controlling serum potassium levels while causing fewer adverse effects. These drugs enable the use of RAASi medications and spironolactone. Patiromer, first approved in 2015, is a potassium binder that works in the colon reducing the amount of potassium available for absorption [31]. Patiromer is more effective at higher potassium concentrations, allowing the medication to adapt to diets with more varied levels of potassium [30].

Patiromer's main benefit is allowing patients to continue taking lifesaving medications commonly discontinued to avoid hyperkalemia in patients with renal conditions. The Eplerenone in Mild Patients Hospitalization and in Survival Study in Heart Failure (EMPHASIS) trial negated the practice of discontinuing eplerenone in mild hospitalized patients with hyperkalemia, stating that eplerenone had favorable effects on all-cause death irrespective of worsening renal function and hyperkalemia [32, 33].

A potential rare side effect of patiromer is hypercalcemia [32]. Patiromer binds potassium in the gut as well as other cations, occasionally causing bound calcium to be released into the gut. This calcium that is absorbed is generally excreted in the urine. This can lead to hypercalciuria; however, in cases where kidney function is not optimal, the ability to excrete calcium can be blunted, therefore raising the levels of calcium in plasma.

The other new agent in management of hyperkalemia is Lokelma (sodium zirconium cyclosilicate). It works throughout the GI tract, and the median time to take effect is 2.2 hours. Unlike patiromer, Lokelma does not affect magnesium or calcium levels. The mechanism of Lokelma is trapping potassium in the gut. The ZS-003 trial was the first trial to highlight the efficacy of Lokelma in maintaining normokalemia [34].

Treating electrolyte abnormalities in a hospital setting can be complex and variable, especially in the setting of renal disease. Over the last few decades, there have been consistent improvements made to dialysis; however, few medications to manage hyperkalemia have been discovered [24]. Patiromer and Lokelma are a couple medications that show promise in allowing patients to manage serious electrolyte disturbances while allowing them to continue taking medications that have been shown to decrease mortality. These medications, though beneficial, do have a high price tag – often too expensive for patients to afford. More research and development of medications related to electrolyte management would have a huge impact on hospital medicine [35].

Hyponatremia

Flowcharts, such as Table 3.1, are often used in hospital settings to diagnose electrolyte abnormalities. Though there are hundreds of sources for flowcharts that help categorize electrolyte abnormalities, many trainees continue to find it difficult to interpret and manage patients in a hospital setting [4]. The next section outlines a

Table 3.1 Etiologies of hypotonic hyponatremia with varied urine sodium (urine Na) in milliequivalents per liter(mEq/L) and urine osmolarity (UOsm) in mOsmol/kg

Urine Na mEq/L	UOsm mOsmol/kg	Hypovolemia	Euvolemia	Hypervolemia
<20	<200		Primary polydipsia Tea and toast diet Beer potomania	
<20	>200	GI loss third spacing belongs here		HF Liver cirrhosis Nephrosis
>20	>200	Vomiting Adrenal insufficiency Renal salt wasting	SIADH Adrenal insufficiency Hypothyroidism	

HF heart failure, *SIADH* syndrome of inappropriate antidiuretic hormone, primary, secondary

few tips to help interpret some of the more common labs and techniques currently used in this setting.

- Step 1: Measure serum osmolality (MO), urine osmolality (UOsm), and urine sodium prior to starting management of any kind.
  Interpretation of osmolality: MO is generally measured in the lab. Osmolality of the serum can also be calculated using this equation [36]:
  2 X Na + urea/2.8 + glucose/18.
  The normal range for MO is 275–290 milliosmoles per kilogram (mOsmol/kg). Occasionally, there is a difference of greater than 10 mOsmol/kg H_2O in MO and CO, which is referred to as an osmolar gap (OG) [37]. The etiology is often dependent on osmotically active compounds such as glucose, mannitol, or alcohol. Recently, there has been some debate on the validity of calculating the OG and whether differences in MO and CO may just be related equipment accuracy [38]. The next step is to find the underlying etiology. If MO indicates hypotonic hyponatremia, then proceed to interpret the UOsm.

  Interpretation of UOsm: In a patient with healthy kidneys, one would expect a concurrent decrease in UOsm with hypotonic hyponatremia. If UOsm is less than 100, the etiology is likely extrarenal. The most common causes include primary polydipsia, malnutrition, and alcoholism. For a patient with no other underlying conditions, this level of sodium dilution would require drinking 12 liters or more of water [39]. If a patient has elevated UOsm, then proceed to examine the urine sodium. Urine sodium is typically low in the setting of poor effective circulatory volume such as in volume depletion and poor cardiac output states. Thus, hyponatremia from volume depletion and poor effective circulatory volume (heart failure, cirrhosis) present with similar abnormalities in urine sodium and UOsm. Thus, history and physical ultimately should dictate the diagnosis in those scenarios. On the other hand, the combination of high UOsm (i.e., >200 mOsm/kg) and high UNa should prompt to consider the diagnosis of syndrom of inappropriate secretion of antidiuretic hormone (SIADH).

- Step 2: Determine volume status
  Determining volume status is arguably one of the most difficult parts of managing a patient with hyponatremia. The section below discusses the evolution of tools and techniques utilized in determining a patient's volume status. Once a patient has been categorized as hypovolemic, euvolemic, and hypervolemic, urine sodium levels should be interpreted. If a patient is euvolemic with increased UOsm, consider history that could increase the pretest probability for specific endocrine disorders such as SIADH, glucocorticoid deficiency, and hypothyroidism [40].

Tools to Assess Volume Status

Evaluation of volume status is challenging, especially in ESRD patients. There is a need for objective assessment as fluid overload is associated with worse outcomes in hemodialysis patients, and there are no universally accepted standards to assess volume status in ESRD. Traditional methods for determining volume status in ESRD patients include blood pressure monitoring and targeting the patient's "dry weight," which is generally considered the body weight at which blood pressure is adequately controlled and the patient experiences minimal symptoms of volume overload or depletion. Conventional physical examination findings for fluid overload include crackles at the lung bases and the presence of peripheral edema. Although these are classic clinical signs, it has been suggested that these signs poorly reflect the severity of interstitial lung edema in ESRD patients [41].

Other methods to measure volume overload include the use of laboratory markers, particularly brain natriuretic peptide (BNP), pro-brain natriuretic peptide (pro-BNP), and atrial natriuretic peptide (ANP). While these biomarkers are inexpensive, have good correlation with volume status, and show a direct association with adverse outcomes in ESRD patients, they lack specificity. These biomarkers may be affected by the dialytic membranes used in hemodialysis patients and can also remain high due to other conditions including cardiovascular conditions, stroke, sepsis, anemia, and cirrhosis [42].

Bioelectrical impedance analysis (BIA) or bioimpedance is an inexpensive, non-invasive method that can estimate total body water, intracellular water, and extracellular water. It can also be used to estimate dry weight. BIA is often used in patients on hemodialysis; however, studies suggest that it overestimates fluid overload in the presence of intra-abdominal fluid, which can be seen in patients undergoing peritoneal dialysis [43]. Studies also suggest that its accuracy may be affected by edema, ascites, or water loss [44].

Volume status can also be assessed using ultrasonography through various measurements, such as the inferior vena cava (IVC) collapse index, lung ultrasound to estimate extravascular lung water, and carotid artery Doppler. The IVC collapse index is a highly sensitive measurement that assesses fluid status by IVC collapsibility and can be used to assess fluid responsiveness. Lung ultrasound estimates extravascular lung water through visual identification of Kerley B-lines. It can be used to quantify pulmonary vascular congestion and can be measured serially to assess volume status during dialysis. Carotid artery Doppler is used to calculate corrected flow time, which directly correlates with intravascular volume status. Overall, some of the benefits of using ultrasound are that it is noninvasive, is radiation-free, and can dynamically assess volume status [41, 43].

Novel Therapeutics in CKD: SGLT2 Inhibitors

Diabetic kidney disease (DKD), often in combination with hypertensive nephropathy, is the number one leading cause of ESRD [45]. As approximately 50% of patients with CKD have diabetes, medications used to treat diabetes should be assessed specifically in the context of CKD patients [46]. Traditional diabetic medications have not shown to protect kidney function; however, newer medications have changed the field. The sodium-glucose transport inhibitors (SGLT2i) are a class of medications that have not only shown to significantly improve diabetes but have also been shown to combat vascular disease as well as the development and progression of chronic kidney disease [47, 48].

Sodium-glucose cotransporters are a class of proteins involved in glucose absorption in the intestinal tract and reabsorption of glucose from the proximal tubule of the kidney. Their action is driven by the electrochemical gradient of sodium which allows for the absorption of glucose against its concentration gradient across apical cell membranes [49]. The SGLT2i inhibits the SGLT2 protein, leading to the increased excretion of glucose.

There are many isoforms of SGLTs, but the one targeted by this new class of drugs is the SGLT2 isoform as demonstrated by Fig. 3.3. This isoform is mainly localized to the proximal tubule of the nephron. SGLT2 is responsible for reabsorbing more than 90% of filtered glucose in the proximal tubule.

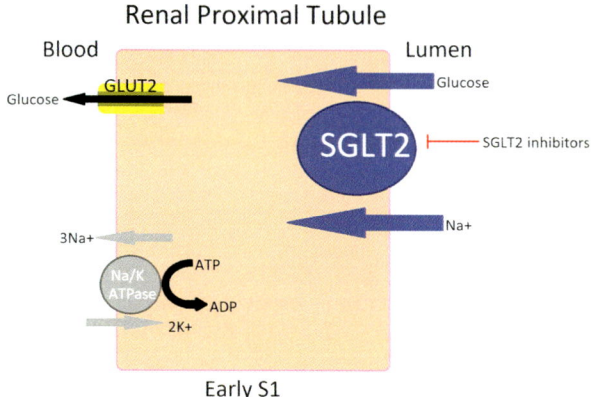

Fig. 3.3 SGLT2 inhibitor mechanism in the proximal tubule of the nephron

The renal threshold for reabsorption of glucose in the proximal tubule is 180 mg/dL. Once serum glucose levels rise above this threshold, the kidneys excrete glucose in the urine [50]. Lowering this threshold by inhibiting reabsorption via SGLT2 inhibitors results in many downstream changes. First, the increased glucose in the tubule increases the hydrostatic pressure in the Bowman's capsule. This increased pressure upregulates the tubuloglomerular feedback at the macula densa, sending signals to decrease the overall work of the kidneys. This not only decreases the inflammatory effects on the kidneys but also has an added benefit of decreasing blood pressure by disrupting the renin-angiotensin system [51].

Canagliflozin (Invokana®) was the first SGLT2 inhibitor to be approved by the FDA in 2013 for the treatment of type 2 diabetes mellitus. Two additional SGLT2 inhibitors are approved by the FDA: dapagliflozin (Farxiga®) and empagliflozin (Jardiance®). These drugs have also been developed in combination with other classes of diabetes drugs. These include canagliflozin/metformin (Invokamet®), dapagliflozin/metformin (Xigduo XR®), empagliflozin/metformin (Synjardy®), and empagliflozin/linagliptin (Glyxambi®) [50]. SGLT2 inhibitors are very effective diabetes medications, replacing other well-known medications like sulfonylureas. Primary care physicians prefer gliflozins due to beneficial side effects of weight loss and decreased systolic blood pressure (with an average decrease of 1.66–6.9 mmHg) [52].

Recently, dapagliflozin (Farxiga) was approved by the FDA for use in kidney disease, specifically to reduce the risk of kidney failure. Previously, this class of drugs have been shown to be efficacious in controlling blood glucose levels, reducing the risk of cardiovascular events, and decreasing hospitalization rates for heart failure. The Dapagliflozin and Prevention of Adverse outcomes in Chronic Kidney Disease (DAPA-CKD) trial was the first double-blind randomized control trial that evaluated Farxiga solely in the setting of kidney injury, and the results were impressive. The multicenter trial studied 4304 patients, assigning them to either a control group receiving placebo or a study group receiving Farxiga. Researchers used certain metrics such as a composite decline in glomerular filtration rate (GFR) of 50%, development of ESRD, and deaths from renal or cardiovascular events to compare the two groups. The positive outcomes in the dapagliflozin group were so significant that the trial was terminated early. The trial also noted that the differences were not attributable to better diabetic control.

The Canagliflozin and Renal Outcomes in Type 2 Diabetes and Nephropathy (CREDENCE) trial, done in 2019, had similarly impressive findings resulting in an early conclusion of the trial. The trial showed improvement in mortality when patients with type 2 diabetes-related renal disease were given canagliflozin. This double-blind randomized control trial observed kidney function in 4401 patients with histories of type 2 diabetes and microalbuminuria. After a median follow-up of 2.62 years, the trial concluded that canagliflozin was effective in reducing the event rate of ESRD, doubling of serum creatinine, and cardiovascular death by approximately 30% [53].

Prior to these studies, there had been evidence of SGLT2 inhibitors having renal protective effects as seen in the Canagliflozin Cardiovascular Assessment Study (CANVAS). The CANVAS study primarily assessed cardiovascular outcomes in patients with type 2 diabetes. The CKD patients in this study were excluded if found to have an eGFR below 30 mL/min/1.73 m^2. On the other hand, DAPA-CKD and CREDENCE were the first studies of their kind to examine a population with both diabetic and nondiabetic patients, in addition to CKD patients with an estimated GFR (eGFR) below 30 mL/min/1.73 m^2. These trials confirm that the renal-protective effects of SGLT2 inhibitors can be extended to broader populations. The results are likely to make this drug class more common among patients who have CKD and/or cardiovascular disease and therefore more frequently seen by hospital medicine physicians [54].

While SGLT2 inhibitors are shown to have benefits, there are side effects as with any drug class. The most well-known adverse effect of SGLT2 inhibitors is urinary tract infections (UTI). These are caused by increased amounts of glucose in the urine promoting mycotic growth. In addition, because of the osmotic diuresis induced by glycosuria, volume depletion and associated urinary frequency, thirst, and orthostatic hypotension are possible adverse effects. Risk factors for these adverse effects include age greater than 75, eGFR less than 60 mL/min/1.73 m^2, or concomitant use of a loop diuretic [55]. Some patients may have an initial drop in GFR and/or albuminuria, but a study in 2019 showed that after 42 months, patients taking may actually have more stable GFRs compared to their baselines [53].

Euglycemic diabetic ketoacidosis (DKA) is a more serious adverse effect of SGLT2 inhibitors. A full-dose SGLT2 inhibitor induces a rapid urinary excretion of glucose, ranging from 5 to 100 g per day. This decline in blood glucose levels may cause diabetic ketoacidosis, even in patients with diabetes. Most patients in the initial case series who presented with diabetic ketoacidosis due to SGLT1 inhibitors were unaware of being in ketosis [56]. Education on this potentially life-threatening complication is important [56].

Conclusion

Nephrology is prevalent in nearly every aspect of hospital medicine. Nephrology in the hospital setting provides its own challenges; however, utilizing tools like urine microscopy can make the process of identifying diagnoses simpler. Consulting a nephrology specialist early for patients with renal conditions and ensuring that they have outpatient follow-up have been shown to improve mortality and quality of life [9]. The American Society of Nephrology, KDIGO, and other nephrology organizations are continuously updating guidelines and creating initiatives to educate fellow medical professionals on some of the most challenging in hospital conditions and complications [57].

References

1. Zhou Y, Yang J. Chronic kidney disease: overview. In: Chronic kidney disease: diagnosis and treatment. Singapore: Springer Singapore; 2020. p. 3–12. https://doi.org/10.1007/978-981-32-9131-7_1.
2. Inker LA, Astor BC, Fox CH, Isakova T, Lash JP, Peralta CA, Tamura MK, Feldman HI, Rocco MV, Berns JS. KDOQI US commentary on the 2012 KDIGO clinical practice guideline for the evaluation and management of CKD. Am J Kidney Dis. 2014;63(5):713–35. https://doi.org/10.1053/j.ajkd.2014.01.416.
3. Calderon K, Jhaveri K. Innovative teaching tools in medicine. In: 3rd international conference on education and new learning technologies (EDULEARN), Barcelona, SPAIN, Jul 04–06 2011. EDULEARN Proceedings; 2011. p. 1093–4.
4. Jhaveri KD, Sparks MA, Shah HH, Khan S, Chawla A, Desai T, Iglesia E, Ferris M, Parker MG, Kohan DE. Why not nephrology? A survey of US internal medicine subspecialty fellows. Am J Kidney Dis. 2013;61(4):540–6. https://doi.org/10.1053/j.ajkd.2012.10.025.
5. Pavkov ME, Harding JL, & Burrows NR. Trends in Hospitalizations for Acute Kidney Injury - United States, 2000–2014. MMWR. 2018;67(10);289–93. https://doi.org/10.15585/mmwr.mm6710a2.
6. Sawhney S, Fraser SD. Epidemiology of AKI: utilizing large databases to determine the burden of AKI. Adv Chronic Kidney Dis. 2017;24(4):194–204. https://doi.org/10.1053/j.ackd.2017.05.001.
7. Mohamed MMB, Lukitsch I, Torres-Ortiz AE, Walker JB, Varghese V, Hernandez-Arroyo CF, Alqudsi M, LeDoux JR, Velez JCQ. Acute kidney injury associated with coronavirus disease 2019 in urban New Orleans. Kidney360. 2020;1(7):614. https://doi.org/10.34067/KID.0002652020.
8. Acosta-Ochoa I, Bustamante-Munguira J, Mendiluce-Herrero A, Bustamante-Bustamante J, Coca-Rojo A. Impact on outcomes across KDIGO-2012 AKI criteria according to baseline renal function. J Clin Med. 2019;8(9). https://doi.org/10.3390/jcm8091323.
9. Liu KD, Goldstein SL, Vijayan A, Parikh CR, Kashani K, Okusa MD, Agarwal A, Cerda J, Amer AKINI. AKI!Now initiative: recommendations for awareness, recognition, and management of AKI. Clin J Am Soc Nephrol. 2020;15(12):1838–47. https://doi.org/10.2215/cjn.15611219.
10. Macedo E, Bihorac A, Siew ED, Palevsky PM, Kellum JA, Ronco C, Mehta RL, Rosner MH, Haase M, Kashani KB, Barreto EF. Quality of care after AKI development in the hospital: consensus from the 22nd Acute Disease Quality Initiative (ADQI) conference. Eur J Intern Med. 2020;80:45–53. https://doi.org/10.1016/j.ejim.2020.04.056.

11. Yassin AR, Sherif HM, Mousa AY, Esmat A. Comparison between fractional excretion of sodium and fractional excretion of urea in differentiating prerenal from renal azotemia in circulatory shock. Egyp. J Crit Care Med. 2013;1(2):69–77. https://doi.org/10.1016/j.ejccm.2013.05.001.
12. Bagshaw SM, Bellomo R. Urine abnormalities in acute kidney injury and sepsis. Cardiorenal Syndr Crit Care. 2010;165:274–83. https://doi.org/10.1159/000313767.
13. Bellomo R, Kellum JA, Ronco C. Acute kidney injury. Lancet (London, England). 2012;380(9843):756–66. https://doi.org/10.1016/s0140-6736(11)61454-2.
14. Kanbay M, Kasapoglu B, Perazella MA. Acute tubular necrosis and pre-renal acute kidney injury: utility of urine microscopy in their evaluation- a systematic review. Int Urol Nephrol. 2010;42(2):425–33. https://doi.org/10.1007/s11255-009-9673-3.
15. Chaumont M, Pourcelet A, van Nuffelen M, Racape J, Leeman M, Hougardy JM. Acute kidney injury in elderly patients with chronic kidney disease: do angiotensin-converting enzyme inhibitors carry a risk? J Clin Hypertens. 2016;18(6):514–21. https://doi.org/10.1111/jch.12795.
16. Ronco C, Reis T, Husain-Syed F. Management of acute kidney injury in patients with COVID-19. Lancet Respir Med. 2020;8(7):738–42. https://doi.org/10.1016/s2213-2600(20)30229-0.
17. Zheng XZ, Zhao YL, Yang L. Acute kidney injury in COVID-19: the Chinese experience. Semin Nephrol. 2020;40(5):430–42. https://doi.org/10.1016/j.semnephrol.2020.09.001.
18. Velez JCQ, Caza T, Larsen CP. COVAN is the new HIVAN: the re-emergence of collapsing glomerulopathy with COVID-19. Nat Rev Nephrol. 2020;16(10):565–7. https://doi.org/10.1038/s41581-020-0332-3.
19. Giordano M, Ciarambino T, Castellino P, Malatino L, Di Somma S, Biolo G, Paolisso G, Adinolfi LE. Diseases associated with electrolyte imbalance in the ED: age-related differences. Am J Emerg Med. 2016;34(10):1923–6. https://doi.org/10.1016/j.ajem.2016.05.056.
20. Betts KA, Woolley JM, Mu F, McDonald E, Tang WX, Wu EQ. The prevalence of hyperkalemia in the United States. Curr Med Res Opin. 2018;34(6):971–8. https://doi.org/10.1080/03007995.2018.1433141.
21. Mushiyakh Y, Dangaria H, Qavi S, Ali N, Pannone J, Tompkins D. Treatment and pathogenesis of acute hyperkalemia. J Community Hosp Intern Med Perspect. 2012;1(4). https://doi.org/10.3402/jchimp.v1i4.7372.
22. Mann JFE. Cardiovascular risk in patients with mild renal insufficiency: implications for the use of ACE inhibitors. Presse Med. 2005;34(18):1303–8. https://doi.org/10.1016/s0755-4982(05)84178-8.
23. Epstein M, Pitt B. Recent advances in pharmacological treatments of hyperkalemia: focus on patiromer. Expert Opin Pharmacother. 2016;17(10):1435–48. https://doi.org/10.1080/14656566.2016.1190333.
24. Hoskote SS, Joshi Sr Fau - Ghosh AK, Ghosh AK. Disorders of potassium homeostasis: pathophysiology and management. (0004-5772 (Print)).
25. Collins AJ, Pitt B, Reaven N, Funk S, McGaughey K, Wilson D, Bushinsky DA. Association of serum potassium with all-cause mortality in patients with and without heart failure, chronic kidney disease, and/or diabetes. Am J Nephrol. 2017;46(3):213–21. https://doi.org/10.1159/000479802.
26. Sterns RH, Rojas M, Bernstein P, Chennupati S. Ion-exchange resins for the treatment of hyperkalemia: are they safe and effective? J Am Soc Nephrol. 2010;21(5):733–5. https://doi.org/10.1681/asn.2010010079.
27. Flinn RB, Merrill JP, Welzant WR. Treatment of the oliguric patient with a new sodium-exchange resin and sorbitol; a preliminary report. (0028-4793 (Print)).
28. Noel JA, Bota SE, Petrcich W, Garg AX, Carrero JJ, Harel Z, Tangri N, Clark EG, Komenda P, Sood MM. Risk of hospitalization for serious adverse gastrointestinal events associated with sodium polystyrene sulfonate use in patients of advanced age. (2168-6114 (Electronic)).
29. Greene SJ, Butler J, Albert NM, DeVore AD, Sharma PP, Duffy CI, Hill CL, McCague K, Mi X, Patterson JH, Spertus JA, Thomas L, Williams FB, Hernandez AF, Fonarow GC. Medical

therapy for heart failure with reduced ejection fraction: the CHAMP-HF registry. (1558-3597 (Electronic)).
30. Picard K, Griffiths M, Mager DR, Richard C. Handouts for low-potassium diets disproportionately restrict fruits and vegetables. J Ren Nutr. 2021;31(2):210–4. https://doi.org/10.1053/j.jrn.2020.07.001.
31. Pitt B, Bakris GL, Bushinsky DA, Garza D, Mayo MR, Stasiv Y, Christ-Schmidt H, Berman L, Weir MR. Effect of patiromer on reducing serum potassium and preventing recurrent hyperkalemia in patients with heart failure and chronic kidney disease on RAAS inhibitors. Eur J Heart Fail. 2015;17(10):1057–65. https://doi.org/10.1002/ejhf.402.
32. Ferreira JP, Abreu P, McMurray JJV, van Veldhuisen DJ, Swedberg K, Pocock SJ, Vincent J, Lins K, Rossignol P, Pitt B, Zannad F. Renal function stratified dose comparisons of eplerenone versus placebo in the EMPHASIS-HF trial. Eur J Heart Fail. 2019;21(3):345–51. https://doi.org/10.1002/ejhf.1400.
33. Rossignol P, Dobre D, McMurray JJ, Swedberg K, Krum H, van Veldhuisen DJ, Shi H, Messig M, Vincent J, Girerd N, Bakris G, Pitt B, Zannad F. Incidence, determinants, and prognostic significance of hyperkalemia and worsening renal function in patients with heart failure receiving the mineralocorticoid receptor antagonist eplerenone or placebo in addition to optimal medical therapy: results from the Eplerenone in Mild Patients Hospitalization and Survival Study in Heart Failure (EMPHASIS-HF). Circ Heart Fail. 2014;7(1):51–8. https://doi.org/10.1161/circheartfailure.113.000792.
34. Packham DK, Kosiborod M. Pharmacodynamics and pharmacokinetics of sodium zirconium cyclosilicate ZS-9 in the treatment of hyperkalemia. Expert Opin Drug Metab Toxicol. 2016;12(5):567–73. https://doi.org/10.1517/17425255.2016.1164691.
35. Lepage L, Desforges K, Lafrance JP. New drugs to prevent and treat hyperkalemia. Curr Opin Nephrol Hypertens. 2016;25(6):524–8. https://doi.org/10.1097/mnh.0000000000000272.
36. Worthley LIG, Guerin M, Pain RW. For calculating osmolality, the simplest formula is the best. Anaesth Intensive Care. 1987;15(2):199–202. https://doi.org/10.1177/0310057x8701500214.
37. Liamis G, Filippatos TD, Liontos A, Elisaf MS. Serum osmolal gap in clinical practice: usefulness and limitations. Postgrad Med. 2017;129(4):456–9. https://doi.org/10.1080/00325481.2017.1308210.
38. Kar E, Kocaturk E, Kiraz ZK, Demiryurek B, Alatas IO. Comparison of measured and calculated osmolality levels. Clin Exp Nephrol. 2020;24(5):444–9. https://doi.org/10.1007/s10157-020-01848-1.
39. Feehally J, Khosravi M. Effects of acute and chronic hypohydration on kidney health and function. Nutr Rev. 2015;73:110–9. https://doi.org/10.1093/nutrit/nuv046.
40. Verbalis JG, Goldsmith SR, Greenberg A, Korzelius C, Schrier RW, Sterns RH, Thompson CJ. Diagnosis, evaluation, and treatment of hyponatremia: expert panel recommendations. Am J Med. 2013;126(10):S5–S41. https://doi.org/10.1016/j.amjmed.2013.07.006.
41. Torino C, Gargani L, Sicari R, Letachowicz K, Ekart R, Fliser D, Covic A, Siamopoulos K, Stavroulopoulos A, Massy ZA, Fiaccadori E, Caiazza A, Bachelet T, Slotki I, Martinez-Castelao A, Coudert-Krier M-J, Rossignol P, Gueler F, Hannedouche T, Panichi V, Wiecek A, Pontoriero G, Sarafidis P, Klinger M, Hojs R, Seiler-Mussler S, Lizzi F, Siriopol D, Balafa O, Shavit L, Tripepi R, Mallamaci F, Tripepi G, Picano E, London GM, Zoccali C. The agreement between auscultation and lung ultrasound in hemodialysis patients: the LUST study. Clin J Am Soc Nephrol. 2016;11(11):2005–11. https://doi.org/10.2215/CJN.03890416.
42. Koratala A, Ronco C, Kazory A. Need for objective assessment of volume status in critically ill patients with COVID-19: the tri-POCUS approach. Cardiorenal Med. 2020;10(4):209–16. https://doi.org/10.1159/000508544.

43. Ekinci C, Karabork M, Siriopol D, Dincer N, Covic A, Kanbay M. Effects of volume overload and current techniques for the assessment of fluid status in patients with renal disease. Blood Purif. 2018;46(1):34–47. https://doi.org/10.1159/000487702.
44. Ugras S. Evaluating of altered hydration status on effectiveness of body composition analysis using bioelectric impedance analysis. Libyan J Med. 2020;15(1):1741904. https://doi.org/10.1080/19932820.2020.1741904.
45. Afkarian M, Zelnick LR, Hall YN, Heagerty PJ, Tuttle K, Weiss NS, de Boer IH. Clinical manifestations of kidney disease among US adults with diabetes, 1988-2014. JAMA. 2016;316(6):602–10. https://doi.org/10.1001/jama.2016.10924.
46. Thomas MC, Cooper ME, Zimmet P. Changing epidemiology of type 2 diabetes mellitus and associated chronic kidney disease. Nat Rev Nephrol. 2016;12(2):73–81. https://doi.org/10.1038/nrneph.2015.173.
47. Alicic RZ, Rooney MT, Tuttle KR. Diabetic kidney disease: challenges, progress, and possibilities. Clin J Am Soc Nephrol. 2017;12(12):2032–45. https://doi.org/10.2215/cjn.11491116.
48. Tomita I, Kume S, Sugahara S, Osawa N, Yamahara K, Yasuda-Yamahara M, Takeda N, Chin-Kanasaki M, Kaneko T, Mayoux E, Mark M, Yanagita M, Ogita H, Araki SI, Maegawa H. SGLT2 inhibition mediates protection from diabetic kidney disease by promoting ketone body-induced mTORC1 inhibition. Cell Metab. 2020;32(3):404–419.e406. https://doi.org/10.1016/j.cmet.2020.06.020.
49. Poulsen SB, Fenton RA, Rieg T. Sodium-glucose cotransport. Curr Opin Nephrol Hypertens. 2015;24(5):463–9. https://doi.org/10.1097/mnh.0000000000000152.
50. Hsia DS, Grove O, Cefalu WT. An update on sodium-glucose co-transporter-2 inhibitors for the treatment of diabetes mellitus. Curr Opin Endocrinol Diabetes Obes. 2017;24(1):73–9. https://doi.org/10.1097/MED.0000000000000311.
51. Vallon V, Thomson SC. Targeting renal glucose reabsorption to treat hyperglycaemia: the pleiotropic effects of SGLT2 inhibition. (1432-0428 (Electronic)).
52. Cefalu WT, Stenlöf K, Leiter LA, Wilding JP, Blonde L, Polidori D, Xie J, Sullivan D, Usiskin K, Canovatchel W, Meininger G. Effects of canagliflozin on body weight and relationship to HbA1c and blood pressure changes in patients with type 2 diabetes. (1432–0428 (Electronic)).
53. Perkovic V, Jardine MJ, Neal B, Bompoint S, Heerspink HJL, Charytan DM, Edwards R, Agarwal R, Bakris G, Bull S, Cannon CP, Capuano G, Chu P-L, de Zeeuw D, Greene T, Levin A, Pollock C, Wheeler DC, Yavin Y, Zhang H, Zinman B, Meininger G, Brenner BM, Mahaffey KW. Canagliflozin and renal outcomes in type 2 diabetes and nephropathy. N Engl J Med. 2019;380(24):2295–306. https://doi.org/10.1056/NEJMoa1811744.
54. Neal B, Perkovic V, Mahaffey KW, Fulcher G, Erondu N, Desai M, Shaw W, Law G, Walton MK, Rosenthal N, de Zeeuw D, Matthews DR, Grp CPC. Optimizing the analysis strategy for the CANVAS program: a prespecified plan for the integrated analyses of the CANVAS and CANVAS-R trials. Diabetes Obes Metab. 2017;19(7):926–35. https://doi.org/10.1111/dom.12924.
55. Garofalo C, Borrelli S, Liberti ME, Andreucci M, Conte G, Minutolo R, Provenzano M, De Nicola L. SGLT2 inhibitors: nephroprotective efficacy and side effects. Medicina (Kaunas). 2019;55(6). https://doi.org/10.3390/medicina55060268.
56. Peters AL, Buschur EO, Buse JB, Cohan P, Diner JC, Hirsch IB. Euglycemic diabetic ketoacidosis: a potential complication of treatment with sodium-glucose cotransporter 2 inhibition. Diabetes Care. 2015;38(9):1687–93. https://doi.org/10.2337/dc15-0843.
57. Braden GL, Chapman A, Ellison DH, Gadegbeku CA, Gurley SB, Igarashi P, Kelepouris E, Moxey-Mims MM, Okusa MD, Plumb TJ, Quaggin SE, Salant DJ, Segal MS, Shankland SJ, Somlo S. Advancing nephrology division leaders advise ASN. Clin J Am Soc Nephrol. 2021;16(2):319–27. https://doi.org/10.2215/CJN.01550220.

Chapter 4
Heart Failure Management for the Inpatient Provider

Tripti Gupta, Vishak Venkataraman, and Sunny Dengle

Epidemiology

The prevalence of heart failure (HF) is on the rise. Currently, there are 6.2 million Americans living with heart failure, with an estimated 64 million people living with it worldwide [1, 2]. The incidence of heart failure increases exponentially with older age. The prevalence of heart failure can also be stratified by ethnicity as the rate of hospitalization for Black patients is 2.5 times higher than that of White patients [3]. With the rise in the prevalence comes an increase in emergency room visits and hospitalizations, which then leads to increased health-care expenditure. In 2012, it was estimated that 31 billion dollars was directed toward heart failure, with projections expecting an increase of 127% by 2030 [4].

Heart failure can be categorized into two subtypes: heart failure with reduced ejection fraction (HFrEF) and heart failure with preserved ejection fraction (HFpEF). Over the last 10 years, HFpEF has become more prevalent, accounting for over half of all hospitalizations of heart failure. HFpEF is more common among older patients and women when compared to HFrEF [5]. With the increase in prevalence of hypertension, obesity, and diabetes, the expected prevalence of HFpEF is further projected to increase.

According to the CDC, risk factors for heart failure include coronary artery disease, hypertension, diabetes, and obesity, with modifiable risk factors including

T. Gupta (✉)
Ocshner Health, New Orleans, LA, USA
e-mail: tripti.gupta@ochsner.org

V. Venkataraman (✉) · S. Dengle
University of Queensland School of Medicine, Ochsner Clinical School, New Orleans, LA, USA
e-mail: v-visvenkataraman@ochsner.org; v-sundengle@ochsner.org

tobacco, alcohol use, sedentary lifestyle, hypertension, diabetes, and obesity [2]. With an expected increase in the prevalence of heart failure, it is crucial for the practicing clinician to understand the pathophysiology of heart failure with reduced ejection fraction (HFrEF) and heart failure with preserved ejection fraction (HFpEF) as well as the optimal medical therapy to best take care of their patients.

Pathophysiology

In the clinical setting, there is often variability between providers in terminology used to describe and classify heart failure [6]. This is, in part, due to the complex pathologic and hemodynamic alterations that occur in patients with heart failure, as well as the large number of potential precipitants and comorbidities that may contribute to this condition [7]. The European Society of Cardiologists have suggested stratification of patients with HF based on left ventricular ejection fraction (LVEF), defining HFrEF as LVEF <40%, HF with midrange EF as LVEF of 40 to 49%, and HFpEF ≥50% [8]. With the increasing prevalence of HFpEF as compared to HFrEF, as well as differences in efficacy of available treatments, it is important to accurately describe and understand the pathophysiological and etiological differences underlying and contributing to HF.

In HFrEF, the ejection fraction is reduced due to systolic dysfunction of the left ventricle (LV), i.e., inability of the LV to appropriately contract. LV systolic dysfunction can be precipitated by dilated cardiomyopathy in which focal or global insult to cardiomyocytes may result in varying levels of scar formation, eccentric hypertrophy, ventricular cavity enlargement, and decreased ventricular contractility [9]. In clinical practice, cardiomyopathy resulting from ischemic heart disease is often referred to as ischemic cardiomyopathy, which represents the most common cause of dilated cardiomyopathy and HFrEF [9]. Established risk factors for the development of ischemic heart disease include dyslipidemia, hypertension, diabetes mellitus, smoking, and family history. There are numerous other recognized precipitants of dilated cardiomyopathy and resultant HFrEF, including hypertension, valvular heart disease, viral infection, chemotoxicity, genetics, and alcohol overuse, which are often collectively referred to as nonischemic cardiomyopathies [9, 10]. Despite this broad division into ischemic and nonischemic causes, efforts to elucidate the underlying etiology of dilated cardiomyopathy and resultant heart failure are essential since treatment approaches and prognosis may differ significantly. It is important to note that in dilated cardiomyopathies, the extent of ventricular systolic dysfunction varies and that ventricular systolic dysfunction may be present in the absence of patient-reported symptoms [9].

With the prevalence of HFpEF increasing, greater efforts are being undertaken to understand the pathophysiological basis for the development of this syndrome. As implied by the name, LV systolic function and ejection fraction are preserved in HFpEF. Whereas some may still think of HFpEF and HFrEF as a clinical spectrum of a single disease, the infrequent progression of HFpEF to HFrEF, differing pathophysiological mechanisms, and disproportionate responses to medical therapy warrants consideration of these conditions as distinct disease processes [7, 11]. HFpEF is characterized by LV diastolic dysfunction or rather impairment of ventricular relaxation and an increase in wall stiffness during diastole [7, 11]. Clinicians often use the terms HFpEF and diastolic heart failure interchangeably; however, this is not wholly accurate as diastolic dysfunction is not exclusive to HFpEF and may also occur in HFrEF [7]. Although the ejection fraction at rest is normal in HFpEF, there is decreased chronotropic reserve resulting in an insufficient increase in ejection fraction in response to stress [5, 7, 11, 12]. This likely contributes to rapid decompensation in these patients. Traditionally, the development of diastolic dysfunction and resultant HFpEF has been associated with concentric hypertrophy, fibrosis, and remodeling of the LV due to systemic hypertension [7, 11, 12]. Emerging models have emphasized the contribution of microvascular endothelial inflammation to increases in oxidative stress, cardiomyocyte signaling disruptions, and myocardial fibrosis [7, 11, 12]. Some of the proposed proinflammatory comorbidities that may precipitate microvascular inflammation include hypertension, diabetes mellitus, iron deficiency, COPD, obstructive sleep apnea, obesity, chronic kidney disease, and smoking [7, 11]. In HFpEF, cardiac remodeling due to hypertrophy, stiffening, and fibrosis ultimately interfere with the ability of the ventricle to relax and fill appropriately in diastole. Since medical therapies for HFrEF have not been shown to be effective in HFpEF thus far, further research into the pathophysiological changes unique to HFpEF is necessary to inform developments in diagnosis and treatment of this condition.

Restrictive cardiomyopathy represents another broad category of myocardial disorders which may result in HF. These conditions are generally characterized by nondilated ventricular cavities, increased myocardial stiffness, severe diastolic dysfunction, and increased ventricular filling pressures [13, 14]. The left or right ventricle may be affected, and patients may exhibit symptoms or signs consistent with left or right HF [14]. Ventricular systolic function and ejection fraction are typically preserved until these disorders have progressed to advanced stages [13, 14]. Restrictive cardiomyopathy is recognized as the rarest form of cardiomyopathy; however, the wide spectrum of inherited and acquired causes and the difficulty in establishing these diagnoses may limit accurate estimations of disease prevalence [14]. Cardiac amyloidosis (CA), an infiltrative disease caused by extracellular deposition of misfolded amyloid protein, is a known precipitant of restrictive cardiomyopathy and HF. However, evolving research suggests that this disease is an underdiagnosed cause of HF [13, 15, 16]. A prospective, single-center analysis of myocardial tissue biopsies from patients with HFpEF showed a CA prevalence of 14% [15]. Another prospective analysis of myocardial tissue biopsies from HFpEF patients showed the prevalence of wild-type transthyretin CA – the most common subtype of CA – to be 13% [17]. These findings hold potentially significant implications for the diagnosis and management of restrictive cardiomyopathies and HF as experimental therapies for transthyretin CA have shown favorable results for slowing decline in functional capacity and reducing all-cause mortality [18].

There are multiple other precipitants of cardiomyopathy not discussed in detail here which may lead to the development of HF, i.e., hypertrophic cardiomyopathy, cardiac sarcoidosis, and cardiac hemochromatosis [14, 19]. Although challenging, it is essential to attempt to elucidate the underlying cause of HF as establishing a definitive pathophysiological mechanism can inform patient prognosis and further management.

Clinical Assessment of Heart Failure

Presentation

HF is a multifaceted clinical syndrome that often presents with wide, case-by-case variability in patient-reported symptomatology, physical examination findings, and investigative results. Detailed history taking, physical examination, and review of patient medical records are essential for appropriate clinical assessment and diagnosis of the patient presenting with suspected HF. Patients with acute decompensated HF may present with symptoms consistent with predominantly right-sided or left-sided heart failure or a combination of both.

Commonly reported symptoms include progressive dyspnea on exertion, fatigue, peripheral edema, unintentional weight gain, orthopnea, paroxysmal nocturnal dyspnea, and abdominal distention or tenderness. In one retrospective study of 99,825 HF admissions, investigators found that the most common presenting symptom was dyspnea on exertion, present in 71.2% of patients [20]. Patients may present with a single reported symptom in the absence of appreciable physical exam findings, warranting investigation of noncardiac differential diagnoses [11]. In the setting of long-standing HF with chronic deconditioning, patients may have trouble differentiating the progression of symptoms [11]. The New York Heart Association (NYHA) classification of patients with HF is regularly used to describe functional status and disease progression. However, the subjective nature of patient-reported symptoms, variability of assessment between clinicians, and similarity in treatment modalities between functional classes might limit the utility of this categorization [6]. The American Heart Association (AHA) and the American College of Cardiology (ACC) have also published staging guidelines designed to be used in conjunction with the NYHA classification scheme in order to stratify the spectrum of clinical HF from those at risk of developing this syndrome to those with advanced HF [6]. Clinicians should hold a high index of suspicion for the presence of HF in patients with identifiable risk factors, symptoms, and signs consistent with this condition.

History

Detailed history is vital to establishing the diagnosis of acute decompensated HF, whether this is a new diagnosis or an exacerbation of chronic HF. Since many HF symptoms are not solely specific to this condition, it is important to consider non-cardiogenic etiologies, i.e., peripheral edema associated with renal disease, dyspnea of primary pulmonary origin, or ascitic abdominal fullness due to hepatic disease. Focused history questions and record review can help to differentiate between likely causes of symptoms and to delineate next steps in investigation.

It is important to characterize the progression of symptoms that led to presentation and to identify symptoms that may point to potential precipitants of HF onset or exacerbation, i.e., chest pain, palpitations, or fever. Assessing the patient's adherence to a low sodium diet, fluid restriction, and measurement of daily weights may also provide useful insight into possible triggers for the patient with HF exacerbation. Ascertaining the patient's current functional status as compared to baseline can provide worthwhile information about symptom progression. It is also essential to review the patient's social history as certain behaviors such as alcohol consumption or substance use may precipitate or exacerbate HF. Reviewing information from previous hospitalizations, carrying out a thorough medication reconciliation to ensure the patient is adherent to an optimized regimen, and performing a thorough review of systems will aid in establishing the diagnosis of HF [11, 20].

Physical Exam

Physical exam can provide important details on the extent and severity of a patient's heart failure. A patient's vital signs and general appearance can suggest the presence of heart failure, especially if it is advanced. Important vitals to assess include heart rate, respiratory rate, blood pressure, and oxygen saturation.

A detailed cardiovascular exam is required to assess volume status in a patient. Examination assessing for volume overload should focus on pulmonary congestion, peripheral edema, elevated jugular venous pressure, and the hepatojugular reflux as these findings suggest high intravascular pressure. Hepatojugular reflex on clinical exam and the presence of orthopnea are two of the most sensitive clinical findings for the presence of advanced heart failure [21]. Pulmonary congestion can clinically manifest as rales and is evident of left-sided heart failure, so a detailed respiratory exam is required. Typically, a patient who is volume overloaded, or "wet," correlates with a pulmonary capillary wedge pressure (PCWP) of greater than 22 mmHg [21].

The clinical assessment of a patient's perfusion status is another aspect of examining a patient with heart failure. A narrow pulse pressure or cold extremities, especially in the presence of hypotension and volume overload, can suggest cardiogenic shock [21]. The patient may have tachycardia or tachypnea at rest, and their extremities will be cold and cyanotic with poor capillary refill due to poor perfusion. In cardiogenic shock due to heart failure, pulsus alternans may also be seen. Pulsus alternans describes an arterial pulse that is characterized by alternate strong and weak beats. This sign is pathognomonic of severe systolic dysfunction and is a sign of poor prognosis.

Investigations

Laboratory testing and various initial investigations can reinforce the diagnosis of heart failure or pave the way toward an alternative diagnosis for the patient's symptoms.

Chest X-Ray

Chest X-ray provides important information to help differentiate heart failure with other primary pulmonary pathology. Important features suggestive of heart failure include a cardiothoracic ratio >50% and pulmonary edema, represented by Kerley B-lines on imaging. When looking at the utility of chest X-ray on diagnosing heart failure, a systematic review of 15 studies showed that it was moderately specific at 76–83% but insensitive at 68% in patients with HFrEF [22]. In patients with HFpEF, the sensitivity of abnormal cardiac findings is even lower than in patients with HFrEF.

Echocardiography

Echocardiography is a widely accepted and readily available confirmatory test for diagnosing heart failure. Echocardiography is a noninvasive method of measuring important clinical parameters for heart failure including left ventricular ejection fraction. The versatility of the echocardiogram makes it a vital imaging modality to assess a patient with heart failure. It has the ability to assess structural or valvular abnormalities as this could be contributing to a patient's disease state. In addition, the use of Doppler can accurately estimate a patient's cardiac output as well as determine important pressure measurements [23]. Echocardiography also has an important role in monitoring disease progression as well as treatment guidance. The combination of BNP and echocardiography results helps determine the severity of the disease as well as the appropriate fluid management in an inpatient setting [23]. The noninvasive nature as well as its importance in both diagnosing as well as treating a patient with heart failure makes it a mainstay in hospital practice.

Biomarkers and Blood Tests

A common biomarker used to evaluate patients with heart failure is BNP or N-terminal pro-BNP. These biomarkers are secreted in the ventricles in response to increased wall tension and myocardial stretch. These biomarkers are often used interchangeably in clinical practice. BNP is commonly increased in patients with

HFrEF, but a normal BNP cannot exclude the diagnosis especially in patients with obesity. Obesity leads to increased neprilysin concentrations, which leads to a decrease in BNP. In addition, obesity leads to an increase in renal filtration which subsequently reduces BNP levels [24]. Patients with HFpEF also commonly have normal BNP levels. BNP levels are increased due to other causes as well, including renal failure, coronary disease, pulmonary hypertension, and sepsis.

Cardiac troponins, a common biomarker measuring myocardial ischemia, can also be used to assess heart failure. It has been seen that patients with chronic or acute heart failure have detectable levels of troponins, with a positive correlation between troponin level and prognosis. This concept demonstrates that there may be multiple mechanisms of troponin release in patients. It is thought that viable cardiomyocytes release troponins in response to myocardial stretch [25]. Therefore, cardiac troponins have a role in measurement as well as prognosis and treatment in patients with heart failure.

In addition to the biomarkers mentioned above, initial blood work is required to help determine the etiology of heart failure. A CBC is important to assess for anemia or an infection that could exacerbate a patient's symptoms. Serum electrolytes and kidney function tests are important to assess as well as patients can have electrolyte abnormalities as well as acute kidney injury due to volume overload. They are important markers for assessing treatment with diuresis as well as fluid restriction. Liver function tests should be measured as well as they can be affected due to hepatic congestion [26].

Management

Guideline-Directed Medical Therapy (GDMT) for Heart Failure

The pharmacological management of HFrEF is an extensively researched and often discussed topic in medical literature. The ACC and AHA have previously outlined specific Guideline-Directed Medical Therapy (GDMT), which consists of optimal medical strategies to control symptoms, limit hospitalizations, and reduce mortality in ambulatory HFrEF patients [26–28]. Notably, the efficacy of these management approaches is based on randomized controlled trials that included only HFrEF patients or rather patients who demonstrated an LVEF ≤40% [26, 27]. Patients with HFpEF and HFrEF may have similar comorbidities and risk factors as HFrEF patients, i.e., hypertension and diabetes mellitus, that serve as alternative indications for the use of GDMT therapies [26, 27]. However, the use of these agents in HFpEF patients has not shown a significant improvement in mortality or rate of hospitalization [11].

The ACC has also published specific algorithms for the initiation and alteration of GDMT in HFrEF to help providers clarify appropriate treatment modalities based on the patient's clinical status. For example, expert consensus from the ACC posits that the initiation of beta-blockers is better tolerated by patients who are clinically euvolemic or "dry" [27]. Conversely, the ACC notes that initiation of medications promoting inhibition of the renin-angiotensin-aldosterone (RAAS) system is often tolerated when patients are clinically volume overloaded or "wet" [27]. It is necessary to assess individual patient characteristics when considering the use of GDMT for HF patients. Each class of medications included in these guidelines may play a role in management depending on patient symptomatology, volume status, contraindications to medication use, NYHA classification, laboratory findings, previously implemented medication regimens, chronicity of HFrEF, and comorbidities [26–28].

Advancements in the Management for Heart Failure

One of the mainstays of pharmacological treatment of HFrEF is the inhibition of the RAAS system. Chronic elevation of angiotensin leads to myocardial hypertrophy [29]. Therefore, over the past 30 years, the use of ACE inhibitors, angiotensin receptor blockers (ARBs), and mineralocorticoid receptor antagonists has been studied and proven to reduce mortality for patients with HFrEF. Specifically, in 1987, results of the CONSENSUS trial showed a decrease in 6-month mortality from severe heart failure from 46 to 25% [30]. In addition, the RALES trial looking at the effect of spironolactone in severe HF showed a decrease in 24-month mortality from 46% to 35% [31].

In the last 5 to 10 years, there have been major advancements in the management of HFrEF. Specifically, this new shift in the treatment stemmed from the addition of neprilysin inhibition to the management. The PARADIGM-HF trial looked at the ARB valsartan combined with the neprilysin inhibitor sacubitril and compared outcomes with treatment with an ACE inhibitor [32]. The results of the study showed that hospitalization and death for patients is 21.8% for the valsartan-sacubitril group and 26.5% for the enalapril group in a 27-month period, demonstrating a significant reduction in CV hospitalization and HF deaths. This study also looked at the secondary outcome of death due to any cause, and the results also showed a significant decrease in mortality with the valsartan-sacubitril group [32]. The PIONEER-HF trial looked specifically at NT-proBNP levels of the two groups. The results of the study showed a significant reduction in the NT-proBNP levels of the valsartan-sacubitril group when compared to the enalapril group, both in week 4 and in week 8 measurement [33]. The use of the combination of ACE inhibitors and neprilysin inhibitors was also tested but resulted in a significant increase in angioedema in patients. The use of RAAS inhibition has also been tested in patients with HfpEF, and there has been no significant evidence pointing to its efficacy in these patients [34].

Cardiovascular disease (CVD) is one of the leading causes of morbidity and mortality for diabetic patients, and there has been much research done looking at cardiovascular outcomes on sodium-glucose cotransporter-2 (SGLT-2) inhibitors. The CVD-REAL 2 study looked at patient records from six different countries in three world regions, amassing over 400,000 patients with type II diabetes, comparing SGLT-2 inhibitors with other glucose-lowering drugs. The results of this study showed that the use of SGLT-2 inhibitors led to significantly lower risk of all-cause death (ACD), heart failure hospitalizations, myocardial infarction, and stroke [35]. With this in mind, the next step was to apply these medications to a broader patient population, specifically ones who do not have type II diabetes. The DAPA-HF trial focused on this patient population [34]. This study looked at the use of dapagliflozin in patients with NYHA II, III, or IV heart failure and an ejection fraction of less than 40%, regardless of whether or not they had type II diabetes. Patients were randomly assigned to dapagliflozin plus recommended therapy or placebo and recommended therapy with the primary outcome being heart failure hospitalization or cardiovascular death. The results showed a significant decrease in the primary outcome in the group with dapagliflozin, confirming its efficacy in patients with HFrEF, regardless of the presence of type II diabetes [35].

With multiple randomized control trials showing identifying the clinical benefit of SGLT-2 inhibitors and angiotensin-receptor neprilysin inhibitors (ARNI) in patients with heart failure, current comprehensive disease-modifying therapy has changed to add these medications. The current quadruple therapy includes an ARNI, beta-blocker, mineralocorticoid receptor antagonist (MRA), and an SGLT-2 inhibitor. A study from JAMA looking at the efficacy of quadruple therapy shows a 73% relative risk reduction in mortality [36]. With the implementation of the new quadruple therapy, there are many challenges associated with the treatment. With the addition of new medications to the standard HF therapy that have overlapping side effects (hypotension, acute kidney injury, electrolyte disturbances), there is some worry with regard to compounding those side effects [37]. The idea of polypharmacy as well as medication compliance and cost also comes to play when adding a new medication. However, with optimal medical management, there is hope for improved quality of life and reduced hospitalization in patients with chronic heart failure.

Addressing Barriers to Health Care

Social determinants of health are very important factors to address when assessing the efficacy of medical therapy in patients with heart failure. Financial barriers are present for many patients resulting in the inability to afford lifesaving medical treatment. In addition, lack of housing or transportation can prevent patients from accessing a nearby hospital. Inadequate health literacy also provides a barrier toward medication compliance as well as complex management of a chronic condition. A meta-analysis looked at the relationship between health literacy and mortality, ED visits, and hospitalization. The results of the study showed that marginal health literacy led to an increase in mortality, hospitalizations, and ED visits for heart failure [38]. It is likely that this measurement of health literacy involves other social determinants of health. Therefore, as hospitalists, it is vital to not only understand the social determinants and cultural differences involved in a patient's health care, but also incorporate these into addressing management of chronic heart failure.

References

1. Groenewegen A, Rutten F, Mosterd A, Hoes A. Epidemiology of heart failure. Eur J Heart Fail. 2020;22:1342–56. https://doi.org/10.1002/ejhf.1858.
2. Heart Failure | cdc.gov. In: Centers for Disease Control and Prevention. 2021. https://www.cdc.gov/heartdisease/heart_failure.htm. Accessed 23 Aug 2021.
3. Nayak A, Hicks A, Morris A. Understanding the complexity of heart failure risk and treatment in black patients. Circ Heart Fail. 2020; https://doi.org/10.1161/circheartfailure.120.007264.
4. Savarese G, Lund L. Global public health burden of heart failure. Cardiac Failure Review. 2017;03(7) https://doi.org/10.15420/cfr.2016:25:2.
5. Paulus W. Unfolding discoveries in heart failure. N Engl J Med. 2020;382:679–82. https://doi.org/10.1056/nejmcibr1913825.
6. Hunt S, Baker D, Chin M, et al. ACC/AHA guidelines for the evaluation and Management of Chronic Heart Failure in the adult: executive summary a report of the American College of Cardiology/American Heart Association task force on practice guidelines (committee to revise the 1995 guidelines for the evaluation and Management of Heart Failure). Circulation. 2001;104:2996–3007. https://doi.org/10.1161/hc4901.102568.
7. Borlaug B, Paulus W. Heart failure with preserved ejection fraction: pathophysiology, diagnosis, and treatment. Eur Heart J. 2010;32:670–9. https://doi.org/10.1093/eurheartj/ehq426.
8. Ponikowski P, Voors A, Anker S, et al. 2016 ESC guidelines for the diagnosis and treatment of acute and chronic heart failure. Eur Heart J. 2016;37:2129–200. https://doi.org/10.1093/eurheartj/ehw128.
9. McNally E, Mestroni L. Dilated cardiomyopathy. Circ Res. 2017;121:731–48. https://doi.org/10.1161/circresaha.116.309396.
10. Bozkurt B, Colvin M, Cook J, et al. Current diagnostic and treatment strategies for specific dilated Cardiomyopathies: A Scientific Statement From the American Heart Association. Circulation. 2016; https://doi.org/10.1161/cir.0000000000000455.
11. Redfield M. Heart failure with preserved ejection fraction. N Engl J Med. 2016;375:1868–77. https://doi.org/10.1056/nejmcp1511175.
12. Borlaug B. The pathophysiology of heart failure with preserved ejection fraction. Nat Rev Cardiol. 2014;11:507–15. https://doi.org/10.1038/nrcardio.2014.83.
13. Pereira N, Grogan M, Dec G. Spectrum of restrictive and infiltrative cardiomyopathies. J Am Coll Cardiol. 2018;71:1130–48. https://doi.org/10.1016/j.jacc.2018.01.016.
14. Muchtar E, Blauwet L, Gertz M. Restrictive cardiomyopathy. Circ Res. 2017;121:819–37. https://doi.org/10.1161/circresaha.117.310982.
15. Hahn V, Yanek L, Vaishnav J, et al. Endomyocardial biopsy characterization of heart failure with preserved ejection fraction and prevalence of cardiac amyloidosis. JACC: Heart Failure. 2020;8:712–24. https://doi.org/10.1016/j.jchf.2020.04.007.
16. Witteles R, Bokhari S, Damy T, et al. Screening for transthyretin amyloid cardiomyopathy in everyday practice. JACC: Heart Failure. 2019;7:709–16. https://doi.org/10.1016/j.jchf.2019.04.010.
17. González-López E, Gallego-Delgado M, Guzzo-Merello G, et al. Wild-type transthyretin amyloidosis as a cause of heart failure with preserved ejection fraction. Eur Heart J. 2015;36:2585–94. https://doi.org/10.1093/eurheartj/ehv338.
18. Yamamoto H, Yokochi T. Transthyretin cardiac amyloidosis: an update on diagnosis and treatment. ESC Heart Failure. 2019;6:1128–39. https://doi.org/10.1002/ehf2.12518.
19. Marian A, Braunwald E. Hypertrophic cardiomyopathy. Circ Res. 2017;121:749–70. https://doi.org/10.1161/circresaha.117.311059.
20. Kapoor J, Kapoor R, Ju C, et al. Precipitating clinical factors, heart failure characterization, and outcomes in patients hospitalized with heart failure with reduced, borderline, and preserved ejection fraction. JACC: Heart Failure. 2016;4:464–72. https://doi.org/10.1016/j.jchf.2016.02.017.

21. Thibodeau J, Drazner M. The role of the clinical examination in patients with heart failure. JACC: Heart Failure. 2018;6:543–51. https://doi.org/10.1016/j.jchf.2018.04.005.
22. Mant J, Doust J, Roalfe A, et al. Systematic review and individual patient data meta-analysis of diagnosis of heart failure, with modelling of implications of different diagnostic strategies in primary care. Health Technol Assess. 2009; https://doi.org/10.3310/hta13320.
23. Kirkpatrick J, Vannan M, Narula J, Lang R. Echocardiography in heart failure. J Am Coll Cardiol. 2007;50:381–96. https://doi.org/10.1016/j.jacc.2007.03.048.
24. Maisel A, McCord J, Nowak R. Bedside B-type natriuretic peptide in the emergency diagnosis of heart failure with reduced or preserved ejection fraction. Results from the breathing not properly multinational study. ACC Curr J Rev. 2003;12(46) https://doi.org/10.1016/j.accreview.2003.08.071.
25. Kociol R, Pang P, Gheorghiade M, et al. Troponin elevation in heart failure. J Am Coll Cardiol. 2010;56:1071–8. https://doi.org/10.1016/j.jacc.2010.06.016.
26. Yancy C, Jessup M, Bozkurt B, et al. 2013 ACCF/AHA guideline for the Management of Heart Failure. Circulation. 2013; https://doi.org/10.1161/cir.0b013e31829e8776.
27. Maddox T, Januzzi J, Allen L, Breathett K, Butler J, Davis L, Fonarow G, Ibrahim N, Lindenfeld J, Masoudi F, Motiwala S, Oliveros E, Patterson J, Walsh M, Wasserman A, Yancy C, Youmans Q. 2021 update to the 2017 ACC expert consensus decision pathway for optimization of heart failure treatment: answers to 10 pivotal issues about heart failure with reduced ejection fraction. J Am Coll Cardiol. 2021;77(6):772–810.
28. Biglane J, Becnel M, Ventura H, Krim S. Pharmacologic therapy for heart failure with reduced ejection fraction: closing the gap between clinical guidelines and practice. Prog Cardiovasc Dis. 2017;60(2):187–97.
29. Leong D, McMurray J, Joseph P, Yusuf S. From ACE inhibitors/ARBs to ARNIs in coronary artery disease and heart failure (part 2/5). J Am Coll Cardiol. 2019;74:683–98. https://doi.org/10.1016/j.jacc.2019.04.068.
30. Effects of Enalapril on Mortality in Severe Congestive Heart Failure. N Engl J Med. 1987:316:1429–35. https://doi.org/10.1056/nejm198706043162301.
31. Pitt B, Zannad F, Remme W, et al. The effect of spironolactone on morbidity and mortality in patients with severe heart failure. N Engl J Med. 1999;341:709–17. https://doi.org/10.1056/nejm199909023411001.
32. McMurray J, Packer M, Desai A, et al. Angiotensin–Neprilysin inhibition versus Enalapril in heart failure. N Engl J Med. 2014;371:993–1004. https://doi.org/10.1056/nejmoa1409077.
33. Velazquez E, Morrow D, DeVore A, et al. Angiotensin–Neprilysin inhibition in acute decompensated heart failure. N Engl J Med. 2019;380:539–48. https://doi.org/10.1056/nejmoa1812851.
34. McMurray J, Solomon S, Inzucchi S, et al. Dapagliflozin in patients with heart failure and reduced ejection fraction. N Engl J Med. 2019;381:1995–2008. https://doi.org/10.1056/nejmoa1911303.
35. Kosiborod M, Lam C, Kohsaka S, et al. Cardiovascular events associated with SGLT-2 inhibitors versus other glucose-lowering drugs. J Am Coll Cardiol. 2018;71:2628–39. https://doi.org/10.1016/j.jacc.2018.03.009.
36. Bassi N, Ziaeian B, Yancy C, Fonarow G. Association of Optimal Implementation of sodium-glucose cotransporter 2 inhibitor therapy with outcome for patients with heart failure. JAMA Cardiol. 2020;5:948. https://doi.org/10.1001/jamacardio.2020.0898.
37. Greene S, Khan M. Quadruple medical therapy for heart failure. J Am Coll Cardiol. 2021;77:1408–11. https://doi.org/10.1016/j.jacc.2021.02.006.
38. Fabbri M, Murad M, Wennberg A, et al. Health literacy and outcomes among patients with heart failure. JACC: Heart Failure. 2020;8:451–60. https://doi.org/10.1016/j.jchf.2019.11.007.

Chapter 5
Advances in the Evaluation and Treatment of Sepsis and Shock

Kevin Conrad and Emily Kelsoe

Introduction

Over the past few decades, the term "sepsis" has evolved through many definitions, treatment algorithms, and approaches. The definition itself, which was originally confined to the basic terms of positive blood cultures, has now transitioned in definition to a dysregulated host response to an infection [1, 2]. However, one constant has remained true throughout the years: the rapid treatment focus on reducing the morbidity and mortality of sepsis. Sepsis is considered a time-sensitive medical emergency, akin to myocardial infarction or stroke, and should be treated accordingly [3]. Sepsis leads to approximately 11 million deaths worldwide each year and, even when not fatal, can have lasting impacts on patients' lives, the health-care system, and antimicrobial stewardship efforts [4].

Defining Sepsis and Septic Shock

The institution of the 2016 Surviving Sepsis Campaign brought about new definitions for sepsis and septic shock [5]. The focus of this update was on the cellular and organ dysfunction associated with sepsis. The systemic inflammatory response syndrome (SIRS) definition was determined to be ineffective in distinguishing a case of

---

K. Conrad (✉)
Ochsner Health, New Orleans, LA, USA
e-mail: kconrad@ochsner.org

E. Kelsoe
The University of Queensland School of Medicine, Ochsner Clinical School,
New Orleans, LA, USA

sepsis from an undetermined host response and was thus replaced with the current definition with this update [6].

The Third International Consensus Definition for Sepsis (Sepsis-3) defines sepsis as life-threatening organ dysfunction caused by a dysregulated host response to infection, whereas septic shock is a subdivision of sepsis which includes the presence of circulatory and cellular/metabolic dysfunction and carries a higher risk of mortality [1, 5]. Along with the new definitions, a new scoring system was instituted for a more rapid assessment and action plan in sepsis. The original SOFA score, as demonstrated in Table 5.1, guides the clinician in the identification of sepsis in an intensive care unit (ICU) patient [7].

However, the institution of the "quick" SOFA score (qSOFA) in 2016 allowed for this clinical score to be used outside of the ICU setting and provided physicians with a quantitative and qualitative metric to act upon [6]. Patients that are outside of the ICU setting are at risk of having sepsis if they have any two of the three components of the qSOFA score, as seen in Table 5.2 [6].

The score allows for the risk of sepsis to be determined in a fastidious manner so that the management approach can be swiftly instituted. This clinical approach and required sepsis workup are provided by the Surviving Sepsis Campaign. In this publication, a series of statements are recorded with varying levels of evidence. The best practice statements and strong recommendations are summarized below:

Table 5.1 The original SOFA score for use of sepsis identification in the critically ill ICU patient [7]

Sequential organ failure assessment score (SOFA)					
System		1	2	3	4
Respiratory: P_aO_2/FiO_2 mmHg (kPa)	≥400 (53.3)	<400 (53.3)	<300 (4)	<200 (26.7) with respiratory support	<100 (13.3) with respiratory support
Coagulation: Platelet count	≥150	<150	<100	<50	<20
Hepatic: Bilirubin mg/dL	<1.2	1.2–1.9	2.0–5.9	6.0–11.9	<12.0
Cardiovascular	MAP ≥70 mmHg	MAP <70 mmHg	Dopamine <5 or dobutamine (any dose)	Dopamine >5 or norepinephrine ≤0.1	Dopamine >15 or norepinephrine >0.1
Central nervous system: Glasgow Coma Score (GCS)	15	13–14	10–12	6–9	<6
Renal: Creatinine mg/dL (umol/L) or urine output (mL)	<1.2 (110)	1.2–1.9 (110–170)	2.0–3.4 (171–299)	3.5–4.9 (300–440) <500 urine output	>5.0 (440) <200 urine output

Table 5.2 Additional sequential organ assessment score for patients outside of the ICU setting who are at risk for or suspected of having sepsis [6]

Components of qSOFA score
1. Elevated respiratory rate ≥ 22 breaths per minute
2. Altered mental status (Glasgow Coma Score< 15)
3. Systolic blood pressure of 100 mmHg or less

Initial Resuscitation: Sepsis is considered a medical emergency.

- Fluid resuscitation: Immediate 30 ml/kg crystalloid fluid bolus within first 3 hours. Frequent reassessment of hemodynamic fluid status including heart rate, respiratory rate, urine output, temperature, and other available metrics [5]
- Initial target arterial pressure of 65 mmHg in patients needing vasopressor support [5]

Screening

- Hospitals and hospital systems should have performance and quality improvement protocols for sepsis, including, but not limited to, screening programs for sepsis in acutely ill patients [5].

Diagnosis

- Routine microbiological cultures are to be obtained before antimicrobial initiation, including at least two sets of blood cultures (aerobic and anaerobic) [5].

Antimicrobial Therapy

- IV empiric antimicrobials should be initiated within 1 hour for both sepsis and septic shock to cover all possible pathogens. After identification and sensitivities of pathogen are identified and/or once sufficient clinical improvement is seen, therapies should be refined [5].
- Recommend against use of systemic antimicrobial prophylaxis in individuals with severe inflammation of noninfectious origin (i.e., burns, pancreatitis) [5].
- If combination, empiric therapy is initially used for septic shock, it should be de-escalated and combination therapy discontinued in the first few days of clinical improvement or evidence of infection resolution. Daily reassessment of potential de-escalation opportunities in patients with sepsis and septic shock should be completed [5].

Source Control

- A specific anatomic source for infection should be identified or excluded as quickly as possible in patients with sepsis or septic shock. An intervention to eliminate a specific source of infection should be initiated as soon as possible after diagnosis is made [5].
- Once alternate vascular access is obtained, remove any intravascular devices that may be sources of infection [5].

Fluid Therapies

- A fluid challenge technique should be utilized when fluid administration is continued, contingent upon the consistent improvement of hemodynamic factors [5].
- Crystalloids should be used as the initial fluid resuscitation and intravascular volume replacement in patients with sepsis and septic shock. Hydroxyethyl starches should not be used in intravascular volume replacement in patients with septic shock [5].

Vasoactive Medications

- First-choice vasopressor in sepsis and septic shock should be norepinephrine [5].
- Low-dose dopamine should not be used for renal protection in patients with sepsis and septic shock [5].

Blood Products

- The threshold for RBC transfusion in sepsis or septic shock should be when hemoglobin is less than 7.0 g/dL, unless underlying conditions of myocardial ischemia, acute hemorrhage, or severe hypoxemia coexist [5].
- Erythropoietin should not be used for the treatment of anemia related to sepsis [5].

Anticoagulants

- Antithrombin should not be used in the treatment of sepsis and septic shock [5].

Mechanical Ventilation

- 6 mL/kg of predicted body weight should be used as the target tidal volume in adults with sepsis-induced acute respiratory distress syndrome (ARDS) [5].
- The maximum plateau pressure goals should be with an upper limit of 30 cm H_2O in adults with sepsis-induced ARDS [5].
- Prone positioning should be used in patients with sepsis-induced ARDS and a Pao_2/Fio_2 ratio < 150 [5].
- High-frequency oscillatory ventilation should not be used in adult patients with sepsis-induced ARDS [5].
- A conservative fluid approach should be used in patients with sepsis-induced ARDS without evidence of tissue hypoperfusion [5].
- Beta-2 agonists should not be used in the treatment of sepsis-induced ARDS without bronchospasm [5].
- Pulmonary artery catheters should not be used routinely in patients with sepsis-induced ARDS [5].
- Head of bed should be elevated to between 30 and 45 degrees to minimize aspiration risk and prevent ventilator-associated pneumonia in mechanically ventilated patients with sepsis [5].
- Spontaneous breathing trials should be utilized in patients with sepsis who are mechanically ventilated and ready for weaning. A weaning protocol should be used to wean ventilated patients [5].

Sedation and Analgesia

- Continuous or intermittent sedation should be minimized, and target titration endpoints should be used in mechanically ventilated patients with sepsis [5].

Glucose Control

- Protocols should be used for glucose management in ICU patients with sepsis. Insulin should be initiated after two consecutive glucose levels >180 mg/dL. The upper limit of glucose management goal should be ≤180 mg/dL rather than ≤110 mg/dL [5].
- In patients on insulin infusions, glucose should be monitored every 1–2 hours until glucose levels and infusion rates are stable and every 4 hours following that [5].
- Capillary blood point-of-care glucose measurements should be considered with caution as they may not reflect actual arterial or plasma glucose levels [5].

Venous Thromboembolism Prophylaxis

- Pharmacologic prophylaxis with low-molecular-weight heparin or unfractionated heparin should be used in patients with sepsis in the absence of contraindications [5].
- Low-molecular-weight heparin should be used in lieu of unfractionated heparin for pharmacologic prophylaxis if no contraindications to its use exist [5].

Stress Ulcer Prophylaxis

- Ulcer prophylaxis should be administered to patients with sepsis or septic shock who have gastrointestinal (GI) bleeding risk factors. Prophylaxis should not be used in patients without GI bleed risk factors [5].

Nutritional Support

- Exclusive use of early parenteral nutrition or the combination of parenteral and enteral feedings should not be utilized in sepsis patients who are critically ill due to the lack of mortality benefit. Instead, early enteral nutrition initiation should be the goal [5].
- If patients are not candidates for early enteral nutrition, IV glucose should be initiated rather than parenteral nutrition, and enteral feeds should be advanced as tolerated [5].
- Omega-3 fatty acids should not be used as immune support in critically ill patients [5].
- The use of glutamine or IV selenium as treatment in patients with sepsis and septic shock is not recommended [5].

Goals of Care

- Prognosis and goals of care should be discussed with the patient and their families or support persons. The determined goals should then be integrated into the treatment plan and potential end-of-life care plans [5].

These statements are provided to guide clinicians' actions in the treatment and workup of patients with sepsis; however, many iterations of such treatments exist. They serve as a guide for best practice care and evidence-driven treatments that should be followed to the best of any physicians' ability. In actual practice, however, following all such guidelines may prove to be a difficult task.

The 1-Hour Bundle

In 2018, the 1-Hour Bundle, as outlined in Table 5.3, was developed by the Surviving Sepsis Campaign in response to evidence that with every hour's delay of antibiotic initiation, there is an increase in mortality, even after adjusting for other variables such as hypotension, multiple organ failures, location of patient, source of infection, and need for mechanical ventilation [8, 9]. Implementation of bundles has allowed for fast-paced, urgent delivery of diagnostics and treatments in a systematic way. The aim of this bundle is to initiate care and assessment within 1 hour of time of presentation, otherwise known as "time zero," which is described as the initial time of triage in the emergency department or the initial chart documentation of confirmed or suspected sepsis. This bundle establishes a combination of the previous 3- and 6-hour bundles into a single protocol, allowing for rapid measures to be further emphasized and the emergence of sepsis to be placed at the forefront [3].

Blood cultures should be collected prior to the initiation of antimicrobials given that sensitivity of blood cultures significantly decreases 1 hour after antibiotic administration [10]. However, obtaining cultures should not delay antimicrobial initiation [10]. Proper blood culture technique should include the collection of a minimum of two sets of cultures [3]. Immediate administration of broad-spectrum antibiotics should appropriately follow the collection of cultures and should cover for the most likely pathogens involved in infection [3]. Fluid status must be addressed within 1 hour of presentation with the administration of a 30 mL/kg of crystalloid fluids [3]. Clinicians should aim to complete this bolus within the first 3 hours [3]. The measurement of lactate serves as an alternate gauge of tissue perfusion, and an increase in lactate may reflect hypoxia and is a predictor of poor outcomes [3]. If there is an initial elevated lactate level, it must then be measured 2–4 hours later to monitor perfusion [3].

Table 5.3 The 2018 1-Hour Bundle that serves as a guide to treating sepsis as a medical emergency requiring intervention within 1 hour of presentation [3]

Bundle element	Grade of recommendation and level of evidence
Obtain blood cultures prior to initiating antibiotics	Best practice statement
Administer broad-spectrum antibiotics	Strong recommendation, moderate quality of evidence
Rapid administration of 30 mL/kg crystalloid fluid for hypotension or lactate ≥4 mmol/L	Strong recommendation, low quality of evidence
Give vasopressors if patient is hypotensive during or after fluid resuscitation to maintain mean arterial pressure ≥65 mmHg	Strong recommendation, low quality of evidence
Measure lactate level. Remeasure if initial lactate is >2 mmol/L	Weak recommendation, low quality of evidence

Sepsis and Antimicrobial Stewardship

As the threat of antimicrobial resistance (AMR) continues to rise, it is of utmost importance that clinicians follow prescribing guidelines while also implementing safe protocols for the treatment of sepsis. However, antimicrobial stewardship and sepsis protocol implementation can often be treated as contending entities in hospital medicine [11]. Initiatives for antimicrobial stewardship and sepsis are often executed by separate teams, and communication between such efforts has been lacking [11].

Proper execution of sepsis rapid response requires the administration of broad-spectrum antibiotics, which carries the threat of antimicrobial resistance [8]. However, emphasis on additional patient review and narrowing the spectrum of antimicrobials is key to protecting against resistance [11]. Even with this knowledge, a physician's focus and concern for the patient in front of them may inhibit them from following these vital guidelines. A sense of urgency to treat the patient and provide the best immediate morbidity and mortality results may overpower the unseen threat of antimicrobial resistance as clinicians are reluctant to modify an effective antibiotic regimen [11]. This is where antimicrobial de-escalation must come into play. To achieve proper antimicrobial stewardship, the short-term benefits of a targeted approach to prescribing must be emphasized, such as the decrease in risk of multidrug-resistant infections in individual patients [12]. Other benefits of proper de-escalation include the reduction in adverse events associated with antibiotic use, such as superinfections or infections with Clostridium difficile [12].

Antibiotic de-escalation, as noted in Table 5.4, relies on proper antimicrobial stewardship modeling, and treatment paradigms exist to guide the clinician.

The implementation of this paradigm, as outlined in Figs. 5.1 and 5.2, guides the clinician toward a goal of de-escalation within the first 3 days [12].

In order to achieve this, a causative organism must be identified, which is particularly difficult to do when 40% of patients with sepsis have negative cultures [8]. The generation of a quick biological report or test is a future direction that will change this facet of sepsis treatment, allowing for a definitive diagnosis within the first 6 hours of presentation [8]. The ideal sepsis test would be one that has rapid results within 3 hours, tests for a wide variety of pathogens, is minimally invasive, can distinguish contaminants from disease-causing pathogens, can give results of

Table 5.4 Antibiotic treatment paradigm in the management of sepsis or septic shock [12]

Principles of the antibiotic treatment paradigm					
Aim for initial correct antibiotic choice.	Base antibiotic choice on local susceptibility patterns for both empiric and narrow coverage.	Immediate use of broad-spectrum antibiotics	Optimization of dose and route of antibiotic administration	Shortest possible duration of antibiotic administration	Discontinue or change antibiotic regimen to properly target pathogen as soon as possible.

5 Advances in the Evaluation and Treatment of Sepsis and Shock

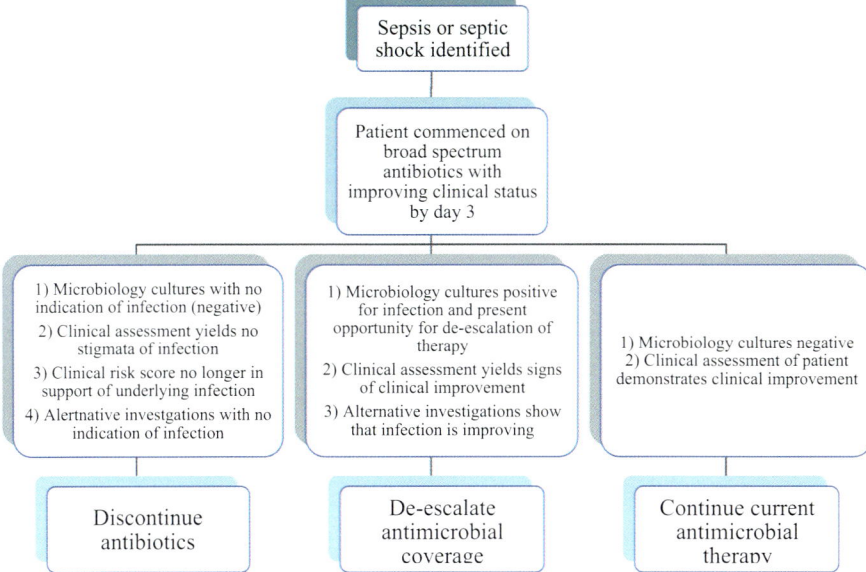

Fig. 5.1 Recommendations for the approach to antibiotic de-escalation for patients with improving clinical status within 3 days of treatment initiation [12]

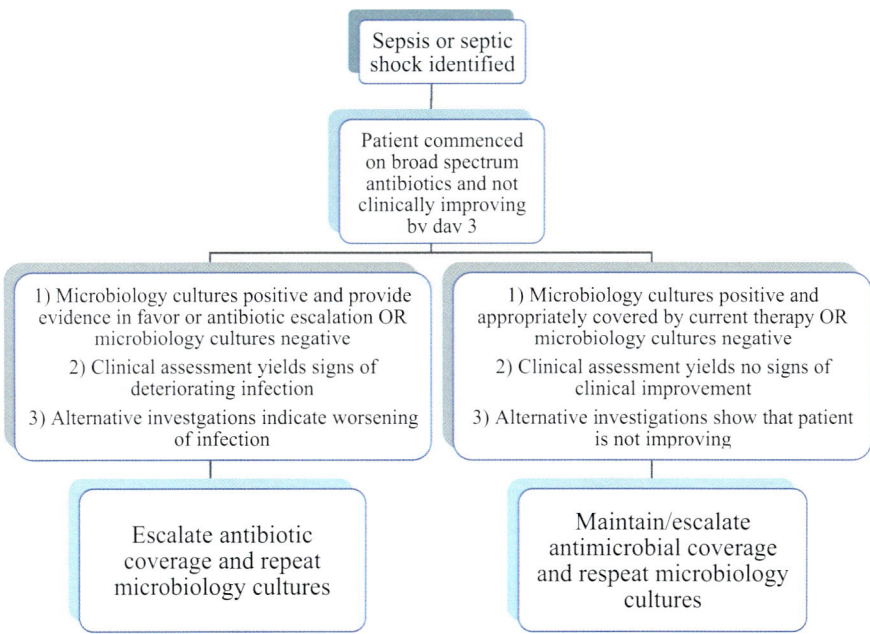

Fig. 5.2 Recommendations for the approach to antibiotic management in patients with sepsis and with no signs of clinical improvement within the first 3 days of treatment initiation [12]

Table 5.5 Clinical approach to de-escalation of antimicrobials in patients who are diagnosed with sepsis and staying as an inpatient in the wards of the hospital [12]

Bedside clinical approach to antibiotic de-escalation in sepsis
1. Every patient with severe sepsis on antibiotic therapy should have therapy considered and formally documented every day

2. Full assessment of results and clinical status should be re-evaluated no later than day 3 and a decision made regarding:
   Cessation of treatment (if no infection is present)
   Narrowing the spectrum of the treatment
   Reducing the number of antimicrobials being used, i.e., redundancy in therapies or increasing clinical improvement that suggests that multiple agents for the same organisms are no longer necessary
   OR no de-escalation, only if the specific reason for not de-escalating is properly documented (i.e., lack of microbiology results or lack of clinical improvement)

3. Reevaluation should take place daily thereafter, and a decision to stop, change, or continue the therapy should be made with specific reasons
4. Goal at every reassessment should be to discontinue the therapy, or parts of the therapy, unless a reason for continuation exists

drug sensitivities, and is easily adapted to the workflow of the specific hospital setting [13]. Though some polymerase chain reaction (PCR)-based tests exist in countries outside of the United States that can test for a number of specific organisms, these tests have mixed results when compared to the sensitivity and specificity of gold standard blood cultures and are not widely used [13]. While these technologies mark future horizons, we must utilize the testing that is available now. Current guidelines, as noted in Table 5.5, recommend reevaluation of patients' antibiotics by the third day of admission for sepsis [8]. This clinical approach to de-escalation relies on daily reevaluation of patients' antibiotic regime with goals of stopping or narrowing the coverage [12]. This practice, according to many studies, provides a similar, if not improved, clinical outcome and does not harm the individual patient [12].

Sepsis and COVID-19

Worldwide, the coronavirus disease 2019 (COVID-19) outbreak has changed the way clinicians approach critically ill patients. Initially, only 5% of patients show severe lung disease/injury or multiple organ dysfunction, and this disease has wreaked havoc worldwide and has brought about requirements to rethink clinical judgment [14].

Patients infected with the SARS-CoV-2 virus show signs of a dysregulated host response to the infection with inflammation, coagulation parameter deviations, and immune response disturbances [14]. As mentioned above, sepsis is defined as a dysregulated host response to infection [1]. Thus, patients who are severely affected by SARS-CoV-2 have elevations in the Multiple Organ Dysfunction Score (MODS) and meet the Sepsis-3 criteria [14]. This pattern differs by age group. Patients with severe COVID-19 and patients with sepsis from a respiratory source both have potential for diffuse alveolar damage resulting in acute respiratory distress syndrome (ARDS), pulmonary inflammation, thick mucus secretions, and increased levels of inflammatory cytokines with potential for microthrombi [15]. Similarly, sepsis due to COVID-19 can present with dyspnea, altered mental status, increased heart rate, weak pulses, and decreased urine output, which are all features of patients with septic shock [14]. Along with these findings, an elevated serum lactate and thrombocytopenia are also features of both the known entity of septic shock and sepsis due to COVID-19 [16]. As new variants of COVID-19 emerge, different symptom patterns are being recognized. As with much of the COVID-19 pandemic, our knowledge continues to evolve.

In response to this crisis, the Surviving Sepsis Campaign created a subcommittee for COVID-19 to determine recommendations [17]. These recommendations are categorized as strong recommendations or best practice statements, which implies that almost all patients in the specified situation would desire the advised treatment and only a few would not want it [17]. There is also the category of weak recommendation, which indicates that the majority of persons in the specified situation would desire the advised treatment; however, many would not [17].

Much of the guidelines pertain to measures taken to ensure the safety of healthcare personnel and is an ongoing process. Measures taken during the start of the pandemic have been modified as father information is obtained.

With these recommendations in place, and with continued research to come, we are better prepared to manage patients with COVID-19 and resultant sepsis.

Conclusion

Sepsis has been an ongoing threat known to medicine since as early as 700 BC [2]. However, with growing treatment modalities and increasing research in the field, it has been redefined and recommendations have changed with consistent updates. First and foremost, sepsis should be treated as a life-threatening medical emergency, with emphasis on treatment and assessment in the first hour [3]. Clinicians should focus on the collection of cultures, administration of antibiotics, assessment and management of fluid and perfusion status, and monitoring of serum lactate levels, all included in the 1-Hour Bundle [3]. The approach to sepsis should be in a protocolized manner with frequent reassessments along the way to ensure proper implementation. As the novel coronavirus continues to threaten the health of the world, new guidelines stand to direct the care of patients with sepsis due to COVID-19 and will most likely evolve in the coming years.

Key Points
- Sepsis is a life-threatening medical emergency that should be recognized and treated within the first hour of presentation [3].
- The 1-Hour Bundle should be implemented for fastidious care and effective emergent management [3].
- Blood cultures should be obtained, if possible, prior to the initiation of antimicrobials [3, 10].
- A fluid bolus of 30 mL/kg should be administered within the first hour and completed within 3 hours in a patient with suspected sepsis [3].
- Vasopressors should be administered if hypotension persists during or after fluid bolus administration [3].
- Daily reassessment of microbiological cultures and clinical status should be done to effectively implement antimicrobial stewardship [11].
- Antibiotic de-escalation protocols should be in place for every patient with sepsis or septic shock [12].
- A severe respiratory infection due to COVID-19 often meets criteria for sepsis. Evolving guidelines exist for the distinct treatment of sepsis due to COVID-19 [14].

References

1. Seymour CW, Liu VX, Iwashyna TJ, Brunkhorst FM, Rea TD, Scherag A, Rubenfeld G, Kahn JM, Shankar-Hari M, Singer M, Deutschman CS, Escobar GJ, Angus DC. Assessment of clinical criteria for sepsis: for the third international consensus definitions for sepsis and septic shock (Sepsis-3). JAMA. 2016;315(8):762–74. https://doi.org/10.1001/jama.2016.0288.
2. Abraham E. New definitions for sepsis and septic shock: continuing evolution but with much still to be done. JAMA. 2016;315(8):757–9. https://doi.org/10.1001/jama.2016.0290.
3. Levy MM, Evans LE, Rhodes A. The surviving sepsis campaign bundle: 2018 update. Crit Care Med. 2018;46(6):997–1000. https://doi.org/10.1097/ccm.0000000000003119.
4. Rudd KE, Johnson SC, Agesa KM, Shackelford KA, Tsoi D, Kievlan DR, Colombara DV, Ikuta KS, Kissoon N, Finfer S, Fleischmann-Struzek C, Machado FR, Reinhart KK, Rowan K, Seymour CW, Watson RS, West TE, Marinho F, Hay SI, Lozano R, Lopez AD, Angus DC, Murray CJL, Naghavi M. Global, regional, and national sepsis incidence and mortality, 1990-2017: analysis for the global burden of disease study. Lancet. 2020;395(10219):200–11. https://doi.org/10.1016/s0140-6736(19)32989-7.
5. Rhodes A, Evans LE, Alhazzani W, Levy MM, Antonelli M, Ferrer R, Kumar A, Sevransky JE, Sprung CL, Nunnally ME, Rochwerg B, Rubenfeld GD, Angus DC, Annane D, Beale RJ, Bellinghan GJ, Bernard GR, Chiche JD, Coopersmith C, De Backer DP, French CJ, Fujishima S, Gerlach H, Hidalgo JL, Hollenberg SM, Jones AE, Karnad DR, Kleinpell RM, Koh Y, Lisboa TC, Machado FR, Marini JJ, Marshall JC, Mazuski JE, McIntyre LA, McLean AS, Mehta S, Moreno RP, Myburgh J, Navalesi P, Nishida O, Osborn TM, Perner A, Plunkett CM, Ranieri M, Schorr CA, Seckel MA, Seymour CW, Shieh L, Shukri KA, Simpson SQ, Singer M, Thompson BT, Townsend SR, Van der Poll T, Vincent JL, Wiersinga WJ, Zimmerman JL, Dellinger RP. Surviving sepsis campaign: international guidelines for Management of Sepsis and Septic Shock: 2016. Intensive Care Med. 2017;43(3):304–77. https://doi.org/10.1007/s00134-017-4683-6.
6. Plevin R, Callcut R. Update in sepsis guidelines: what is really new? Trauma Surgery & Acute Care Open. 2017;2(1):e000088. https://doi.org/10.1136/tsaco-2017-000088.

7. Jones AE, Trzeciak S, Kline JA. The sequential organ failure assessment score for predicting outcome in patients with severe sepsis and evidence of hypoperfusion at the time of emergency department presentation. Crit Care Med. 2009;37(5):1649–54. https://doi.org/10.1097/CCM.0b013e31819def97.
8. Seok H, Jeon JH, Park DW. Antimicrobial therapy and antimicrobial stewardship in sepsis. Infect Chemother. 2020;52(1):19–30. https://doi.org/10.3947/ic.2020.52.1.19.
9. Ferrer R, Martin-Loeches I, Phillips G, Osborn TM, Townsend S, Dellinger RP, Artigas A, Schorr C, Levy MM. Empiric antibiotic treatment reduces mortality in severe sepsis and septic shock from the first hour: results from a guideline-based performance improvement program. Crit Care Med. 2014;42(8):1749–55. https://doi.org/10.1097/ccm.0000000000000330.
10. Rand KH, Beal SG, Rivera K, Allen B, Payton T, Lipori GP. Hourly effect of pretreatment with IV antibiotics on blood culture positivity rate in emergency department patients. Open forum. Infect Dis. 2019;6(5) https://doi.org/10.1093/ofid/ofz179.
11. Fitzpatrick F, Tarrant C, Hamilton V, Kiernan FM, Jenkins D, Krockow EM. Sepsis and antimicrobial stewardship: two sides of the same coin. BMJ Quality & Safety. 2019;28(9):758–61. https://doi.org/10.1136/bmjqs-2019-009445.
12. Masterton RG. Antibiotic de-escalation. Crit Care Clin. 2011;27(1):149–62. https://doi.org/10.1016/j.ccc.2010.09.009.
13. Sinha M, Jupe J, Mack H, Coleman TP, Lawrence SM, Fraley SI. Emerging Technologies for Molecular Diagnosis of sepsis. Clin Microbiol Rev. 2018;31(2):e00089–17. https://doi.org/10.1128/cmr.00089-17.
14. Beltrán-García J, Osca-Verdegal R, Pallardó FV, Ferreres J, Rodríguez M, Mulet S, Ferrando-Sánchez C, Carbonell N, García-Giménez JL. Sepsis and coronavirus disease 2019: common features and anti-inflammatory therapeutic approaches. Crit Care Med. 2020;48(12):1841–4. https://doi.org/10.1097/ccm.0000000000004625.
15. Barnes BJ, Adrover JM, Baxter-Stoltzfus A, Borczuk A, Cools-Lartigue J, Crawford JM, Daßler-Plenker J, Guerci P, Huynh C, Knight JS, Loda M, Looney MR, McAllister F, Rayes R, Renaud S, Rousseau S, Salvatore S, Schwartz RE, Spicer JD, Yost CC, Weber A, Zuo Y, Egeblad M. Targeting potential drivers of COVID-19: neutrophil extracellular traps. J Exp Med. 2020;217(6) https://doi.org/10.1084/jem.20200652.
16. Wujtewicz M, Dylczyk-Sommer A, Aszkiełowicz A, Zdanowski S, Piwowarczyk S, Owczuk R. COVID-19 - what should anaesthesiologists and intensivists know about it? Anaesthesiol Intensive Ther. 2020;52(1):34–41. https://doi.org/10.5114/ait.2020.93756.
17. Alhazzani W, Møller MH, Arabi YM, Loeb M, Gong MN, Fan E, Oczkowski S, Levy MM, Derde L, Dzierba A, Du B, Aboodi M, Wunsch H, Cecconi M, Koh Y, Chertow DS, Maitland K, Alshamsi F, Belley-Cote E, Greco M, Laundy M, Morgan JS, Kesecioglu J, McGeer A, Mermel L, Mammen MJ, Alexander PE, Arrington A, Centofanti JE, Citerio G, Baw B, Memish ZA, Hammond N, Hayden FG, Evans L, Rhodes A. Surviving sepsis campaign: guidelines on the management of critically ill adults with coronavirus disease 2019 (COVID-19). Intensive Care Med. 2020;46(5):854–87. https://doi.org/10.1007/s00134-020-06022-5.

Chapter 6
Current Trends in Stroke Management

Mohammad Moussavi and Kiana Moussavi

Epidemiology of Stroke

Every 40 seconds, there is a stroke in the United States, equating to approximately 795,000 strokes each year [1]. The most recent data from the Center of Disease Control and Prevention (CDC) demonstrates that within the United States, stroke is the third leading cause of death in women and fifth in men [1]. The data also indicates that 1 in 4 of the strokes in the United States happen in those who have previously had a stroke [2].

The CDC has also provided some more specific statistics in regard to the prevalence of strokes between different race and ethnical backgrounds. The data suggest that the risk of having a first-time stroke is twice as high among the African-American population compared to white patients and that death rates secondary to stroke are highest among African-American people [1]. The data also indicates that there has been an increase in death rates due to stroke in the Hispanic population since 2013 [1]. In the United States alone, the cost of stroke-related care, including medications, health care services, and missed workdays, has been estimated at approximately 46 billion dollars between the years of 2014 and 2015 [1].

This data reiterates the importance of providing the most efficient management to those suffering from new strokes and also the prevention of primary and secondary strokes. It shines a light on the importance of being more aware of some institutional and individual biases that perhaps affect the quality of care distributed among

M. Moussavi (✉)
Neurovascular Surgery, Northwell Health, Staten Island, NY, USA
e-mail: mmoussavi@northwell.edu

K. Moussavi
The University of Queensland School of Medicine, Ochsner Clinical School, New Orleans, LA, USA

different races and ethnicities in order to make the best effort to overcome these biases and provide the best care to all patients irrespective of their ethnical background.

Types of Stroke

Stroke can be divided into two large categories: ischemic and hemorrhagic. Ischemic stroke makes up approximately 85% of strokes [3]. Ischemic and hemorrhagic strokes can be divided into further subcategories that will be discussed below.

Ischemic strokes occur secondary to a blockage within the brain's arterial vasculature, which then cuts off oxygen and nutrients to a specific region of the brain [4]. The two main types of ischemic stroke are thrombotic and embolic [3]. Thrombotic strokes occur due to thrombus formation within the arterial vasculature directly supplying specific regions of the brain, whereas embolic strokes occur secondary to emboli that break off from a thrombus in a distant site, such as the carotid arteries, the heart, or less commonly, the extremities [3].

Hemorrhagic strokes occur as a result of rupture or leakage of brain vasculature [5]. The two major subcategories of hemorrhagic strokes include intracerebral hemorrhage (ICH) and subarachnoid hemorrhage (SAH) [5]. Intracerebral or intraparenchymal hemorrhage occurs most commonly due to elevated blood pressure, which causes weakening of the blood vessels in the brain over time and leakage of blood directly into the brain parenchyma [5]. Other risk factors for intracerebral hemorrhage include bleeding disorders, connective tissue disorders, injury or trauma, and blood vessel deformities such as aneurysms [5]. Subarachnoid hemorrhages occur as a result of rupture of an aneurysm or outpouching of blood vessels on the surface of the brain [5].

Ischemic Stroke Management

There is a reason the term "time is brain" is so widely emphasized in the management of stroke [6]. It is estimated that 1.9 million neurons are lost for every minute of stroke due to occlusion of large vessels, such as the internal carotid artery (ICA) or middle cerebral artery (MCA) [6]. Therefore, the most important factor when it comes to the management of stroke is early intervention [6]. This is why it is imperative for the public to know the signs of acute stroke. The most common sign of acute ischemic stroke is focal loss of brain function; however, acute stroke can present in a variety of ways [6].

When evaluating a patient for a possible stroke, first and foremost it is most important to determine whether it is an ischemic or hemorrhagic event as the management differs significantly. This is determined by getting a non-contrast CT as soon as possible, which is known as door-to-imaging time. Door-to-imaging time is defined as the time from which the patient enters the hospital to the time they are imaged for a possible stroke. National guidelines have established that the ideal door-to-imaging time (DIT) is 25 minutes for suspected acute stroke patients [7]. If the stroke is ischemic, the physician must then determine whether the patient qualifies for intravenous thrombolytic therapy, endovascular thrombectomy, or both. The National Institutes of Health Stroke Scale (NIHSS) score is part of the assessment that helps determine if a patient is a candidate for intravenous thrombolysis and/or mechanical thrombectomy [8]. The NIHSS score ranges from 0 to 42 and has 11 categories, including the level of consciousness (LOC), visual, facial palsy, motor arm, motor leg, limb ataxia, sensory, language, dysarthria, extinction, and inattention [3]. The baseline NIHSS score can also be used as a predictive indicator for long-term stroke outcomes [8].

IV Thrombolysis Guidelines

Establishing the exact time of onset of symptoms due to an ischemic event is the most important factor in determining eligibility for intravenous tissue plasminogen activator (tPA) or thrombectomy. The door-to-needle time describes the time from the arrival of a patient into the hospital until the administration of intravenous thrombolytics, such as tissue-type plasminogen activator (tPA) in the setting of an acute ischemic stroke [9]. The national guidelines have determined ideal door-to-needle time to be less than 60 minutes and the therapeutic window for tPA therapy to be less than 4.5 hours since symptom onset [9].

Mechanical Thrombectomy Guidelines

It is estimated that every 1-min reduction in the interval between stroke onset and start of mechanical thrombectomy results in an additional week of healthy living [10]. The recent guidelines for mechanical thrombectomy are based on several major trials entitled MR CLEAN, ESCAPE, EXTEND-IA, REVASCAT, SWIFT PRIME, THRACE, and most recently DAWN and DEFUSE 3 trials [11]. The guidelines state that patients 18 years of age and older can undergo mechanical thrombectomy with a stent retriever if they have minimal prestroke disability, have an occlusion of the internal carotid artery (ICA) and main branch of middle cerebral artery (MCA), have an NIHSS score of ≥6 and Alberta Stroke Program Early CT Score (ASPECT) ≥6, and have a last seen normal of less than 6 hours prior to thrombectomy [11]. The guidelines also state that in selected patients who are 6–24 hours within their last known normal and who have evidence of anterior circulation large vessel occlusion and would otherwise be eligible for DAWN or DEFUSE 3, perfusion imaging or MRI with diffusion-weighted imaging should be obtained in order to determine whether the patient is a candidate for mechanical thrombectomy [11]. Trials indicate that the best long-term outcome for patients treated with thrombectomy is within the first 6 hours of symptom onset [12]. Data also suggest that in certain patients with perfusion-imaging, treatment can be beneficial up to 24 hours after stroke onset [12].

However, there are many factors that have yet to be studied in detail and may lead to expansion of inclusion criteria and relaxation of exclusion criteria for mechanical thrombectomy. In following the above-mentioned trials, there are many ongoing trials which focus on the benefit of thrombectomy in patients with mild cognitive impairment with large vessel occlusions and recanalization of more distal vessel and other large vessels (such as basilar artery or its main branches), and if successful they will greatly expand the use of mechanical thrombectomy [13, 14].

The Role of Collateral Blood Flow

When a large vessel is occluded in an acute ischemic stroke event, the brain tissue that is fed exclusively by the occluded vessel dies at a much faster rate than the peripheral tissue due to blood flow from the neighboring vessels, also known as collaterals. Not all patients suffering from acute ischemic stroke due to large vessel occlusion have the same rate of progression of stroke. This progression has a spectrum of slow to fast. Fast progression refers to those in which the rate of brain cell death is much higher than average, and the opposite is true for the slow-progression ischemic strokes. Progression of acute ischemic stroke depends on many factors, especially collateral blood flow to the ischemic area, patient's age, individual's oxygen-carrying capacity, and other cerebrovascular comorbidities [15, 16]. The number, caliber, and sustainability of collaterals vary greatly among each patient. In most cases, these collaterals cannot survive for a long time. Therefore, the sooner the occluded vessel is recanalized, the less cell death is observed. The current guidelines for intravenous thrombolytics and especially mechanical thrombectomy are based on relatively new trials which have very strict exclusion criteria. However, based on these trials, many acute ischemic stroke patients who may potentially benefit from treatment are excluded. For example, time cutoffs, baseline function, size of already-infarcted tissue, and size and location of vessels are all used as exclusion parameters. Therefore, it is important to note that the majority of current required parameters and scoring systems for treatment of ischemic stroke are arbitrary, and as stroke knowledge continues to expand, the treatment of stroke will become more individualized and the exclusion criteria will be less strict [13].

The degree and speed of ischemic injury can be minimized by collateral blood flow to the ischemic territory as well as the collaterals supplying the large vessels [17]. Therefore, it may be of benefit for endovascular therapy to be tailored to those with better collateral flow, allowing for a more personalized approach to ischemic stroke management on a case-by-case basis. Stroke neurologists or interventionalists do not usually focus on the pretreatment collateral flow to the region of infarct and tend to focus more on restoring anterograde flow more aggressively if the patient has poor retrograde flow through collateral vessels [15]. All patients presenting with ischemic stroke have a varying range of collaterals. Despite this fact, collaterals at the time of angiography are not typically factored into the decision-making process in the management of stroke [15]. In a study conducted by Bang et al., the relationship between baseline collaterals and recanalization results after endovascular therapy was evaluated [15]. All patients within the study underwent cerebral angiography and subsequently angiographic collateral grade was determined based on the ASITN/SIR collateral flow grading system [15]. The ASITN/SIR grading system assigns a value ranging from 0 indicating no visible collaterals to grade 4 indicating rapid and complete retrograde perfusion of entire ischemic territory via collateral blood flow [15]. The study found that in patients with higher ASITN/SIR scores indicating greater pretreatment collaterals, recanalization rates were higher post-endovascular therapy [15]. The data collected also demonstrated that among the variables studied, collateral status was the strongest predictor for positive revascularization results [15]. The authors suggested that by selecting patients for endovascular therapy based on collateral assessment, more favorable results are achieved and the need for other time-consuming tests is decreased [15].

Neuroprotection

Another important discussion in the management of ischemic stroke is the use of neuroprotection in order to achieve better functional outcomes [18]. Neuroprotective agents are used in hopes of preventing irreversible injury to ischemic neurons [18]. There have been several studies demonstrating improvements in outcomes post-recanalization after administration of neuroprotection or hypothermia. Neuroprotective agents such as N-methyl-D-aspartate receptor (NMDA) antagonists and magnesium have shown promising potential and are continued to be studied. There have also been studies showing the benefit of cooling ischemic stroke patients by decreasing the temperature by 2 degree Celsius in order to decrease ischemic damage [19]. Hypothermia reduces damage to the brain by reducing the generation of free radicals and inflammatory response, decreasing excitotoxicity, inhibiting neuron cell apoptosis, and reducing the basal metabolic rate of the brain [19, 20]. A recent phase III clinical trial (ESCAPE-NA1) on the novel drug candidate Nerinetide has brought much attention and provides a promising future for the use of neuroprotection in the treatment of acute ischemic stroke (AIS) [21]. Nerinetide is a neuroprotective eicosapeptide that suppresses the interaction of NMDA receptors with the postsynaptic density protein 95 (PSD-95) and thereby prevents the neurotoxic signaling of neuronal NO synthase (nNOS) in AIS [22]. The trial demonstrated that in those who had not received intravenous alteplase, better clinical outcomes with Nerinetide were achieved versus placebo [21]. Additional trials are necessary in order to further evaluate the efficacy of neuroprotective agents and to determine whether the use of neuroprotection can improve the outcome of patients with large vessel occlusion especially after mechanical thrombectomy [14].

Stroke and Women

As discussed earlier, the time it takes from the onset of stroke symptoms to the time of treatment is the most important factor in the prognosis of stroke. Unfortunately, a major delay to seeking treatment has been proven to be lack of recognition of traditional signs of stroke at the time of onset [23]. There appears to be a significant gender disparity in recognition of the early signs of stroke and therefore a delay in seeking medical attention in women.

Zrelak et al. conducted a study designed to evaluate sex-based differences in symptom perception [23]. The results indicated that men arriving within 4.5 hours of symptom onset had a higher NIHSS score at the time of presentation (7.7 versus 4.8 respectively) and were significantly more likely to be treated with alteplase compared with their female counterparts [23]. The study also demonstrated that most patients enrolled in the study were unaware of the importance of getting to the hospital quickly, and interestingly women with prior strokes were slower to seek medical help, with the majority presenting late (defined as greater than 4.5 hours since the time of symptom onset) [23].

Several other studies have demonstrated that women present with "nontraditional" signs of stroke. Jerath et al. conducted a study in which symptoms in 449 first-time stroke patients were evaluated in order to determine the most common neurological symptoms among both men and women [24]. The study indicated that generalized weakness and mental status changes were among the most commonly presenting symptoms in women compared to men who presented with paresthesia, ataxia, and double vision [24]. Men presented with signs of ischemic stroke such as nystagmus and sensory abnormalities, whereas women presented with fatigue, disorientation, and fever [24].

It is also established that women have experienced longer delays in door-to-needle and door-to-image times after presenting to the emergency department with signs and symptoms of stroke [24]. Gargano et al. further established that this delay is not attributed to the previously mentioned difference in signs and symptoms, pointing to more complex causes [25].

The term "availability heuristic" refers to the act of making judgments about a certain scenario based on available examples in your mind [26]. The tendency to treat women in an inferior manner when they present with nontraditional signs of stroke can to an extent be explained by this heuristic. It is therefore imperative that the general public as well as healthcare workers learn to recognize the "nontraditional" signs and symptoms of stroke in both men and women.

COVID and Stroke

Epidemiology

There is limited data thus far in regard to the incidence of stroke among patients with COVID-19. Preliminary data suggest that the majority of neurological complications include myalgia, headaches, and encephalopathy, with a minority of patients suffering from ataxia, movement disorders, motor and sensory deficits, and stroke [27].

The incidence of stroke is approximately 2.5 to 5 percent among patients hospitalized for COVID-19 [28]. In the setting of COVID-19, onset of stroke symptoms was 9 days after the onset of other COVID symptoms [29].

The most common subtype of stroke presentation in the setting of COVID-19 is ischemic stroke, with less frequent presentation of venous sinus thrombosis, intracerebral hemorrhage, and subarachnoid hemorrhage [27].

Effects of COVID-19 on Stroke Admissions

According to data collected in stroke centers throughout China, in the first half of 2020, there were fewer admissions due to stroke [30]. This could potentially be attributed to fear of exposure to COVID-19 among those with more mild stroke symptoms; however, it was found that those who did present for hospital evaluation had more severe strokes [30].

Proposed Mechanisms of COVID-19-Induced Stroke

Hypercoagulability

As previously stated, COVID-19 is associated with a higher prevalence of stroke compared with the general population [31]. Though most proposed mechanisms of stroke in the setting of COVID-19 remain hypothetical, one proposed mechanism is hypercoagulability [31]. COVID-19 is associated with a hypercoagulable state that is confirmed by elevated levels of D-dimer, elevated fibrinogen, and normal or slightly increased prothrombin time, which are more markedly elevated in patients with ischemic stroke [32].

Cerebral Endotheliopathy

Another proposed mechanism of stroke in the setting of COVID-19 infection is endotheliopathy of brain vasculature. Endotheliopathy describes the inflammatory process within the endothelial lining of blood vessels associated with high levels of certain cytokines, including interleukin-6 [33, 34].

There have also been several studies designed with the primary objective of analyzing hemostatic factors as well as markers of endothelial cell and platelet activation in critically ill COVID-19 patients admitted to the ICU as well as a possible correlation between the aforementioned markers and clinical outcomes [32, 33]. These studies demonstrated an elevated level of von Willebrand factor (vWF), soluble P-selectin, and soluble thrombomodulin in patients critically ill with COVID-19 compared to non-critically ill patients [32, 33]. It was determined that among patients in a hyperinflammatory state, the cascade of events that leads to the release of soluble thrombomodulin began with direct injury to endothelial cells [32, 33]. It was also concluded that vWF antigen and thrombomodulin were both correlated with increased mortality risk among all patients [32, 33]. Goshua et al. determined that based on the findings of elevated vWF, plasminogen activator inhibitor-1 (PAI-1), soluble thrombomodulin, soluble P-selectin, and sCD40L endotheliopathy and platelet activation may be the underlying cause of the coagulopathy associated with COVID-19 [34].

Additional Risk Factors

The traditional risk factors for stroke are still applicable to the development of stroke in the setting of COVID-19. Cardiac dysfunction as a result of myocarditis, arrhythmias, heart failure, and myocardial infarction and cardiac injury as a direct result of critical illness in the setting of COVID-19 have all been associated with potential embolic stroke mechanisms [35]. However, in a study evaluating 100 consecutive COVID-19 patients, only 10 percent demonstrated any left ventricular dysfunction, making cardiac embolism as a cause of stroke in the setting of COVID-19 infection less likely [35].

Retrospective data has also found that prognosis for stroke in patients with COVID-19 is worse among African Americans compared to other racial ethnicities. The data also showed that on admission, the severity of stroke as determined by the National Institutes of Health and Stroke score was similar for African Americans when compared to other races; however, the mortality rate was significantly higher for African-American patients [36].

Post-stroke Depression

Prevalence

A study conducted by Ayerbe et al. found that following a stroke, the prevalence of depression was 29 percent [37]. It has also been established that depression after stroke is associated with poorer outcomes. Consequently, the study proposed a positive correlation between depression and 12- to 24-month mortality [37]. A separate case-control study conducted by Jorgensen et al. comparing stroke patients with no prior history of depression to controls established that the incidence of depression during the first two years following hospitalization was significantly higher among stroke patients compared to control [38].

Risk Factors and Assessment of Post-stroke Depression

The possible risk factors for post-stroke depression (PSD) include, but are not limited to, physical disability, cognitive changes, inadequate social support, and prior history of depression or mental illness [39].

The biggest challenge with PSD is the ability to recognize the signs and symptoms [39]. Due to the possible effects of stroke on patients including aphasia, aprosodia, or flat affect, it may be difficult for healthcare providers to pick up on signs of depression. It is therefore important for providers to have a high clinical suspicion in order to properly treat patients suffering from PSD. Although there are many resources and depression scales that can assess possible depression, the single most important question to directly ask is whether the patient "feels sad or depressed" [39]. A positive answer to this question has been found to have a sensitivity and specificity of 86 and 78 percent, respectively [39].

Treatment

Thus far, the most effective treatment for PSD has focused on a multidisciplinary approach, including regularly scheduled patient follow-up and effective inter-professional communication among all healthcare providers within the team [39].

Post-stroke Care

Of the 795,000 patients with strokes annually within the United States, approximately two-thirds survive and require rehabilitation [40]. The amount of rehabilitation necessary varies from person to person and depends on the severity and extent of damage to the brain [40]. Evidence suggests that the earlier patients are started on rehabilitation and the longer they are able to participate in each session, the better are their long-term outcomes [40]. Rehabilitation therapy is focused on helping the brain relearn the skills that it has lost as a consequence of the stroke and is usually started within the first 48 hours after the stroke once the patient has stabilized [40]. This is in order to increase natural brain neuroplasticity in response to the damage caused [40]. Neuroplasticity or neural plasticity describes the process of brain "rewiring" by creating new neural pathways and synapses in order to compensate for the ones that were destroyed as a consequence of the stroke [4].

Key Points
1. Stroke can be divided into two large categories: ischemic and hemorrhagic. Ischemic stroke makes up approximately 85% of strokes.
2. The most important factor when it comes to the management of stroke is early intervention. The national guidelines have established that the ideal door-to-imaging time (DIT) is within 25 minutes for suspected acute stroke patients.
3. The national guidelines have determined ideal door-to-needle time to be less than 60 minutes and the therapeutic window for tPA therapy to be less than 4.5 hours since symptom onset. The guidelines have also indicated the best long-term outcomes for patients treated with thrombectomy within the first 6 hours of symptom onset. In certain patients with perfusion-imaging, treatment can be beneficial up to 24 hours after stroke onset.
4. Progression of acute ischemic stroke depends on many factors, especially collateral blood flow to the ischemic area, patient's age, individual's oxygen-carrying capacity, and other cerebrovascular comorbidities.
5. Studies suggest that collateral status was the strongest predictor for positive revascularization results and that by selecting patients for endovascular therapy based on collateral assessment, more favorable results are achieved and the need for other time-consuming tests is decreased [15].
6. Neuroprotective agents are used in hopes of preventing irreversible injury to ischemic neurons. There have been several studies demonstrating improvements in outcomes post-recanalization after administration of neuroprotection or hypothermia. Most recently, a phase III clinical trial (ESCAPE-NA1) focusing on the use of the novel drug Nerinetide (neuroprotective eicosapeptide) has shown a promising future for the use of neuroprotection in the treatment of acute ischemic stroke (AIS) [21].
7. Women often present with "nontraditional" signs of stroke and data has shown that women experience longer delays in door-to-needle and door-to-image times after presenting to the emergency department with signs and symptoms of stroke.

8. Current and ongoing research suggests that endotheliopathy and platelet activation may be the underlying cause of the coagulopathy associated with COVID-19.
9. Following a stroke, the prevalence of depression has been reported as 29 percent, and consequently it has been established that depression after stroke is associated with poorer functional outcomes.
10. Evidence suggests that the earlier patients are started on rehabilitation post-stroke and the longer they are able to participate in each session, the better are their long-term outcomes.

References

1. Stroke Facts | cdc.gov. In: Cdc.gov. https://www.cdc.gov/stroke/facts.htm. 2021. Accessed 2 Mar 2021.
2. Kamel H, Zhang C, Kleindorfer D, et al. Association of Black Race with Early Recurrence after Minor Ischemic Stroke or transient ischemic attack. JAMA Neurol. 2020;77:601. https://doi.org/10.1001/jamaneurol.2020.0010.
3. Hui C, Tadi P, Patti L. Ischemic Stroke. [Updated 2021 Apr 29]. In: StatPearls [Internet]. Treasure Island (FL): StatPearls Publishing; 2021 Jan. Available from: https://www.ncbi.nlm.nih.gov/books/NBK499997/.
4. Sharma N, Classen J, Cohen LG. Neural plasticity and its contribution to functional recovery. Handb Clin Neurol. 2013;110:3–12. https://doi.org/10.1016/B978-0-444-52901-5.00001-0.
5. Unnithan AKA, Mehta P. Hemorrhagic Stroke. [Updated 2021 Jan 16]. In: StatPearls [Internet]. Treasure Island (FL): StatPearls Publishing; 2021 Jan-. Available from: https://www.ncbi.nlm.nih.gov/books/NBK559173/.
6. Saver J. Time is brain—quantified. Stroke. 2006;37:263–6. https://doi.org/10.1161/01.str.0000196957.55928.ab.
7. Reznek MA, Murray E, Youngren MN, Durham NT, Michael SS. Door-to-imaging time for acute stroke patients is adversely affected by emergency department crowding. Stroke. 2017;48(1):49–54. https://doi.org/10.1161/STROKEAHA.116.015131.
8. Oliveira-Filho J, Samuels OB. Intravenous thrombolytic therapy for acute ischemic stroke: therapeutic use. Uptodate. (2020, December 9). https://www-uptodate-com.ezproxy.library.uq.edu.au/contents/intravenous-thrombolytic-therapy-for-acute-ischemic-stroke-therapeutic-use?search=nihss&topicRef=14084&source=see_link.
9. Fonarow GC. Improving door-to-needle times in acute ischemic stroke. Am Heart Associat. 2011, September 1; https://doi.org/10.1161/STROKEAHA.111.621342.
10. Seah H, Burney M, Phan M, et al. CODE STROKE ALERT—concept and development of a novel open-source platform to streamline acute stroke management. Front Neurol. 2019; https://doi.org/10.3389/fneur.2019.00725.
11. 2018 AHA/ASA Stroke Early Management Guidelines. In: American College of Cardiology.
12. Snelling B, Mccarthy D, Chen S, et al. Extended window for stroke Thrombectomy. Journal of Neurosciences in Rural Practice. 2019;10:294–300. https://doi.org/10.4103/jnrp.jnrp_365_18.
13. Fisher M, Xiong Y. Evaluating patients for thrombectomy. Brain circulation. 2018;4(4):153–9. https://doi.org/10.4103/bc.bc_27_18.
14. Kwak HS, Hyo Sung Kwak Department of Radiology (H.S.K.), Park JS, et al. Mechanical Thrombectomy in basilar artery occlusion. In: Stroke. 2020. https://www.ahajournals.org/doi/full/10.1161/STROKEAHA.120.029861. Accessed 18 Jul 2021.

15. Bang OY, Saver JL, Kim SJ, Kim GM, Chung CS, Ovbiagele B, Lee KH, Liebeskind DS. Collateral flow predicts response to endovascular therapy for acute ischemic stroke. Stroke. 2011;42(3):693–9. https://doi.org/10.1161/STROKEAHA.110.595256.
16. Raoult H, Eugène F, Ferré JC, Gentric JC, Ronzière T, Stamm A, Gauvrit JY. Prognostic factors for outcomes after mechanical thrombectomy with solitaire stent. Journal of neuroradiology = Journal de neuroradiologie. 2013;40(4):252–9. https://doi.org/10.1016/j.neurad.2013.04.001.
17. Jung S, Wiest R, Gralla J, McKinley R, Mattle H, Liebeskind D. Relevance of the cerebral collateral circulation in ischaemic stroke: time is brain, but collaterals set the pace. Swiss Med Wkly. 2017 Dec 11;147:w14538. https://doi.org/10.4414/smw.2017.14538.
18. Helmi L Lutsep MD. In: neuroprotective agents in stroke: overview of neuroprotective agents, prevention of early ischemic injury, prevention of reperfusion injury. 2021. https://emedicine.medscape.com/article/1161422-overview#a2. Accessed 17 Jul 2021.
19. Onwuekwe I, Ezeala-Adikaibe B. Ischemic stroke and neuroprotection. Ann Med Health Sci Res. 2012;2(2):186–90. https://doi.org/10.4103/2141-9248.105669.
20. Sun Y-J, Zhang Z-Y, Fan B, Li G-Y. Neuroprotection by therapeutic hypothermia. In: Frontiers in neuroscience. https://www.ncbi.nlm.nih.gov/pmc/articles/PMC6579927/. 2019. Accessed 18 Jul 2021.
21. Hill MD, Goyal M, Menon BK, Nogueira RG, McTaggart RA, Demchuk AM, Poppe AY, Buck BH, Field TS, Dowlatshahi D, van Adel BA, Swartz RH, Shah RA, Sauvageau E, Zerna C, Ospel JM, Joshi M, Almekhlafi MA, Ryckborst KJ, Lowerison MW, Heard K, Garman D, Haussen D, Cutting SM, Coutts SB, Roy D, Rempel JL, Rohr AC, Iancu D, Sahlas DJ, Yu AYX, Devlin TG, Hanel RA, Puetz V, Silver FL, Campbell BCV, Chapot R, Teitelbaum J, Mandzia JL, Kleinig TJ, Turkel-Parrella D, Heck D, Kelly ME, Bharatha A, Bang OY, Jadhav A, Gupta R, Frei DF, Tarpley JW, McDougall CG, Holmin S, Rha JH, Puri AS, Camden MC, Thomalla G, Choe H, Phillips SJ, Schindler JL, Thornton J, Nagel S, Heo JH, Sohn SI, Psychogios MN, Budzik RF, Starkman S, Martin CO, Burns PA, Murphy S, Lopez GA, English J, Tymianski M; ESCAPE-NA1 Investigators. Efficacy and safety of nerinetide for the treatment of acute ischaemic stroke (ESCAPE-NA1): a multicentre, double-blind, randomised controlled trial. Lancet. 2020;395(10227):878–87. https://doi.org/10.1016/S0140-6736(20)30258-0. Epub 2020 Feb 20.
22. Cao J, Viholainen JI, Dart C, Warwick HK, Leyland ML, Courtney MJ. The PSD95-nNOS interface: a target for inhibition of excitotoxic p38 stress-activated protein kinase activation and cell death. J Cell Biol. 2005;168(1):117–26. https://doi.org/10.1083/jcb.200407024.
23. Zrelak PA. Sex-based differences in symptom perception and care-seeking behavior in acute stroke. Perm J. 2018;22:18–042. https://doi.org/10.7812/TPP/18-042.
24. Jerath NU, Reddy C, Freeman WD, Jerath AU, Brown RD. Gender differences in presenting signs and symptoms of acute ischemic stroke: a population-based study. Gend Med. 2011;8(5):312–9. https://doi.org/10.1016/j.genm.2011.08.001.
25. Gargano, J. W., Reeves, M. J., & Paul Coverdell National Acute Stroke Registry Michigan Prototype Investigators. Sex differences in stroke recovery and stroke-specific quality of life: results from a statewide stroke registry. Stroke. 2007;38(9):2541–8. https://doi.org/10.1161/STROKEAHA.107.485482.
26. Klein JG. Five pitfalls in decisions about diagnosis and prescribing. BMJ (Clinical research ed). 2005;330(7494):781–3. https://doi.org/10.1136/bmj.330.7494.781.
27. Tsivgoulis G, Palaiodimou L, Zand R, Lioutas VA, Krogias C, Katsanos AH, Shoamanesh A, Sharma VK, Shahjouei S, Baracchini C, Vlachopoulos C, Gournellis R, Sfikakis PP, Sandset EC, Alexandrov AV, Tsiodras S. COVID-19 and cerebrovascular diseases: a comprehensive overview. Ther Adv Neurol Disord. 2020;13:1756286420978004. https://doi.org/10.1177/1756286420978004.
28. Wang Z, Yang Y, Liang X, Gao B, Liu M, Li W, Chen Z, Wang Z. COVID-19 associated ischemic stroke and hemorrhagic stroke: incidence, potential pathological mechanism, and management. Front Neurol. 2020;11:571996. https://doi.org/10.3389/fneur.2020.571996.

29. Valencia-Enciso N, Ortiz-Pereira M, Zafra-Sierra MP, Espinel-Gómez L, Bayona H. Time of stroke onset in coronavirus disease 2019 patients around the globe: a systematic review and analysis. J Stroke Cerebrovasc Dis. 2020;29(12):105325. https://doi.org/10.1016/j.jstrokecerebrovasdis.2020.105325.
30. Wang J, Chaudhry SA, Tahsili-Fahadan P, Altaweel LR, Bashir S, Bahiru Z, Fang Y, Qureshi AI. The impact of COVID-19 on acute ischemic stroke admissions: analysis from a community-based tertiary care center. J Stroke Cerebrovasc Dis. 2020;29(12):105344. https://doi.org/10.1016/j.jstrokecerebrovasdis.2020.105344.
31. Rosa K. Endotheliopathy: a marker of progression to critical illness in COVID-19. In: OncLive. 2021. https://www.onclive.com/view/endotheliopathy-a-marker-of-progression-to-critical-illness-in-covid-19. Accessed 2 Mar 2021.
32. Grobler C, Maphumulo SC, Grobbelaar LM, Bredenkamp JC, Laubscher GJ, Lourens PJ, Steenkamp J, Kell DB, Pretorius E. Covid-19: the rollercoaster of fibrin(Ogen), D-dimer, Von Willebrand factor, P-selectin and their interactions with endothelial cells, platelets and erythrocytes. Int J Mol Sci. 2020;21(14):5168. https://doi.org/10.3390/ijms21145168.
33. Stancu P, Uginet M, Assal F, et al. COVID-19 associated stroke and cerebral endotheliitis. J Neuroradiol. 2021; https://doi.org/10.1016/j.neurad.2021.01.012.
34. Goshua G, Pine AB, Meizlish ML, Chang CH, Zhang H, Bahel P, Baluha A, Bar N, Bona RD, Burns AJ, Dela Cruz CS, Dumont A, Halene S, Hwa J, Koff J, Menninger H, Neparidze N, Price C, Siner JM, Tormey C, et al. Endotheliopathy in COVID-19-associated coagulopathy: evidence from a single-Centre, cross-sectional study. The Lancet Haematology. 2020;7(8):e575–82. https://doi.org/10.1016/S2352-3026(20)30216-7.
35. Elkind MIn: UpToDate. https://www.uptodate.com/contents/covid-19-neurologic-complications-and-management-of-neurologic-conditions/print?sectionName=Guillain-Barr%C3%A9+syndrome&search=ORAPRED&topicRef=128323&anchor=H740526394&source=see_link. Accessed 11 Jul 2021.
36. Cummings C, Cori Cummings Department of Neurology, Almallouhi E, et al. Blacks are less likely to present with strokes during the COVID-19 pandemic. In: Stroke. 2020. https://www.ahajournals.org/doi/10.1161/STROKEAHA.120.031121. Accessed 11 Jul 2021.
37. Ayerbe L, Ayis S, Wolfe CD, Rudd AG. Natural history, predictors and outcomes of depression after stroke: systematic review and meta-analysis. The British Journal of Psychiatry: The Journal of Mental Science. 2013;202(1):14–21. https://doi.org/10.1192/bjp.bp.111.107664.
38. Jørgensen TS, Wium-Andersen IK, Wium-Andersen MK, Jørgensen MB, Prescott E, Maartensson S, Kragh-Andersen P, Osler M. Incidence of depression after stroke, and associated risk factors and mortality outcomes, in a large cohort of Danish patients. JAMA Psychiat. 2016;73(10):1032–40. https://doi.org/10.1001/jamapsychiatry.2016.1932.
39. Towfighi A, Ovbiagele B, El Husseini N, et al. Poststroke. A Scientific Statement for Healthcare Professionals From the American Heart Association/American Stroke Association. Stroke: Depression; 2017. https://doi.org/10.1161/str.0000000000000113.
40. Post-Stroke Rehabilitation Fact Sheet | National Institute of Neurological Disorders and Stroke. 2020, May 13. National Institute of Neurological Disorders and Stroke. https://www.ninds.nih.gov/Disorders/Patient-Caregiver-Education/Fact-Sheets/Post-Stroke-Rehabilitation-Fact-Sheet.

Chapter 7
Co-management of Orthopedic Patients

Allison Leonard, James Mautner, and Andrew Bennie

What Is Co-management?

The concept of internal medicine–trained physicians being involved in the care of surgical post-operative patients, otherwise known as co-management, was first identified in the 1950s within the United Kingdom [1]. This system was primarily established as part of a combined orthopedic-geriatric service. However, this model only became popular in the United States during the last few decades, where it has been deployed most often in the specialties of orthopedics and neurosurgery [2].

Hospitalists have always co-managed patients, as they frequently collaborate with primary care physicians when a patient is admitted to the hospital, so in theory hospitalists are the perfect co-management partners for surgeons. The 2015 American Hospital Association survey found that of hospitals with over two hundred beds, ninety-two percent of them utilized hospitalists [3]. The recent growth in hospitalist positions can be explained by the installation of numerous co-management programs. Medicine physicians co-managing surgical patients increased from 33.3% in 1996 to 40.8% in 2006 and orthopedic co-management rose from 28.6% to 41.7% in the same time frame [4]. This new trend has allowed for a myriad of improved outcomes for the patients, hospital, and staff.

A. Leonard (✉)
Hospital Medicine, Ochsner Health, New Orleans, LA, USA
e-mail: allison.leonard@ochsner.org

J. Mautner
Orthopedics, Ochsner Health, New Orleans, LA, USA

A. Bennie
The University of Queensland Faculty of Medicine, Ochsner Clinical School, New Orleans, LA, USA

Traditionally, surgeons manage their own patients postoperatively and consult other services as needed if complications arise. This has resulted in a reactive, rather than proactive, approach, eliminating the ability for hospitalists to prevent complications from occurring and instead managing problems after the fact. In a value-based healthcare setting, this can be detrimental to the hospital's bottom line. With co-management, hospitalists can be involved from the beginning of care, helping to prevent these potential complications in a more proactive fashion.

Co-management has no set definition and therefore comprises a variety of tasks including managing chronic medical comorbidities, addressing daily acute postoperative complications, organizing discharge from the hospital, and communicating with the surgery team [4]. Given the lack of a true definition, co-management programs can vary dramatically based on the needs of the hospital and staff. These co-management systems are built individually by the hospital, implementing agreements between the surgeons, hospitalists, and hospital executives to streamline the patient flow, maximize the efficiency of the available resources, and coordinate responsibilities.

Co-management Roles

Due to the ambiguity surrounding co-management, it is essential for hospitals to design programs that help delineate the roles of every health care provider involved. Without clear protocols, there is potential for miscommunication between the hospitalist and surgeon leading to suboptimal patient care. When integrating hospitalists into a co-management system, there are two central theories. In the first scenario, the hospitalist acts as the primary attending physician for the patient with the surgeon as a consultant. Alternatively, the surgeon maintains the attending physician role and the hospitalist works purely as a consultant [3].

Co-management began with hospitalists intervening postoperatively on surgical patients, but recently has evolved to include some programs where hospitalists provide peri-operative care. This has been installed with the hope of optimizing comorbidities and assessing risk prior to the surgical procedure to provide the best possible outcome for the patient. The Department of Orthopedic Surgery at the Cleveland Medical Center began an orthopedic/hospitalist fellowship position with this aim. Since beginning the program, the department has seen significant improvements in hospital length of stay, complication rate, 30 day readmission rate, and percentage of patients discharged home [5]. The Society of Hospital Medicine has subsequently acknowledged that perioperative medicine is a core requirement in becoming a hospitalist [6].

One of the most significant concerns when beginning a co-management program is ensuring that the scope of practice aligns with each provider's clinical training and expertise. When establishing practice guidelines, developing a comprehensive policy known as a co-management agreement is key. This outlines roles, establishes work flow, and helps answer questions, e.g., who is responsible for prescribing deep

7 Co-management of Orthopedic Patients

Table 7.1 Allocation of hospitalist versus orthopedic roles and responsibilities (Whinney 2012)

Hospitalist	Orthopedics
Meet with orthopedic surgeons and review preoperative assessments and new admissions to identify potential patients for co-management	Utilize the current system of residents with physician's assistant and nurse practitioner positions
Evaluate new patients in co-management program and record pertinent findings	Daily rounding and examinations with progress notes for postoperative orthopedic patients
Follow-up on results of labs and imaging ordered by the hospitalist team	The first avenue of support for nursing when issues with patients arise. Defer to hospitalist for more complex medical decisions
Be available to provide pre- and postoperative medical consultation as needed	Continue as primary attending for patients that do not require co-management (less medically complicated)
Teach residents on orthopedic surgery as to important perioperative medical topics	Along with the medicine resident, provide coverage of patients on holidays, weekends, and nights
Complete daily multidisciplinary rounds with nursing, allied health staff, and case management	Follow-up on results from labs or imaging ordered by the orthopedics team
	Manage basic postoperative orders, including: Blood and fluids Pain and routine PRN medications DVT prophylaxis Wound care and perioperative antibiosis Admission to co-management program Discharge plan Allocation of discharge prescriptions Family communication

vein thrombosis (DVT) prophylaxis or which provider decides when discharge from the hospital is appropriate.

These clinical boundaries help define the specific duties for the hospitalist and surgeon, allowing for the benefits of co-management to emerge. Table 7.1 demonstrates an example of the divided tasks between the hospitalist and orthopedic surgeon, from a recognized co-management program [7]. In this setup, it is important to note that multi-disciplinary rounds occur daily incorporating the hospitalist, orthopedics, nursing, and case managers. This allows for better communication and more thorough patient care. In addition, orthopedics is responsible for most of the surgically related postoperative management here. From pain control to fluid management to DVT prophylaxis and even discharge, orthopedic physicians are the drivers in this particular program, but other hospitals may opt to place more onus on the hospitalist in order to ease the orthopedic responsibilities.

Patients without significant medical complexity were followed only by the orthopedics team. Hospitalists were brought into co-management for their expertise in treating complicated patients with multiple comorbidities; therefore, young and healthy patients undergoing a surgical procedure do not require co-management as their potential for post-operative complications will be minimal. Table 7.2 lists

Table 7.2 Conditions eliciting referral to co-management program (Whinney 2012)

Medical co-morbidities requiring co-management
Coronary artery disease (CAD)
Congestive heart failure (CHF)
Hypertension (HTN)
History of stroke
Peripheral vascular disease (PVD)
Chronic obstructive pulmonary disease (COPD)
Current antibiotic treatment for pneumonia
History of gastrointestinal bleed in last three months
Chronic enteral tube feedings
Diabetes mellitus, type 1 or 2
Psychiatric illnesses
Chronic anti-coagulation
Anti-coagulation for deep vein thrombosis or pulmonary embolism in last 6 months
Chronic immunosuppression
Physiologic glucocorticoid treatment within past year (>two weeks duration)
Medical issues that require medical evaluation, monitoring, or treatment
Atypical chest pain
Shortness of breath (SOB)
Acute deep vein thrombosis (DVT) or pulmonary embolism (PE)
Baseline anemia
Urinary tract infection (UTI)
Acute delirium
Electrolyte disorders
Hyperglycemia without evidence of diabetic ketoacidosis or hyperosmolar state
Acute renal failure
Others

chronic medical conditions that initiate co-management in the same program that is represented in Table 7.1 [7]. This is not an exhaustive list and may fluctuate depending on the hospital, but provides a guide to selecting patients that might require a higher level of care following their surgery.

Orthopedic Patients

Disorders of the musculoskeletal system are one of the principal causes of disability in the United States. In fact, just over 25% of Americans have a musculoskeletal issue that will necessitate a visit to a physician, resulting in a major cost burden to the healthcare system. Throughout developed countries, musculoskeletal injuries represent a majority of chronic diseases in patients over 50 years old [7]. While not all musculoskeletal disorders require an orthopedic surgeon, 40% of Caucasian women in the United States over the age of 50 will endure either a wrist, spine, or hip fracture at some point in their lives [8]. Most of those fractures will be repaired surgically by orthopedic physicians.

Orthopedic injuries predominately affect the elderly population, with nine out of every ten hip fractures occurring in patients aged 65 years or older; this is why orthopedic co-managed care began in conjunction with geriatric services [9]. In addition, the population of individuals over the age of 65 is estimated to be roughly 20% of the world's population by 2030 [10]. This means that the patients at most risk of an orthopedic condition will be a significant portion of the population. Given the excessive costs orthopedic surgery already brings to the table, adding more could be detrimental to the healthcare system.

Within the American healthcare system alone, there were 208,600 registered total hip arthroplasties in 2005. With current projections, it is thought that roughly 572,000 total hip arthroplasties will be completed in 2030, indicating a growth of 174%. For total knee arthroplasties, the year 2005 saw roughly 450,000 procedures, whereas by 2030, it is expected that 3.48 million will be required, a staggering 673% increase [11]. Similar proliferation can be seen for hip fractures, with over 21 million projected worldwide by 2050 [12]. However, hip fractures can result in more long-term impairment. Of the patients that were previously living independently prior to their hip fracture, about one in every four will need some type of long-term nursing home care. Of the patients that do return to their home following surgical repair of their hip fracture, approximately 60% will demand assistance in one or more of their activities of daily living [12]. Furthermore, only half of the hip fracture patients ever recuperate to their full pre-fracture ability [9]. The orthopedic needs of the aging population will strain the healthcare system from several angles: first by increasing the operative workload of orthopedic surgeons, then by bottlenecking the already-crowded nursing homes, and lastly by placing a heavier stress on the at-home services sector of medicine.

These patients are also becoming more complex to manage. With a longer life span, patients are accumulating more and more medical comorbidities which can complicate the postoperative period [7]. As these convoluted patients continue to push the boundaries of the expertise of orthopedic surgeons in their medical management, it is beneficial to introduce a physician who routinely treats patients with multiple serious comorbidities, hence the addition of hospitalist in orthopedic co-management.

With the high prevalence of chronic conditions in the elderly in addition to their increased susceptibility to hip fractures, it follows that frailty is common in this group. Frailty can be explained as a syndrome consisting of reduced physiologic functioning which results in individuals becoming more vulnerable to increased levels of dependency or even death [13]. Because of this, lower energy injuries can produce a more drastic effect on a 70 year old patient with diabetes, osteoporosis, and malnutrition than a 22 year old healthy individual. A fall from standing height may only result in some mild ecchymosis in the latter, whereas it may cause a hip fracture in the former. With frail patients, the risk of falls and subsequent fractures increases two times [14]. To summarize, orthopedic patients are getting older and more complex, and in addition they are at increased risk of sustaining a fracture due to their frail baseline. Therefore, hospitalists are needed in order to help support orthopedic surgeons in managing these patients and improving their outcomes.

Benefits of Orthopedic Co-management

When hospitalists enter a co-management agreement with surgeons, it has been demonstrated that outcomes are superior compared to the previous model of practice which included surgeons only consulting hospitalists once a complication had already presented. In fact, the American Academy of Orthopedic Surgeons has claimed that communication between providers and synchronization of care are vital elements when managing patients undergoing surgery for hip fractures [9]. Therefore, the Society of Hospital Medicine released a guideline for measuring the success of an orthopedic co-management program. A committee formed by the Society of Hospital Medicine detailed a list of factors that must be evaluated which comprises length of stay, mortality rate, admissions to intensive care unit, venous thromboembolism prophylaxis, infection rate, patient/provider satisfaction, readmission rate, discharge disposition, and hospital finances [15]. To explore some of these measures, the findings of several orthopedic co-management programs are discussed below.

Hospital Length of Stay

Numerous studies have elicited that when co-management of orthopedic patients is started, the total length of stay within the hospital is significantly decreased [4]. In a co-managed geriatric fracture center in Germany, the overall length of stay for femoral neck fractures in patients over the age of 60 was discovered to be 4.9 days less than for similar patients treated prior to the beginning of co-management. These patients' time in the hospital consisted of a preoperative segment, from admission to surgery, and then a postoperative portion, the time from the surgical procedure to discharge. This German study revealed that the preoperative interval was also reduced from an average of 3.1 days before co-management to 2.1 days [16]. Although fractures represent a large portion of orthopedics, this diminished time in hospital was also displayed in patients undergoing total knee replacements [5]. These significant decreases in hospital length of stay validate the addition of hospitalists to the care team of orthopedic patients as they have impacts both pre- and postoperatively.

As seen in Table 7.1 earlier, co-management is a multi-disciplinary approach. With regard to reducing patients' length of stay in the hospital, incorporating social workers earlier in the process has been shown to result in earlier discharges [1]. Avoiding unnecessary prolonged stays in the hospital prevents nosocomial infections, among other benefits. Consequently, it is critical that co-management includes specialties, such as social work, to expedite discharge planning.

Mortality Rate

Mortality rate can be high following orthopedic surgery, with one year death rates as high as 25–30% after a hip fracture repair [17]. These staggering numbers represent a burden for orthopedic surgeons when caring for these patients. However, a meta-analysis by Komadina et al. found that, in 18 different studies with the introduction of co-managed care, there was significantly reduced mortality after hip fracture surgery both in-hospital and long term [18]. This argues that the addition of a hospitalist for these patients can have a life-saving effect, but by how much? An orthogeriatric center in Germany demonstrated that following their addition of a co-management intervention, mortality rates dropped by 5.3% in hip fracture patients at one year after surgery [17].

The chief causes of death for orthopedic patients within the hospital setting are cardiac disease and sepsis [14]. These are common conditions that hospitalists treat on a daily basis. Therefore, adding hospitalists in a co-management environment allows for prevention or recognition of the early signs/symptoms seen in these major mortality drivers. A massive study incorporating over 50,000 patients across 828 hospitals in Europe revealed that orthogeriatric co-management was responsible for an attributable fraction of approximately 30 avoided deaths for every 1000 hip fracture patients treated [19]. In addition, a study on the implementation of an orthogeriatric co-management program in China found that the decrease in one year mortality rates was a fundamental driver of cost-effectiveness within the program [20]. Thus, hospitalists functioning in a co-management environment can increase survival rates for orthopedic patients which will then benefit the hospital financially.

Discharge Disposition

Given the nature of orthopedic surgery, with many patients getting joints replaced or receiving surgically placed nails, screws, and plates, the majority of patients will need significant rehabilitation both in the hospital and after discharge. Patients that undergo an orthopedic procedure who are later discharged to either a rehabilitation center or a skilled nursing facility have an increased possibility of readmission to the hospital within the first 90 days. Additionally, these facilities lead to an increased cost to patients of nearly 30% more than those who are discharged directly home [21]. These rates of readmission and surplus expenses can be prohibitive for the patients and detrimental to the healthcare system.

In order to allow more of these patients to be discharged home, efficiency in the postoperative period is key. To aid hip fracture patients in achieving their pre-fracture condition, time spent in bed following the procedure must be curtailed [14]. Studies have shown that early mobilization and weight-bearing postoperatively have led to improved outcomes for orthopedic patients [21]. Incorporating a multidisciplinary team – physical therapy, occupational therapy, and nursing – is of utmost importance. Patients who have enrolled in an orthopedic co-management program have progressed to more intense physical therapy exercises compared to traditional orthopedic care [17]. This may allow for more effective rehabilitation while in the hospital. Geriatric hip fracture patients have demonstrated that when co-management is implemented, patients have significantly increased ambulatory distance at discharge [22]. Furthermore, the improved functional status brought on by co-management has led to these patients having less fear of experiencing falls upon discharge [23]. This impacts the patients' ability to return home as orthogeriatric co-management has led to reduced requirements for further care in either a rehabilitation center or skilled nursing facility [18].

Normally, only 11% of hip fracture patients are discharged directly home, with the majority being placed in skilled nursing facilities or centers for extra rehabilitation. After introducing co-management, this proportion of patients discharged home after orthopedic surgery rises to 25% [23]. With the large number of hip fractures occurring annually, this has the potential to lighten the burden of both the nursing and rehabilitation centers. Although the percentage of patients discharged home is higher following total knee or hip arthroplasty, co-management still revealed a statistically significant increase [5]. As discussed earlier, avoiding discharge to another facility reduces the financial impact of this process for patients and shrinks the possibility they will be readmitted.

Readmission Rate

Readmission to the hospital in general is viewed as a failure for the hospital system as many insurance companies will refuse to reimburse full amounts if the patient requires treatment again in such a short period of time. Among those patients on Medicare who undergo any type of surgical procedure, 70.5% are rehospitalized for a medical disease rather than a surgical issue [4]. This stresses the significance of managing these patients' chronic medical conditions during their initial admission to the hospital. The trend is apparent in orthopedics as approximately three out of every ten hip fracture patients are readmitted within one year. Again, the most common reasons for these presentations include infections or exacerbations of underlying pulmonary disease, heart failure, and renal failure [14], none of which are related to a surgical problem but rather to poor medical management.

After installing a co-management program, a center focusing on geriatric hip fracture repair found that the 6 month readmission rate of their patients had significantly decreased [22]. Avoiding rehospitalization for these patients can be lifesaving, as mortality rates during readmission are nearly double when compared to patients who are not hospitalized again [14]. Most orthopedic patients end up spending time in the hospital postoperatively to recover and regain function regardless of baseline medical function, so introducing a hospitalist to use that interval to manage chronic conditions will ultimately decrease the possibility of readmission for medical comorbidities.

Total Cost of Care

Many of the improved outcome metrics of co-management programs have secondary benefits, including financial savings. For hip fracture patients, approximately 44% of the cost of their care is represented by charges from the hospital [9]. This means that a reduced time spent in hospital would directly result in significant decreased costs for the patient. The decreased length of stay paired with lower rehospitalization rates can also represent improved profit margins for the hospital. Within surgical comanagement programs, the average funds saved have been estimated to range from $2642 to $4303 per individual [24]. Given the future of orthopedics, with case numbers forecast to skyrocket over the next few decades, these financial consequences may result in massive savings for the whole healthcare system. Potentially, this will allow investment into other areas to develop future advances in medicine.

Satisfaction

In addition to enhancing outcomes for patients, orthopedic co-management can have positive effects on hospital staff. For example, significant improvements in nurse communication and a general trend toward better physician communication were noted when co-management was begun for orthopedics [25]. With the multidisciplinary method of co-management, the staff are more accustomed to their role. Furthermore, confidential surveys of participants in the co-management program described drastically improved job satisfaction for the orthopedic surgeons, hospitalists, and nurses involved [4].

In addition to staff satisfaction with co-management, exploring how satisfied the patients are with their experience can be informative and lead to positive changes. The Press-Ganey Hospital Consumer Assessment of Healthcare Providers and Systems (HCAHPS) is a tool to monitor patient satisfaction and has eight main categories: communication with doctors, communication with nurses, overall rating, responsiveness of hospital staff, hospital environment, pain management, communication about medications, and discharge information. This survey is sent to patients recently discharged from the hospital, where "top box" scores represent the highest possible rating. After introducing hospitalists into an orthopedic joint replacement co-management center, six of those eight categories received more "top box" scores, with statistically significant increases in three categories (hospital environment, overall rating, and staff responsiveness) [5]. Outside of the physical benefits of co-management, such as superior readmission and mortality rates, the happiness of the staff and patients that is part of these programs is important to keep in mind.

QALYs

Quality-adjusted life years, or QALYs as they are usually referred to, is a common metric used to help quantify the burden a disease or condition may represent for a patient. A study evaluating hip fracture patients in the Chinese population demonstrated that with the implementation of co-management, these individuals gained 0.07 QALYs [20]. Although this may not appear to be significant for patients, hip fracture mortality is quite high, so any improvement following surgery is beneficial. In a separate study exploring hip fractures in the German community, co-management revealed that one year following their surgery, patients believed they had a superior health status compared to their pre-fracture condition [17]. While this is subjective data, the trend is consistent for objective results as well. When analyzing American hip fracture patients at four and twelve months after their procedure, co-managed adults exhibited increased quality of life and functional status at both time points, improved physical performance at four months, and lastly enhanced cognitive status at twelve months [23]. All of these quality metrics add to the value that co-management brings to these orthopedic patients.

Pain Management

It is well known that orthopedic injuries are among the most painful. When treating these patients, failure to control pain has been associated with prolonged recovery, leading to increased expenses and longer length of stay [26]. Patients' pain level following their orthopedic surgery has been discovered to be the single most decisive factor in their satisfaction with the experience. Curtailing their pain during the entire perioperative time is linked with reduced complications postoperatively as well as a lower readmission rate [27]. Co-management programs have been shown to improve these metrics, so incorporating pain management into the multidisciplinary approach is key.

Acute pain experienced by patients can manifest into numerous undesirable complications. The patient's body often responds to sustained pain levels with a neuroendocrine reaction, which then causes several effects including tachycardia, tachypnea, hypercoagulability, hypertension, bowel stasis, and even a decreased immune response. All of these consequences can expand the possibility of a myriad of postoperative complications, such as ileus, respiratory failure, stroke, myocardial infarction, DVT/PE, and confusion. Furthermore, hip fracture patients who feel severe pain are at risk of developing delirium at nine times the rate of patients with appropriate pain control. Pain experienced during dynamic movements like deep inspiration or ambulation can be factors in whether a patient is actively participating in physical therapy exercises or simply getting out of bed. Ensuring proper pain control when these patients are active results in less time in bed, which can reduce consequences correlated with immobility such as pneumonia or DVT and possibly thwart declines in muscle strength or functional baseline [26].

When choosing a treatment plan for pain, opioids are the most frequently prescribed option [28]. Given that orthopedic injuries are extremely painful, opioids have often been the first choice of medication, as demonstrated by the fact that 47% of opioid addicts receive their first dose via a prescription for pain [26]. Unfortunately, America is in the midst of an opioid crisis, with overdose deaths tripling in the last 15 years. Opioids are responsible for a staggering 61% of those deaths. Any patient prescribed opioids, regardless of the duration of the prescription, is at risk for addiction or dependence, with roughly two of every ten patients later getting extra prescriptions and 6% remaining chronic users. In fact, of individuals who consistently take opioids over a three month period, half will continue to use opioids five years later whether prescribed or not, and at that point are prospective lifelong consumers [28]. Keeping in mind the expected rise in orthopedic cases in the near future, better pain control options must be addressed to reduce these preventable overdose deaths.

Apart from the overdose-related deaths, opioids can present more acute problems for staff while the patient remains in the hospital postoperatively. The inherent pharmacology of opioids put patients at increased risk of several issues, including urinary retention, respiratory depression, hypotension, and delirium [27]. Also, patients treated with opioids have been found to ambulate shorter distances on postoperative day one, leading to a slower recovery, which ends with prolonged length of stay and higher chance of being discharged to a skilled nursing facility or rehabilitation center rather than directly home [29]. Most importantly, the odds ratio of in-hospital cardiopulmonary arrest nearly doubles when opioids are prescribed [26]. Eliminating any of these issues with a co-management program would be advantageous in maximizing benefits for orthopedic patients.

Pertinent to orthopedic patients specifically is the effect of opioids on bone healing. In vitro, morphine has been demonstrated to inhibit osteocalcin, a contributor to bone formation. Additionally, in animals opioids were found to result in the formation of a larger callus that was significantly weaker and more disorganized [28]. Although these findings have not been replicated in human subjects, it is worth remembering the implications these pain medications may have on orthopedic patients.

The process of pain optimization must begin prior to the surgical procedure. Educational sessions before surgery explaining what to expect regarding alleviation of pain and outlining a timeline for recovery help influence the patient's perception of pain [27]. This primes the patient's brain for appropriate and expected levels of postoperative pain. To further aid in pain prevention, preoperative analgesia is offered to prevent nociceptors from reaching hyperalgesia [29]. Inhibiting pain can be vital, but some patients who present with fractures or more acute issues will likely already be in pain prior to entering the hospital. In this case, treating the pain as early as possible is key, because the pain signal can intensify with time. Likewise, if tissue is exposed to sustained injury, nerve sensitization can occur [30].

After maximizing pain control in the preoperative period, the focus must be on intra-operative decisions that minimize pain. Traditionally, general anesthesia has been used for both total hip and knee arthroplasties. However, recently the idea of introducing spinal anesthesia for these procedures has become popular. Spinal anesthesia, a specialized regional nerve block, has the ability to inhibit pain signals from reaching the cerebral cortex. Since the brain cannot identify pain in this scenario, the usual physiologic responses that are associated with pain, including tachycardia and hypertension, are minimized [29]. Furthermore, spinal anesthesia has demonstrated better outcomes postoperatively. In a study comparing general anesthesia with oxycodone and celecoxib versus intra-thecal bupivacaine, clonidine, and morphine, the general anesthesia group remained in the hospital longer, reported more pain, and were quicker to their first rescue pain medication [28]. Also, patients who undergo general anesthesia for their hip fracture surgery are placed at higher risk of mortality while they remain in the hospital during the postoperative time [21]. Understanding the impacts that these intraoperative choices hold can have long-lasting effects for the patient.

Lastly, and arguably most importantly, are the postoperative options for pain management. Given the many downfalls of utilizing opioid medications for analgesia, there is a consensus that the multimodal analgesic (MMA) model is superior. MMA involves using a range of different therapies to help control pain from different angles. These can include cryotherapy, psychotherapy, non-steroidal anti-inflammatory drugs (NSAIDs), peri-articular injections, regional nerve blocks, and even transcutaneous electrical stimulation (TENS) [28]. Rather than the traditional analgesia method of as-needed (PRN) medications, the MMA strategy employs scheduled medications to get ahead of the pain [27]. Besides decreased pain levels, MMA has been shown to reduce length of stay and acuity of care in the postoperative stage, as well as improvements in range of motion, mobility, and recovery. With the addition of increased satisfaction for patients receiving MMA, this approach to pain management would work synergistically with a co-management program. When considering all types of surgeries, the most common postoperative complication leading to prolonged hospital admissions is gastrointestinal dysfunction. Since MMA aims to reduce the use of opioids, one of the main causes of intestinal stasis, the decreased incidence of gastrointestinal dysfunction helps promote earlier discharges [26].

One of the main instruments used in MMA is continuous peripheral nerve blocks. As seen with spinal anesthesia utilized intra-operatively, this can prevent pain signals from reaching the brain and, therefore, providing superior analgesia compared to opioids [26]. The most significant consideration for nerve blocks is location. Placing continuous blocks at the femoral nerve risks losing quadriceps muscle function and increases risk of falls, so for total knee arthroplasties, one must insert the nerve block within the adductor canal to avoid the motor portions of the femoral nerve. In general, these peripheral nerve blocks can allow the patient to mobilize more quickly and participate in more vigorous physical therapy, ultimately reducing their stay within the hospital [29]. These functional results extend up to six weeks following surgery with further ambulatory distance and stronger stair-climbing ability [28]. Continuous peripheral nerve blocks have been an effective strategy in MMA, helping to curtail the need for additional pain medications.

Another advantage of MMA is the implementation of regularly scheduled medications to keep pain minimal. Two of the more commonly used options are acetaminophen and celecoxib. COX is believed to play a role in the pain pathway. In fact, higher levels of prostaglandin E2, a product of the COX pathway, have been linked with slower progress in physical therapy [29]. This is why acetaminophen, a COX-3 inhibitor in the thalamus, and celecoxib, a selective COX-2 inhibitor in the dorsal spinothalamic tract of the spinal cord, are used [27]. One of the main medication classes in this pharmacological group is that of non-steroidal anti-inflammatory drugs (NSAIDs); however, these have previously been withheld due to their potentially negative impact on bone healing. In fact, although animal studies have implicated that fracture healing concerns with NSAIDs, a recent meta-analysis determined there had been no quality evidence of this within the human clinical environment [28]. Regardless, since acetaminophen is not considered an NSAID and celecoxib selectively blocks COX-2, physicians can effectively control pain without the concern of impaired bone healing.

Less commonly used methods in MMA include cryotherapy, TENS, and peri-articular injections. Cryotherapy utilizes near-freezing temperatures to provide analgesia for postoperative patients. The extremely low temperatures cause vasoconstriction within the tissue to reduce the presence of inflammatory mediators and lessen the metabolic demand. Furthermore, dropping the temperature of the affected tissue has been proven to increase pain tolerance [28]. Peri-articular injections are often seen in chronic pain clinics and utilize corticosteroids to decrease a patient's pain level both at rest and with dynamic movements, without the negative side effects of opioids [29]. TENS aims to activate opioid receptors via endogenous pathways of inhibition by distributing low-voltage electrical currents to the site of pain. However, due to the use of electricity, this strategy is contraindicated in patients with pacemakers or defibrillators. As noted above, a majority of the orthopedic patient population is elderly with multiple comorbidities and therefore these devices may be more common among them, prohibiting the use of TENS [28].

ICU Admissions

The intensive care unit (ICU) of hospitals requires a higher acuity of care for patients. Due to the fact that these patients are sicker, the ICU also increases costs for the patient and hospital. Given that there are a fixed number of ICU beds available in any hospital, decreasing the number of patients that may require this level of care is immensely valuable. The introduction of co-management to any surgical patient has reduced rates of medical deterioration, causing fewer escalations of care to the ICU [4]. Similar results were found with co-management of orthopedic patients, but also demonstrated that if patients were admitted to the ICU during their postoperative interval, they required a shorter duration before being transferred back to the orthopedic ward [5]. Less admissions to the ICU for orthopedic patients mean a faster recovery and more intensive care beds for other acutely ill patients.

Hospital Medications

Without co-management, surgeons consult other services as needed. When those physicians examine the patient, they order medications that are deemed appropriate; however, they may not be aware of what other providers have already prescribed. The multi-disciplinary strategy of co-management helps to eliminate any confusion as rounds are often completed with other specialties to ensure that all parties are aware of the current treatment plan. This has led to the reduction of polypharmacy for co-managed orthopedic patients [17]. The surgeon's main focus is becoming an expert in surgical techniques and remaining up to date on the best surgical practices. However, hospitalists are more likely to be aware of current guidelines for certain medical conditions. Therefore, co-management has led to the increased use of evidence-based treatments, in an effort to provide the patient optimal care [4].

The most obvious example of this within orthopedic surgery is management of osteoporosis. Osteoporosis is quite common in the United States, affecting nearly 27 million individuals [29]. Despite numerous studies revealing the effectiveness of anti-osteoporotic medications (vitamin D, calcium, and bisphosphonates) in preventing future fractures, the bulk of patients who present with a fracture are never even assessed for osteoporosis at all, let alone treated for it [14]. Given the prevalence of the disease, and the potential impacts on mortality rate and independence that fractures could hold for patients, this is not optimal. If all patients with any type of fracture were to be appropriately managed with anti-osteoporotic therapy, it is estimated that 22% fewer of them would go on to have a future hip fracture [21]. Besides fracture risk, osteoporosis is also of concern postoperatively for orthopedic surgeons. Due to the nature of osteoporosis, the bone is less likely to take the implant and often has higher complication rates, including poor bone healing and difficulty preserving fracture reduction [21]. Also, osteoporosis could hinder activity levels postoperatively and therefore slow progress through a physical therapy program. Co-management has altered this for the better, with the percentage of postoperative patients using anti-osteoporotic therapy increased from 12% without co-management to an astounding 93% [22]. In addition, these patients are reporting improved compliance with the medications compared to before the introduction of co-management [7]. With the high incidence of osteoporosis in the community paired with readily available prevention, appropriate treatment by a co-management team can significantly impact future fracture rates.

Consults

Consulting many specialists for complex patients in the absence of a co-management team can result in disjointed management as these specialties often round and treat each patient separately. Although these specialists are experts within their given specialty, many of them are not familiar with surgical physiology and the problems postoperative patients may present. One example is that of postoperative third spacing and fluid shifts. Third spacing alone can lead to potential pre-renal acute kidney injury, a condition familiar to a nephrologist [21]. However, understanding that these fluid shifts are expected in postoperative patients and how to prevent or manage this requires the nephrologist to have experience working with surgical patients. Therefore, adding hospitalists who strictly manage postoperative patients allows these physicians unique insight into these specific surgical issues. Before co-management, hospitalists were only consulted on 13.8% of orthopedic patients. Optimizing various patient medical comorbidities is not necessarily within the scope of practice for orthopedic surgeons, consequently leading to readmissions for medical exacerbations rather than surgical problems [11]. Another documented benefit of orthopedic co-managed care is that, following its introduction, the proportion of instances where two or more specialties were consulted for an orthopedic postoperative patient significantly decreased [24]. Adding hospitalists devoted to orthopedic postoperative patients ensures not only maximized management of their chronic medical comorbidities but also a decreased workload for consulting specialties.

Complications

Most often, postoperative surgical complications are due to poor medical management rather than suboptimal intraoperative technique. The National Surgical Quality Improvement Project recently discovered that postoperative complications occur at similar rates regardless of the mortality rate observed while in hospital. This implies that top hospitals do not distinguish themselves by avoiding these complications but by their ability to save the patient once the complication has already happened [2]. Therefore, in order to distinguish themselves even further, it would be advantageous to hospitals to prevent these complications from occurring in the first place.

Adding co-managed care has led to significantly reduced percentages of orthopedic patients suffering one or more complications in the postoperative interval [24]. The most common complications seen in orthopedic patients are urinary tract infection (UTI) and delirium [14]. As many postsurgical patients tend to remain with indwelling catheters following anesthesia, being acutely aware of when to remove it and thereby reducing the possibility of developing a UTI is a major benefit that hospitalists have brought to the co-managed setting [18]. On the other hand, delirium was found to be diagnosed up to 15% more once co-management began. This is thought to be due to increased delirium awareness by hospitalists [16]. Recognizing the symptoms earlier can mean quicker initiation of treatment and better outcomes for patients.

Other complications that are often experienced during the postoperative time by orthopedic patients include pneumonia, surgical site infections, and DVT/PE. In 2008, the Centers for Medicaid and Medicare Services added both DVT and PE to their "never event" list for patients undergoing total knee or hip arthroplasties [7]. A "never event" indicates that if the event were to occur in this patient population, reimbursement is withheld from the hospital. Thankfully, a co-management program was able to reduce the rate of venous thromboembolism rates from 4.6% to 1.3% [22]. As discussed earlier, the multi-disciplinary approach of co-management allows for services such as pain management plus physical and occupational therapy to get orthopedic patients to mobilize as fast as possible. Ambulating early in the postoperative period has been associated with fewer DVTs [29] and pulmonary complications [22]. This can be beneficial as pneumonia can complicate the postoperative course in up to 10% of all hip fracture patients [14].

Infections of the surgical site are dreaded setbacks in the postoperative interval for orthopedic surgeons. A nutritionist can have extensive influence on preventing infections when added to the comprehensive co-management team. Malnutrition is prevalent within the geriatric population, which represent a majority of orthopedic patients. Adequate nutritional status can not only impede infection from developing but also improve wound healing [21]. Thus, supplying proper nutrition in these patients has been linked with fewer overall complications and earlier rehabilitation [14]. Utilizing the medical expertise of hospitalists as well as applying the multi-disciplinary concept with applied health services, hospitals can now proactively prevent postoperative complications.

Blending Co-management and Orthopedics

The impact of co-management for orthopedic patients, their providers, and hospitals can be wide ranging. Hip fractures are quite common in the geriatric community and are a devastating problem, resulting in loss of functional independence and increased mortality rates [23]. These fractures drastically increase the risk of falls and future fractures. Even though many co-management programs will not encounter these patients until after their first fracture, by identifying risk factors such as osteoporosis and treating them, in addition to optimizing chronic medical conditions, co-management has been able to reduce secondary fractures by roughly 15% [17]. With the increasingly complex medical patients presenting to orthopedic surgery, hospitalists are necessary to help this vulnerable patient population.

Hospitals prosper financially from co-management as well. Before co-management, the treatment of acute medical issues may have been postponed if the surgeon was still in the operating room [19]. With fewer postoperative patients to manage, orthopedic surgeons in a co-management program can increase their surgical workload. As orthopedic surgery is one of the more profitable specialties for hospitals, the prospect of expanded surgical lists is an incentive for hospital systems.

In academic hospitals, surgeons have traditionally relied on resident physicians to help manage postoperative patients [22]. However, orthopedic residents have little training within internal medicine, making them less than ideal providers for medically complicated patients [7]. With the introduction of hospitalists dedicated to managing these orthopedic postoperative patients, resident physicians are able to gain more experience in the operative setting. Increased time spent in the operating room over their years as resident physicians will groom them into orthopedic surgeons with better practical skills and the ability to offer future patients improved outcomes.

Key Points
- Hospitalists have effectively been co-managers since their inception.
- Co-management consists of a comprehensive multi-disciplinary approach, including physical and occupational therapists, nutritionists, and pain management.
- When developing a co-management program, assigning clear roles helps providers stay within their scope of practice.
- The orthopedic patient population is rapidly aging and becoming more complicated to medically manage.
- Co-management, specifically within orthopedic surgery, has been shown to improve a variety of clinical patient outcomes.
- Apart from superior outcomes for their patients, providers are noticing healthier communication and better job satisfaction.
- With reduced length of stay and less readmissions, co-management has been fiscally advantageous for hospital systems.

References

1. Hempsall VJ, Robertson DR, Campbell MJ, Briggs RS. Orthopaedic geriatric care--is it effective? A prospective population-based comparison of outcome in fractured neck of femur. J R Coll Physicians Lond. 1990;24(1):47–50.
2. Hinami K, Feinglass J, Ferranti DE, Williams MV. Potential role of comanagement in "rescue" of surgical patients. Am J Manag Care. 2011;17(9):e333–9.
3. Vora H, Atchley B, Behnke S, Cockerham C, Pyke ON, Sittig R, Vulgamore P. The evolution of co-management. 2017.
4. Sharma G, Kuo YF, Freeman J, Zhang DD, Goodwin JS. Comanagement of hospitalized surgical patients by medicine physicians in the United States. Arch Intern Med. 2010;170(4):363–8. https://doi.org/10.1001/archinternmed.2009.553.
5. Fitzgerald SJ, Palmer TC, Kraay MJ. Improved perioperative Care of Elective Joint Replacement Patients: the impact of an orthopedic perioperative hospitalist. The. 2018.
6. Pistoria M, Amin A, Dressler D, McKean S, Budnitz T. The core competencies in hospital medicine: a framework for curriculum development by the society of hospital medicine. J Hosp Med. 2006;1(S1):iii–v. https://doi.org/10.1002/jhm.72.

7. Whinney C. Chapter 67. Co-management of orthopedic patients. In: McKean SC, Ross JJ, Dressler DD, Brotman DJ, Ginsberg JS, editors. Principles and practice of hospital medicine. New York, NY: McGraw-Hill Companies; 2012.
8. Gosch M, Hoffmann-Weltin Y, Roth T, Blauth M, Nicholas JA, Kammerlander C. Orthogeriatric co-management improves the outcome of long-term care residents with. 2016.
9. Friedman SM, Mendelson DA, Kates SL, McCann RM. Geriatric co-Management of Proximal Femur Fractures: Total quality management and protocol-driven care result in better outcomes for a frail patient population. J Am Geriatr Soc. 2008;56(7):1349–56. https://doi.org/10.1111/j.1532-5415.2008.01770.x.
10. Vitiello R, Bellieni A, Oliva MS, Di Capua B, Fusco D, Careri S, Colloca GF, Perisano C, Maccauro G, Lillo M. The importance of geriatric and surgical co-management of elderly in muscoloskeletal oncology: a literature review. Orthop Rev (Pavia). 2020;12(Suppl 1):8662. https://doi.org/10.4081/or.2020.8662.
11. Duplantier NL, Briski DC, Luce LT, Meyer MS, Ochsner JL, Chimento GF. The effects of a hospitalist Comanagement model for joint arthroplasty patients in a teaching facility. J Arthroplast. 2016;31(3):567–72. https://doi.org/10.1016/j.arth.2015.10.010.
12. Grigoryan KV, Javedan H, Rudolph JL. Orthogeriatric care models and outcomes in hip fracture patients: a systematic review and meta-analysis. J Orthop Trauma. 2014;28(3):e49–55. https://doi.org/10.1097/BOT.0b013e3182a5a045.
13. Morley JE, Vellas B, van Kan GA, Anker SD, Bauer JM, Bernabei R, Cesari M, Chumlea WC, Doehner W, Evans J, Fried LP, Guralnik JM, Katz PR, Malmstrom TK, McCarter RJ, Gutierrez Robledo LM, Rockwood K, von Haehling S, Vandewoude MF, Walston J. Frailty consensus: a call to action. J Am Med Dir Assoc. 2013;14(6):392–7. https://doi.org/10.1016/j.jamda.2013.03.022.
14. Pioli G, Bendini C, Pignedoli P, Giusti A, Marsh D. Orthogeriatric co-management – managing frailty as well as fragility. Injury. 2018;49(8):1398–402. https://doi.org/10.1016/j.injury.2018.04.014.
15. McKean S, Adair W, Allen K, Fishmann A, Gul F, Gulseth M, Kisuule F, Masters M, Mraz B, Pinzur M, Ruhlen M, Whinney C. A white paper on a guide to hospitalist/orthopedic surgery co-management. 2010.
16. Biber R, Singler K, Curschmann-Horter M, Wicklein S, Sieber C, Bail HJ. Implementation of a co-managed geriatric fracture center reduces hospital stay and time-to-operation in elderly femoral neck fracture patients. Arch Orthop Trauma Surg. 2013;133(11):1527–31. https://doi.org/10.1007/s00402-013-1845-z.
17. Neuerburg C, Förch S, Gleich J, Böcker W, Gosch M, Kammerlander C, Mayr E. Improved outcome in hip fracture patients in the aging population following co-managed care compared to conventional surgical treatment: a retrospective, dual-center cohort study. BMC Geriatr. 2019;19(1):330. https://doi.org/10.1186/s12877-019-1289-6.
18. Komadina R, Wendt KW, Holzer G, Kocjan T. Outcome parameters in orthogeriatric co-management – a mini-review. Wien Klin Wochenschr. 2016;128(7):492–6. https://doi.org/10.1007/s00508-016-1118-2.
19. Rapp K, Becker C, Todd C, Rothenbacher D, Schulz C, König HH, Liener U, Hartwig E, Büchele G. The association between Orthogeriatric co-management and mortality following hip fracture. Dtsch Arztebl Int. 2020;117(4):53–9. https://doi.org/10.3238/arztebl.2020.0053.
20. Peng K, Yang M, Tian M, Chen M, Zhang J, Wu X, Ivers R, Si L. Cost-effectiveness of a multi-disciplinary co-management program for the older hip fracture patients in Beijing. Osteoporos Int. 2020;31(8):1545–53. https://doi.org/10.1007/s00198-020-05393-1.
21. Greenstein AS, Gorczyca JT. Orthopedic surgery and the geriatric patient. Clin Geriatr Med. 2019;35(1):65–92. https://doi.org/10.1016/j.cger.2018.08.007.
22. Whinney C, Michota F. Surgical comanagement: a natural evolution of hospitalist practice. J Hosp Med. 2008;3(5):394–7. https://doi.org/10.1002/jhm.359.

23. Chen P, Hung WW. Geriatric orthopedic co-management of older adults with hip fracture: an emerging standard. Ann Transl Med. 2015;3(16):224. https://doi.org/10.3978/j.issn.2305-5839.2015.07.13.
24. Rohatgi N, Loftus P, Grujic O, Cullen M, Hopkins J, Ahuja N. Surgical Comanagement by hospitalists improves patient outcomes: a propensity score analysis. Ann Surg. 2016;264(2):275–82. https://doi.org/10.1097/sla.0000000000001629.
25. Martin D, Kain M, Bramlett KJ, Brabeck D, Marcantonio A. Toward the triple aim: implementing a hospitalist co-management model for orthopaedic surgical patients in an academic medical Centre. Future Hosp J. 2015;2(Suppl 2):s33. https://doi.org/10.7861/futurehosp.2-2s-s33.
26. Jones J Jr, Southerland W, Catalani B. The importance of optimizing acute pain in the orthopedic trauma patient. Orthop Clin North Am. 2017;48(4):445–65. https://doi.org/10.1016/j.ocl.2017.06.003.
27. Trasolini NA, McKnight BM, Dorr LD. The opioid crisis and the orthopedic surgeon. J Arthroplasty. 2018;33(11):3379–3382.e3371. https://doi.org/10.1016/j.arth.2018.07.002.
28. Hsu JR, Mir H, Wally MK, Seymour RB, Force tOTAMPT. Clinical practice guidelines for pain Management in Acute Musculoskeletal Injury. J Orthop Trauma. 2019;33(5):e158–82. https://doi.org/10.1097/bot.0000000000001430.
29. Gaffney CJ, Pelt CE, Gililland JM, Peters CL. Perioperative pain Management in hip and Knee Arthroplasty. Orthop Clin North Am. 2017;48(4):407–19. https://doi.org/10.1016/j.ocl.2017.05.001.
30. Nischal N, Arulraja E, Shaheen SP. Pain Management for Orthopedic Injuries. Emerg Med Clin North Am. 2020;38(1):223–41. https://doi.org/10.1016/j.emc.2019.09.013.

Chapter 8
Pediatric Hospital Medicine

Alexandra Wright and Margaret Malone

Pediatric Hospital Medicine (PHM) is a relatively new field, proposed by the American Academy of Pediatrics (AAP) as a new subspecialty in 2014 [1] and officially recognized as a subspecialty by the American Board of Medical Specialties (ABMS) in 2016. Pediatric patients in the acute setting have increasingly complex conditions, including chronic disease, mental illness, special or technology-dependent needs, and/or multiple comorbidities. Simultaneously, providers in outpatient community centers have increased requirements for complex care due largely to scientific developments, allowing previously terminal illness to become manageable chronic conditions [1]. A separation of inpatient and outpatient care therefore allows providers to focus their expertise on the differing needs of these two populations.

Clinical practice guidelines exist for many pediatric conditions commonly encountered in hospital medicine, just as in adult hospital medicine. However, the authors have observed that guidelines seem to be applied less frequently than in adult populations, with greater variation in the guidelines that are used and more subjectivity in providers' clinical decisions. We believe this is largely an issue of difference in training practice and lack of awareness of available evidence-based tools and protocols. The following is a summary of some common conditions that have evidence-based guidelines but which are often managed subjectively or in a manner inconsistent with best practice.

A. Wright (✉)
Ochsner Hospital for Children, New Orleans, LA, USA
e-mail: alexandra.wright@ochsner.org

M. Malone
The University of Queensland-Ochsner Clinical School, New Orleans, LA, USA

Management of Bronchiolitis in the Emergency Department and Hospital

Bronchiolitis is the most frequent lower respiratory infection in infants and presents with cough, wheezing, tachypnea, crackles, and/or respiratory distress [2]. The most common underlying pathogens are respiratory syncytial virus (83%) and human rhinovirus (34%) [3]. According to a 2005 retrospective analysis of 17,397 patients published prior to the AAP guidelines, 45% of patients with bronchiolitis received antibiotics and 25% received systemic steroids [4]. Another, more recent analysis published well after the AAP guidelines found even higher rates with 26.5% receiving steroids and 81.6% receiving albuterol [5]. Other treatments that have been used by pediatric providers include inhaled epinephrine, nebulized hypertonic saline, chest physiotherapy, and deep suctioning [6].

The AAP clinical practice guideline (published in 2006 and revised in 2014), in fact, recommends almost none of these common treatment modalities. The strongest/highest quality of evidence recommendations are against the use of albuterol, epinephrine, corticosteroids, and antibiotics [6]. It is important to note that these guidelines do not apply to the management of bronchiolitis in immunocompromised patients or those with underlying respiratory conditions. Here, we will review strong and moderate recommendations – i.e., those with the highest quality of evidence – for management of uncomplicated bronchiolitis cases.

Strong Recommendations

Perhaps the most surprising recommendation from the updated guidelines is that against the use of beta-adrenergic agonist agents such as albuterol [6]. Randomized controlled trials have found that use of these agents does not affect time to disease resolution, need for hospitalization, or length of stay (LOS) for hospitalized patients. However, a retrospective analysis in 2013 found that 32% of infants discharged from emergency departments in the United States were prescribed albuterol – the highest rate of the eight countries studied [7]. Further research and quality improvement initiatives into how best to implement practice change would likely prove helpful in reducing unnecessary albuterol prescription.

The updated guidelines also strongly recommend against the use of systemic corticosteroids or inhaled epinephrine [6]. These treatments have not been found to decrease hospital admissions or LOS. The safety of administering steroids is unclear although there is some evidence that they may increase the duration of viral shedding after an infection [8]. Steroids are prescribed less frequently than beta-agonists at discharge in the United States, at a rate of around 6% [7].

Antibiotics should not be used unless there is a strong suspicion of concomitant bacterial infection. In fact, a child with a distinct viral syndrome such as bronchiolitis has a less than 1% chance of a concurrent bacterial infection with positive cerebrospinal fluid culture or blood culture [9].

The only treatment that is strongly recommended is the administration of fluids either intravenously or via nasogastric tube for patients who are unable to maintain adequate oral hydration. While there are hazards of these interventions including risk of infection, patient discomfort, aspiration with nasogastric tube, and overhydration, the AAP has determined that the benefits of maintaining hydration in these children outweigh the risks [6].

Moderate Recommendations

The use of nebulized hypertonic saline in the emergency department is not recommended as administration over periods of less than 24 hours has not been shown to be of benefit. However, there is a weak recommendation favoring this treatment for patients admitted to the hospital with mild to moderate disease. There is some evidence that continuous administration for longer than 24 hours can shorten LOS, likely via enhancement of mucociliary clearance in these patients [6].

Nonpharmacological management typically includes suctioning of the nasopharynx and chest physiotherapy, e.g., vibration, percussion, and passive expiratory techniques. However, none of these interventions have been shown to have clinical benefit in the management of bronchiolitis, and, in fact, deep suctioning may be associated with increased LOS in infants aged 2–12 months [10]. Formally, there is a moderate recommendation against the use of chest physiotherapy. There remain insufficient data to make a recommendation regarding suctioning, and it is likely that deep suctioning of infants with uncomplicated bronchiolitis should be avoided [6].

Despite AAP clinical practice guidelines that are in place, bronchiolitis management in the emergency department and hospital remains variable and often nonevidence based. The writers propose that much of this problem stems from variance in practice during medical training as well as the timing of when the practice guidelines are implemented. A retrospective chart review in 2013 examined behavioral change in physician practice before and after the release of guidelines. While diagnostic laboratory testing rates did not decline, the number of children receiving racemic epinephrine decreased from 17.8% to 12.2% and those receiving albuterol decreased from 81.6% to 72.6% [5]. Since adherence to these guidelines remains less than ideal in the United States, research should be performed to identify effective interventions that will result in increased compliance to guidelines and decreased use of unnecessary treatment.

Prevention of Neonatal Sepsis

Neonatal sepsis is a feared complication of childbirth, with an estimated 1–5 cases per 1000 live births annually and accounting for approximately 15 percent of neonatal deaths worldwide [11]. In the United States, the incidence is lower at approximately 0.5 in 1000 live births at term and 1 in 1000 for late-preterm births [12]. Early-onset sepsis (EOS), defined here as sepsis with onset in the first 7 days of life (although there is variability in this definition as some experts limit this to infections occurring within the first 72 hours of life), is most commonly due to infection with either Group B *Streptococcus* (GBS) or *Escherichia coli* [12, 13]. Risk factors include duration of rupture of membranes (ROM) >18 hours, maternal intrapartum fever ≥100.4 F, maternal colonization with GBS, maternal chorioamnionitis, and gestational age (GA) <37 weeks [12].

Revisions of a protocol for prevention of neonatal sepsis from the Centers for Disease Control (CDC) have been available since 1996. This approach results in all babies whose mothers are diagnosed with chorioamnionitis, having a blood culture and complete blood count (CBC) drawn and receiving antibiotics, despite any other considerations (i.e., maternal GBS status and/or maximum maternal intrapartum temperature). However, due to the decline in rates of neonatal sepsis with the implementation of maternal intrapartum antibiotic prophylaxis, this results in many asymptomatic infants receiving antibiotics unnecessarily. In addition to the risk of creating antibiotic resistance, perinatal exposure to antibiotics increases risk of necrotizing enterocolitis, invasive fungal infections, and death [14]. This protocol also results in unnecessary blood draws and the risk of false-positive blood cultures with organisms that are commonly found on the skin.

In 2018, the AAP neonatal sepsis guidelines were modified, and a tool called the Neonatal Sepsis Risk Calculator was introduced [15]. The goal of these new guidelines was to decrease antibiotic utilization for asymptomatic newborns and to improve antibiotic stewardship. When implemented in a study by Ellington et al., the tool reduced utilization among asymptomatic infants ≥36 weeks GA by 75%. In this study, only one infant out of 3158 participants had a positive blood culture requiring >48 hours of intravenous antibiotic treatment [16].

The EOS calculator is an open-source tool available without cost online through Kaiser Permanente's website [17]. The required input values are as follows: regional incidence of EOS (or you may select the CDC national statistic of 0.5/1000 live births), GA, highest maternal antepartum temperature, duration of ROM, maternal GBS status, and the administration of any maternal intrapartum antibiotics. Inputting these variables calculates the patient's risk of EOS at birth. A table is generated further stratifying risk based on the clinical appearance of the infant, with a corresponding clinical recommendation: "no culture, no antibiotics" versus "blood culture" versus "strongly consider starting empiric antibiotics" versus "empiric antibiotics." The table also includes recommendations regarding frequency of vital sign monitoring including "routine vitals," "vitals every four hours for 24 hours," or "vitals per NICU." Table 8.1 shows a sample table of recommendations using the CDC incidence for a case of a baby born at GA 38 weeks 0 days to a mother who had a maximum antepartum temperature of 98.0F and a ROM of 8 hours, was GBS positive, and received GBS-specific antibiotics >2 hours prior to birth.

The AAP currently recommends any of the following three approaches: (1) Categorical Risk Assessment, (2) Neonatal EOS Calculator, or (3) Enhanced Observation [18]. Despite the development of the neonatal EOS tool by Kaiser for

Table 8.1 Sample table of recommendations

EOS risk after clinical exam	Risk per 1000 births	Clinical recommendation	Vitals
Well appearing	0.02	No culture, no antibiotics	Routine vitals
Equivocal	0.28	No culture, no antibiotics	Routine vitals
Clinical illness	1.20	Strongly consider empiric antibiotics	Vitals per NICU

Adapted from Kaiser Neonatal Early-Onset Sepsis Calculator [17]

use in infants born ≥35 weeks GA, many practitioners continue to utilize variable older guidelines, often resulting in unnecessary antibiotic use. From the authors' perspective, a reason for this stems from practitioners being more comfortable with the style of management acquired during their initial years of training and work experience, and they may be hesitant to invest the time into learning and trusting a new tool. Furthermore, the providers may not even be aware of modifications to the management guidelines, especially if they are not employed in an academic setting or have not attended a recent conference or remained up to date on reviewing related journal material. Even if the providers do become aware of the updates, their colleagues and/or the institution may be reluctant to change the current management practice.

It remains important for neonatal and pediatric providers to stay informed of updates in clinical practices that may reduce unnecessary harm and risk to vulnerable infants while also making sure to monitor babies clinically in the rare cases where neonatal sepsis may present itself, even in babies with no obvious risk factors.

Management of Neonatal Hyperbilirubinemia

Jaundice is one of the most common clinical signs in neonates. While hyperbilirubinemia is usually benign, left untreated, it can rarely progress to kernicterus or be a harbinger of a serious disorder. Clinical appearance of jaundice is not a reliable indicator of the severity of hyperbilirubinemia [19]. Therefore, it is essential to screen newborns for hyperbilirubinemia so that phototherapy (the mainstay of treatment for the indirect form) as well as other measures can be initiated when necessary. However, we must also bear in mind that treating low-risk infants can lead to unnecessary stress for the family, early cessation of breastfeeding, and/or further unwarranted testing [20].

In 2004, the AAP, in an effort to identify those jaundiced infants born ≥35 weeks GA that were most at risk of complications if their hyperbilirubinemia was left untreated, published a risk curve along with recommendations for treatment [20]. This nomogram assists providers in deciding when to initiate phototherapy or exchange transfusion based on the baby's risk factors, the bilirubin level, and the age of the infant at that time. In the authors' experience, clinicians often use the online user-friendly resource called BiliTool™ [21]. To use this tool, the clinician inputs the patient's age in hours and total bilirubin and then, based on the baby's GA and any other hyperbilirubinemia risk factors, receives guidelines for management, follow-up, and repeat bilirubin testing. An individualized table is also shown for further management guidelines (i.e., whether phototherapy is indicated) based on the infant's bilirubin, GA, and any neurotoxic risk factors.

While the AAP guideline and BiliTool™ provide objective guidelines for the initiation of phototherapy, there is no standardized guidance for when to discontinue phototherapy once it is initiated. This results in variability in practice by medical providers and potentially preventable readmissions for hyperbilirubinemia. Chang et al.'s 2017 research helps to address this gap although the authors recognize that their research has only been internally validated. Their research established three variables that best predicted the risk of rebound hyperbilirubinemia in jaundiced infants and created a simple clinical prediction rule [22]. Two years later, Chang et al. further simplified this rule to two variables – gestational age and difference in bilirubin level (between the starting threshold and the ending serum bilirubin level) – that were shown to reliably predict the risk of rebound hyperbilirubinemia [23].

Based on Chang et al.'s research, there has since been the development of a rebound hyperbilirubinemia risk calculator now available online [24]. This tool allows the clinician to input the variables identified as most important in their research, and, once the values are entered, a score is computed along with the probability of rebound hyperbilirubinemia as a percentage. Depending on the calculated risk of rebound hyperbilirubinemia (<4% was suggested to be acceptable per Chang et al.), the clinician will then be able to determine whether it is reasonable to discontinue phototherapy at that time. It should be noted that this tool does not capture the risk of rebound hyperbilirubinemia after additional rounds of phototherapy; therefore, more research is needed.

While the AAP hyperbilirubinemia guidelines have now existed for nearly two decades and the clinical prediction tool developed by Chang et al. has existed for several years, decisions about when to discontinue phototherapy continue to be made subjectively, resulting in inconsistency in clinical practice. Even within provider groups, there remains variability based on the individual clinician's training history as well as their attention to practice updates, as observed by the authors. Until the AAP publishes relevant guidance, Chang et al.'s clinical prediction rule serves as a quick and easy tool that can be used, with the goal of decreasing the need to reinitiate phototherapy as well as preventing unnecessary hospital readmissions. The authors look forward to when the AAP will provide standardized guidelines about discontinuation of phototherapy to optimize the management of this common condition.

Management of Multisystem Inflammatory Syndrome in Children

Multisystem inflammatory syndrome in children (MIS-C) is an inflammatory syndrome associated with COVID-19 infection in children that was first described in the United Kingdom in April 2020 [25]. While MIS-C can be clinically severe, this syndrome is rare and outcomes with treatment are promising – in a systematic review of 16 studies with 655 participants, the majority of children recovered while 11 (1.7%) of children died [26]. As literature is evolving regarding guideline-based management at this time, here we will describe the guidelines for diagnosis and management used by Ochsner Hospital for Children in Louisiana as well as the AAP's interim guidance. Both sets of recommendations include the disclaimer that as this is a new syndrome, the written guidance should never supersede clinical judgment.

Presentation

The MIS-C definition used by the Centers for Disease Control and Prevention (CDC), AAP, and Ochsner is shown in Table 8.2.

MIS-C should be considered in any pediatric patient presenting with a persistent fever of unknown origin, especially with recent COVID exposure [28]. This syndrome may present like Kawasaki disease (in up to 40–50% either complete or incomplete based on available case series at the time of this writing); therefore, children who present with Kawasaki features should have MIS-C on their differential [29]. Echocardiogram is indicated immediately if there are signs of cardiogenic shock and/or arrythmias; otherwise, it is recommended to obtain one within 12 hours [30]. An echocardiogram is also indicated for all patients with features of Kawasaki disease; however, obtaining an echocardiogram should not delay treatment if this diagnosis is suspected. Pediatric specialists including infectious disease, cardiology, and hematology should be involved in the management of these patients as soon as possible [28].

Table 8.2 Adapted from CDC [27]

An individual age < 21 years presenting with
Fever[a]
Laboratory evidence of inflammation[b]
And evidence of clinically severe illness requiring hospitalization, with multisystem (≥2) organ involvement
And no alternative plausible diagnosis
And
Positive for current or recent SARS-CoV-2 infection by RT-PCR, serology, or antigen test OR exposure to a suspected or confirmed COVID-19 case within the 4 weeks prior to the onset of symptoms

[a]Fever ≥38.0 °C for ≥24 hours or report of subjective fever lasting ≥24 hours
[b]Including, but not limited to, one or more of the following: an elevated C-reactive protein (CRP), erythrocyte sedimentation rate (ESR), fibrinogen, procalcitonin, d-dimer, ferritin, lactic acid dehydrogenase (LDH), or interleukin 6 (IL-6), elevated neutrophils, reduced lymphocytes, and low albumin

Treatment Modalities

The most important initial treatment consideration is the stabilization of patients presenting with shock-like symptoms. This includes aggressive fluid resuscitation with the addition of inotropes if required. Broad-spectrum antibiotics may be considered in patients with signs of septic shock [28].

Following any necessary resuscitation measures, the hallmark treatment for MIS-C is intravenous immunoglobulin (IVIG). Per both Ochsner and AAP guidelines, the dose is 2 g/kg over 1–2 days [28, 30]. IVIG treatment is considered in all MIS-C patients, especially those with evidence of Kawasaki features, coronary artery involvement, or other cardiac involvement.

Systemic steroids should also be considered in all patients; steroids administered in addition to IVIG have been shown to lead to earlier resolution of fever in MIS-C patients than IVIG alone [28]. The AAP recommends methylprednisolone dosed at 2–30 mg/kg/day, depending on the severity of the illness. Ochsner administers 10 mg/kg twice a day for 3 days (with a maximum single dose of 500 mg) [30]. This may be followed by an oral taper at the physician's discretion.

Biologic agents may be part of treatment, especially in patients with large coronary aneurysms, with severe clinical presentation, or who fail to respond to IVIG and steroids alone [28]. Ochsner prefers anakinra, an interleukin-1 receptor agonist, dosed at 2–4 mg/kg (with a maximum of 100 mg per dose) subcutaneously or intravenously twice a day for 5–10 days [30]. Physicians should consider consulting a rheumatology specialist prior to initiating this treatment.

Another important treatment consideration in MIS-C is that of anticoagulation. Per Ochsner protocol, anticoagulation can be considered in all patients with active inflammation, based on clinical judgment and consultation with a pediatric hematologist. Low-molecular-weight heparin (LMWH, e.g., enoxaparin) is preferred if the patient has no renal disease and no procedures are anticipated; otherwise, unfractionated heparin may be used. Due to its anti-inflammatory effects, the AAP recommends that all patients without contraindication initiate prophylactic low-dose aspirin [28]. At Ochsner, patients are given medium-dose aspirin until they have remained afebrile for greater than 48 hours, at which point they receive low dose aspirin for a minimum of 6 weeks [30]. If patients have Kawasaki-like features, providers should initiate high-dose aspirin, unless they have bleeding concerns and/or thrombocytopenia (e.g., platelets <50,000).

Discharge Criteria

Ochsner's protocol states that patients may be discharged when they have remained afebrile for at least 48 hours, have consistently maintained oxygen saturation above 94% for 24–48 hours on room air, have downtrending inflammatory markers, and show overall clinical improvement [30]. In addition to following up with their primary pediatric provider, patients should have outpatient follow-up with cardiology, as well as rheumatology if a biologic treatment was used.

Although the CDC, AAP, and individual hospitals such as Ochsner Hospital for Children have published guidance for the diagnosis and management of MIS-C, clinical judgment combined with staying current on the latest evidence-based recommendations remain the most important factors at the time of this writing. Due to MIS-C being a new phenomenon, the authors suspect that management guidance will continue to evolve as more data become available. Our hope is that the AAP's current "MIS-C Interim Guidance" will be developed into a more specific guideline, enabling us to provide more consistent, quality care for our pediatric patients.

Summary

Pediatric Hospital Medicine is currently recognized as a new subspecialty, guided by the principle that children will be better served by the establishment of this field [1]. The authors propose that PHM will make way for continued developments in evidence-based guidelines with the goal of improving and standardizing the management of common clinical conditions. We have reviewed three of the most common clinical conditions in PHM-based practice –bronchiolitis, neonatal sepsis, and neonatal hyperbilirubinemia – each with an emphasis on the importance of attention to guidelines-based medicine. The authors opted to review the additional topic of MIS-C to emphasize the importance of guidelines to aid in the management of novel and evolving diagnoses as well.

Key Points
- In the management of uncomplicated bronchiolitis, there is strong evidence that nebulized albuterol, systemic steriods, nebulized epinephrine, and antibiotics should not be used. The only medication shown to have effect is nebulized hypertonic saline when used for more than 24 hours, although this remains a weak recommendation.
- An evidence-based calculator exists to determine the necessity of antibiotic administration in neonates at risk of early-onset sepsis which, when used, can reduce use of empiric antibiotics by 75% without causing additional risk of infection.
- For the management of neonatal hyperbilirubinemia, in addition to the commonly used BiliTool™ for initiating treatment, there is also an online calculator available to aid clinicians in determining when to discontinue phototherapy.
- MIS-C is a new COVID-19-related syndrome in children that may present with features of Kawasaki disease; early recognition and attention to the latest evidence-based recommendations remain vital in obtaining best clinical outcomes.

References

1. Barrett DJ, McGuinness GA, Cunha CA, Emans SJ, Gerson WT, Hazinski MF, Lister G, Murray KF, St. Geme JW, Whitley-Williams PN. Pediatric hospital medicine: a proposed new subspecialty. Pediatrics. 2017;139(3):e20161823. https://doi.org/10.1542/peds.2016-1823.
2. Diagnosis and management of bronchiolitis. Pediatrics. 2006;118 (4):1774–93. https://doi.org/10.1542/peds.2006-2223.
3. Skjerven HO, Megremis S, Papadopoulos NG, Mowinckel P, Carlsen KH, Lødrup Carlsen KC. Virus type and genomic load in acute bronchiolitis: severity and treatment response with inhaled adrenaline. J Infect Dis. 2016;213(6):915–21. https://doi.org/10.1093/infdis/jiv513.
4. Christakis DA, Cowan CA, Garrison MM, Molteni R, Marcuse E, Zerr DM. Variation in inpatient diagnostic testing and management of bronchiolitis. Pediatrics. 2005;115(4):878–84. https://doi.org/10.1542/peds.2004-1299.
5. McCulloh RJ, Smitherman SE, Koehn KL, Alverson BK. Assessing the impact of national guidelines on the management of children hospitalized for acute bronchiolitis. Pediatr Pulmonol. 2014;49(7):688–94. https://doi.org/10.1002/ppul.22835.
6. Ralston SL, Lieberthal AS, Meissner HC, Alverson BK, Baley JE, Gadomski AM, Johnson DW, Light MJ, Maraqa NF, Mendonca EA, Phelan KJ, Zorc JJ, Stanko-Lopp D, Brown MA, Nathanson I, Rosenblum E, Sayles S, Hernandez-Cancio S. Clinical practice guideline: the diagnosis, management, and prevention of bronchiolitis. Pediatrics. 2014;134(5):e1474–502. https://doi.org/10.1542/peds.2014-2742.
7. Jamal A, Finkelstein Y, Kuppermann N, Freedman SB, Florin TA, Babl FE, Dalziel SR, Zemek R, Plint AC, Steele DW, Schnadower D, Johnson DW, Stephens D, Kharbanda A, Roland D, Lyttle MD, Macias CG, Fernandes RM, Benito J, Schuh S. Pharmacotherapy in bronchiolitis at discharge from emergency departments within the Pediatric Emergency Research Networks: a retrospective analysis. Lancet Child Adolesc Health. 2019;3(8):539–47. https://doi.org/10.1016/s2352-4642(19)30193-2.
8. Hall CB, Powell KR, MacDonald NE, Gala CL, Menegus ME, Suffin SC, Cohen HJ. Respiratory syncytial viral infection in children with compromised immune function. N Engl J Med. 1986;315(2):77–81. https://doi.org/10.1056/nejm198607103150201.
9. Spurling GK, Doust J, Del Mar CB, Eriksson L. Antibiotics for bronchiolitis in children. Cochrane Database Syst Rev. 2011;(6):Cd005189. https://doi.org/10.1002/14651858.CD005189.pub3.
10. Mussman GM, Parker MW, Statile A, Sucharew H, Brady PW. Suctioning and length of stay in infants hospitalized with bronchiolitis. JAMA Pediatr. 2013;167(5):414–21. https://doi.org/10.1001/jamapediatrics.2013.36.
11. Oza S, Lawn JE, Hogan DR, Mathers C, Cousens SN. Neonatal cause-of-death estimates for the early and late neonatal periods for 194 countries: 2000-2013. Bull World Health Organ. 2015;93(1):19–28. https://doi.org/10.2471/blt.14.139790.
12. Puopolo KM, Benitz WE, Zaoutis TE. Management of neonates born at ≥35 0/7 weeks' gestation with suspected or proven early-onset bacterial sepsis. Pediatrics. 2018;142(6):e20182894. https://doi.org/10.1542/peds.2018-2894.
13. Bizzarro MJ, Raskind C, Baltimore RS, Gallagher PG. Seventy-five years of neonatal sepsis at Yale: 1928-2003. Pediatrics. 2005;116(3):595–602. https://doi.org/10.1542/peds.2005-0552.
14. Esaiassen E, Fjalstad JW, Juvet LK, van den Anker JN, Klingenberg C. Antibiotic exposure in neonates and early adverse outcomes: a systematic review and meta-analysis. J Antimicrob Chemother. 2017;72(7):1858–70. https://doi.org/10.1093/jac/dkx088.
15. Ellington M, Naves E, Williams K, Kasat K. Improving antibiotic stewardship: modifying the AAP sepsis guidelines with the addition of the neonatal early onset sepsis risk calculator. Pediatrics. 2019;144(2 MeetingAbstract):649. https://doi.org/10.1542/peds.144.2_MeetingAbstract.649.
16. Ellington M, Kasat K, Williams K. Improving antibiotic stewardship among asymptomatic newborns born at or greater than 36 weeks using the neonatal early onset risk

calculator. Pediatrics. 2020;146(1 MeetingAbstract):332–4. https://doi.org/10.1542/peds.146.1_MeetingAbstract.332.
17. Probability of Neonatal Early-Onset Sepsis Based on Maternal Risk Factors and the Infant's Clinical Presentation. 2021. Kaiser Permanente Division of Research. https://neonatalsepsiscalculator.kaiserpermanente.org/. Accessed 24 June 2021.
18. Puopolo KM, Lynfield R, Cummings JJ. Management of Infants at risk for group B streptococcal disease. Pediatrics. 2019;144(2):e20191881. https://doi.org/10.1542/peds.2019-1881.
19. Ives NK. Management of neonatal jaundice. Paediatr Child Health. 2011;21(6):270–6. https://doi.org/10.1016/j.paed.2011.02.011.
20. Pediatrics AAo. Management of hyperbilirubinemia in the newborn infant 35 or more weeks of gestation. Pediatrics. 2004;114(1):297–316. https://doi.org/10.1542/peds.114.1.297.
21. Burgos T, Turner S. BiliTool. 2021. https://bilitool.org/. Accessed 24 June 2021.
22. Chang PW, Kuzniewicz MW, McCulloch CE, Newman TB. A clinical prediction rule for rebound hyperbilirubinemia following inpatient phototherapy. Pediatrics. 2017;139(3):e20162896. https://doi.org/10.1542/peds.2016-2896.
23. Chang PW, Newman TB. A simpler prediction rule for rebound hyperbilirubinemia. Pediatrics. 2019;144(1):e20183712. https://doi.org/10.1542/peds.2018-3712.
24. Knitter J. BiliRebound – rebound hyperbilirubinemia calculator. JSCalc. 2014. https://jscalc.io/calc/68NNiFfS7iTMZhZY. 2021.
25. Riphagen, et al. Hyperinflammatory shock in children during COVID-19 pandemic. Lancet. 2020;395(10237):1607. Epub 2020 May 7.
26. Kaushik A, et al. A systematic review of multisystem inflammatory syndrome in children associated with SARS-CoV-2 infection. Pediatr Infect Dis J. 2020;39(11):e340–6. https://doi.org/10.1097/INF.0000000000002888.
27. CDC. Multisystem Inflammatory Syndrome (MIS). Centers for Disease Control and Prevention (CDC). 2020. https://www.cdc.gov/mis/. 2021.
28. AAP. Multisystem Inflammatory Syndrome in Children (MIS-C) Interim Guidance. American Academy of Pediatrics. 2020. https://services.aap.org/en/pages/2019-novel-coronaviruscovid-19-infections/clinical-guidance/multisystem-inflammatory-syndrome-in-children-misc-interim-guidance/. 2021.
29. Son MBF, Friedman K. COVID-19: multisystem inflammatory syndrome in children (MIS-C) clinical features, evaluation, and diagnosis. In *UpToDate*, Fulton DF, et al., editors. upToDate. Waltham. (Accessed on August 19, 2021).
30. Kleinmahon J, et al. Guidance document for multisystem inflammatory syndrome in children (MIS-C). Unpublished manuscript, Ochsner Hospital for Children. Used with permission. 2020.

Chapter 9
Management of Psychiatric Disorders in the Hospital

Shilpa Amara and Brett Pearce

Introduction

Psychiatric disorders are among the most debilitating disorders, and patients with psychiatric conditions are more likely to have increased rates of premature mortality due to causes unrelated to their psychiatric condition [1]. Thus, it is unsurprising that patients with psychiatric conditions are at an increased risk for hospitalizations for general medical conditions. Delirium and psychosis are among the most common psychiatric disorders that present in hospital settings.

Delirium and psychosis are known to have significant impacts on individuals, their caregivers, healthcare systems, as well as the population at large. Though they both are conditions that are difficult to manage due to both the intrinsic pathophysiology and extrinsic psychosocial issues, there are ways to decrease the burden of the diseases, especially within hospital settings. This chapter aims to highlight a few of these mitigating techniques that can aid hospitalists to improve the treatment of delirium and psychosis within hospital settings. It is not intended to be a comprehensive guide regarding the management of psychiatric disorders within the hospital setting, but rather a reference to well-researched, effective, therapies and management advice.

S. Amara (✉)
Ochsner Health, New Orleans, LA, USA
e-mail: shilpa.amara@ochsner.org

B. Pearce
The University of Queensland-Ochsner Clinical School, New Orleans, LA, USA

© The Author(s), under exclusive license to Springer Nature Switzerland AG 2022
K. Conrad (ed.), *Clinical Approaches to Hospital Medicine*,
https://doi.org/10.1007/978-3-030-95164-1_9

Delirium

Delirium is a challenging condition that is highly prevalent within hospital medicine. Due to the variability in presentations, lack of clear identifying symptoms, and variety of settings in which it presents, it can be easily misdiagnosed and, therefore, mismanaged. Within medical education, there is a clear emphasis on differentiating delirium from other primary medical conditions based on timelines (acute versus chronic) and possible fluctuations in attention, but much less importance is placed on the workup and management of a suspected patient with delirium. This section will attempt to provide a concise summation of the etiology, epidemiology, risk factors/precipitating factors, management, and possible complications of delirium.

Etiology

Although it is difficult to quantify the exact percentage of psychiatric admissions in hospitals, there tends to be a general consensus that the management of psychiatric illnesses plays a large role in internal medicine. Unfortunately, the majority of the available research concerning the epidemiology of psychiatric disorders in adult hospital admissions are either outdated or nonspecific. A meta-analysis analyzing emergency department admissions across seven different countries in 18 different studies concluded that psychiatric conditions and mental disorders were responsible for an overall 4% of admissions [1]. Another study corroborated the overall emergency department admission rates (5.4%) and found in their study that the three most common presentations were substance abuse (27%), neurosis (26%), and psychosis (21%) [2]. This chapter aims to highlight a few interesting/relevant management guidelines and interventions regarding psychiatry in the hospital.

Epidemiology

The epidemiology of delirium has fortunately been studied across multiple settings (intensive care unit (ICU), surgical ward, palliative care services) and among multiple different patient populations (elderly, pediatric, adult). Among patients already admitted to the hospital, the prevalence of delirium ranges from 11 to 42% based on risk factors, with older adults having a nearly 30% chance of developing delirium at some point during their hospitalization. In contrast, the prevalence of delirium at the time of admission is 10–30% and has been found to be more common than new onset of delirium during hospitalization [3, 4]. Other studies have found that 7–9.6%

of patients ≥65 of age have delirium on presentation to the ED, with the majority of those coming from frail elderly patients as well as those arriving from nursing homes [3, 5]. While these numbers are impressive, the prevalence of delirium in other acute care settings with sicker patients is even higher. More than 50% of elderly patients admitted to the ICU have delirium at the time of admission and delirium can be found in 80% of all ICU patients during the course of their hospital stay [6, 7]. Similarly, as high as 50% of postoperative elderly patients are diagnosed with delirium depending on the procedure [8, 9]. Furthermore, the risk of delirium has been shown to be higher in hospice units (42%), than in either post-acute care settings (16%) or the emergency department (10%) [10–12]. With delirium seemingly ubiquitous among sick patients, it is increasingly important to be able to spot delirium in a variety of clinical settings.

Risk Factors

To aid in understanding, the etiology of delirium has been historically subdivided into underlying factors that increase an individual's susceptibility to delirium (predisposing factors), factors that may acutely lead to the precipitation of delirium (precipitating factors), and factors that aggravate or prolong the state of delirium (perpetuating factors). However, there is considerable overlap between the three, and these factors might be better thought of as a continuum instead of a binary parameter.

The most commonly identified predisposing factors associated with an increased rate of delirium include underlying neurocognitive disorders, increased age, and the presence/severity of an associated medical illness, with the overall most commonly identified risk factor being underlying neurocognitive disorder [13]. A meta-analysis conducted demonstrated the prevalence of delirium superimposed on dementia to range between 22% and 89% [14].

In contrast to predisposing factors, precipitating factors for delirium include more acute disturbances such as noxious stimuli, dehydration/malnutrition, infection, surgery, loss of stimulation, and environmental exposures (e.g., suprapubic catheters or tethers) [13]. Additionally, medication use (especially that of sedative hypnotics, benzodiazepines, and anticholinergics) can be thought of as an independent risk factor. Drugs that may precipitate delirium and confusion are noted in Table 9.1. Perpetuating or aggravating factors that may prolong the state of delirium include deliriogenic medications (e.g., benzodiazepines or sedatives), physical restraints or tethers, as well as factors that may alter the patient's orientation (e.g., artificial light exposure and sleep deprivation). The predisposing, precipitating, and perpetuating factors are summarized in Fig. 9.1.

Table 9.1 Select medications that may prolong or perpetuate delirium as mentioned in the previous edition of *Clinical Approaches to Hospital Medicine* [15]

Drug Class	Examples of specific drugs within class
Antiarrhythmics	Atropine, digoxin, disopyramide, lidocaine, procainamide, quinidine
Antibiotics and antivirals	Acyclovir, cephalosporins (first, second, and third generation), interferon
Anticholinergic	Antihistamines (diphenhydramine, trihexyphenidyl), antimuscarinics (scopolamine), antispasmodics (benztropine, hydroxyzine), tricyclic antidepressants (amitriptyline, doxepin, imipramine)
Anticonvulsant	Carbamazepine, levetiracetam, phenytoin, valproate, vigabatrin
Antihypertensives	α-methyldopa, clonidine, dihydropyridines, diuretics, propranolol
Dopamine agonists	Amantadine, bromocriptine, levodopa, pramipexole, ropinirole
Herbal supplements	Belladonna extract, henbane, jimson weed, kava kava, mandrake, St John's wort, valerian root
Other	Antiemetics (prochlorperazine), corticosteroids, lithium, muscle relaxants (baclofen, cyclobenzaprine), NSAIDs
Opioids, sedatives, and hypnotics	All opioids but specifically meperidine, barbiturates, benzodiazepines, gabapentin

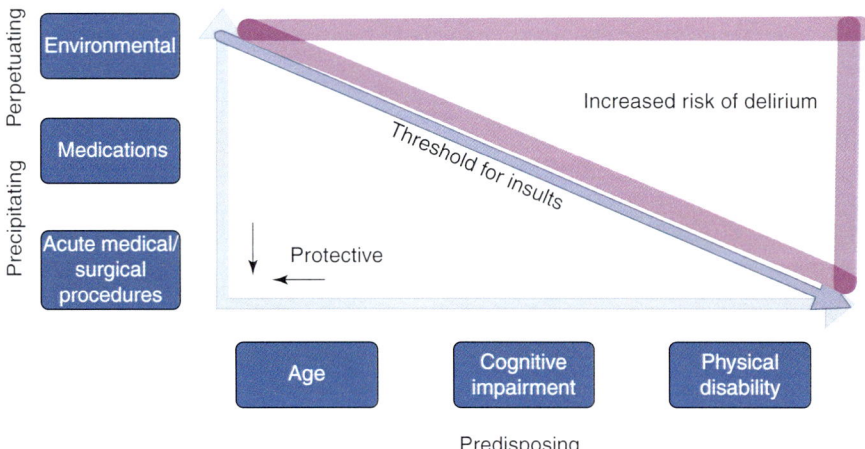

Fig. 9.1 This diagram, adapted from multiple sources, aims to illustrate the multifactorial nature of delirium [15, 16]. The deliriogenic state is a manifestation of the complex interactions between acute inciting (precipitating) events such as infection, surgery, and some medications with inherent (predisposing) patient factors such as age and preexisting medical comorbidities. Additionally, other (perpetuating) factors such as environmental disorientation, pain, and some medications may serve to further maintain the deliriogenic state once established

Diagnostic Criteria

Delirium can be somewhat simplistically thought of as an acute brain dysfunction that is usually reversible. As mentioned earlier, this can be contrasted with dementia which is more analogous to a chronic brain dysfunction, whose effects are less reversible. In terms of actual diagnostic criteria, the DSM-5 considers dementia to have several core components: an acute disturbance in attention and cognition, not better explained by another preexisting neurocognitive disorder, and secondary to either medical condition, medication side effect, intoxication/substance withdrawal, or another acute insult [17]. Attention in this context can be thought of as reduced ability to direct, maintain, and shift focus. Similarly, cognition can be affected by changes in memory, orientation, language, perception, and visuospatial abilities. Other possible variations in presentation that may accompany delirium include disturbances in the sleep–wake cycle, increased sympathetic stimulation, and emotional disturbance or dysregulation [17].

Subtypes

There is a wide spectrum of presentations that have been classified into different subtypes of delirium. It has been shown that certain etiologies as well as patient characteristics and even clinical settings can influence the development of certain motoric symptoms [18, 19]. With these taken into account, there may be different underlying pathophysiological pathways, complications, and even therapeutic treatments attributable to each of the different subtypes [20]. Classifying delirium into subtypes is traditionally done by looking at the motoric symptoms of the patient in combination with their level of arousal and any other non-cognitive symptoms [19]. The two most recognized forms of delirium are that of hyperactive and hypoactive delirium, with an additional subtype termed "mixed" that incorporates features of both subtypes within a relatively short timeline [21]. To date there is an absence of a standardized classification system for assigning subtypes. Acknowledging that in the literature there have been multiple different reported subtypes of delirium such as chronic delirium and subsyndromal delirium, this chapter will specifically address hyperactive, hypoactive, and mixed delirium.

The hyperactive form of delirium tends to present with more positive motor symptoms such as restlessness, increasing agitation, and increased arousal. It was initially thought that hyperactive delirium was more likely to present psychotic features, but recent literature has drawn that association into question [22]. The incidence of hyperactive delirium appears to be correlated with acute precipitating factors, which may factor into the reported relative increase in reversibility of hyperactive delirium compared with hypoactive delirium [23]. In regard to etiology, both the ingestion of toxic substances and the subsequent withdrawal are associated with a hyperactive presentation [24]. Context also matters; hyperactive delirium is more commonly seen in the emergency department, and the term is more often utilized in services such as consult-psychiatry [12, 23].

Conversely, the hypoactive form of delirium is characterized by behavior that could be described as lethargic, drowsy, or sedated. Additionally, patients may be unable to respond to questions or move spontaneously and may demonstrate increased apathy. In comparison to some of the positive motor symptoms present in hyperactive delirium, the subtlety of some hypoactive features may play a role in the increased rates of misdiagnosis and late diagnosis of hypoactive delirium compared to its hyperactive counterpart [22]. Similarly, hypoactive delirium is more likely to be misdiagnosed as dementia or depression than hyperactive delirium. In regard to predisposition and etiologies, studies have suggested that factors such as advanced age, frailty, severe medical illness, malnutrition, and comorbid neurocognitive diseases are associated with increased rates of hypoactive delirium, but much more work is needed to elucidate this association [25]. The clinical setting itself appears to play a role; rates of hypoactive delirium (versus other types) are highest in the ICU and palliative care settings [26]. Lastly, in regard to prognosis, despite inconsistencies among several studies, the general trend indicates that hypoactive delirium carries a worse prognosis than its hyperactive counterpart [23].

Assessment

Given the negative consequences associated with a missed diagnosis of delirium, including both a reduction of quality of care received inside the hospital and increased mortality outside of the hospital, it is important to diagnose delirium as early as possible [12]. Ultimately, while the diagnosis of delirium is made clinically, there are screening tools designed to aid the diagnosis of delirium in multiple clinical settings. The method most commonly used is the Confusion Assessment Method (CAM) has versions that have been verified both inside (CAM-ICU) and outside the ICU (brief Confusion Assessment Method –bCAM). This tool can be taught to healthcare workers within 30 minutes and administered within two minutes, and this has high sensitivity (80%) and specificity (96%) [12]**.** Once delirium is confirmed, there are a number of further screening tools that are more focused on specific etiologies/differential diagnosis (e.g., Mini Mental Status Exam (MMSE) for suspected delirium or Clinical Institute Withdrawal Assessment for Alcohol (cIWA) for alcohol withdrawal).

The assessment of delirium should first begin with an attempt to uncover the possible underlying etiologies of the delirium. This general assessment should include a detailed patient history, focused physical exam, and appropriate auxiliary workup. There are variations between patients, but in general, important details to obtain during the patient history include timeframe of delirium symptoms, drug/alcohol history, history of malnutrition/dehydration, past psychiatric history, baseline functional status (whether able to perform ADLs?), history of delirium, and any recent surgery, procedure, or illness. In addition, a full medication review should be undertaken. Table 17.1 is a list of commonly implicated drugs. In particular, classes of medications to note are opioids (OR 2.5, 95% CI 1.2–52), benzodiazepines (OR 3.0, 95% CI 1.3–6.8), and antihistamines (OR = 1.8, 95% CI 0.7–4.5) [27]. Additionally, when dealing with disorders that affect mentation, it is important to have an adequate understanding of the patient's general cognition, in terms of both their baseline mental status and any recent decline in function. This idea is particularly important when considering that nearly half of delirium occurring in the hospital occurs at the time of admission [4]. This understanding can again be aided by taking a careful patient history as well as utilization of collateral history. The importance of family members in establishing a patient's cognitive baseline cannot be overstated. Even simple screening questions such as "do you think this person has been acting more confused lately" have been shown to be 80% sensitive and 71% specific for a diagnosis of delirium [28]. This idea of understanding a patient's baseline mental status is especially important in older patients in which there might be a concern for possible dementia. In that case understanding a patient's baseline can aid in differentiating transient neurologic dysfunction from a chronic neurocognitive disorder. A focused physical exam should also be conducted that assesses vital signs, major organ systems, and possible precipitants/complications (infections, pressure ulcers, etc.). Additionally, a tailored workup may include complete blood count (CBC), hepatic/renal function tests, blood sugar levels, electrolytes, electrocardiogram (EKG), and urinalysis. If suspicion is high based on history or findings found via workup, then further studies may be warranted including imaging chest X-ray (CXR), head computerized tomography (CT), toxicology screen, lumbar puncture (LP), or autoimmune panels; however, routinely scheduling these studies for every patient undergoing a delirium workup is not advised [16].

Management

Once a diagnosis of delirium is made, it is important to act quickly to prevent deterioration and reverse neurologic dysfunction. As mentioned previously, there is a considerable weight placed upon identifying an underlying etiology so as to provide effective and targeted management. While searching for the underlying etiology, non-pharmacologic interventions should be implemented, symptoms such as pain should be managed appropriately, the patient's clinical status should be monitored, and further complications should be prevented.

Several studies have demonstrated potential benefits of a multicomponent model centered around non-pharmacologic management. These therapies are typically administered via a multidisciplinary team and focus on minimizing any modifiable risk factors and improving cognition, sleep, and sensorimotor orientation [16, 20, 29].

Multicomponent therapies have been demonstrated as cost-effective in delirium prevention when applied to admitted hospital patients deemed at risk. The mainstay of these multicomponent therapies revolves around risk factor mitigation. This may include addressing issues such as cognitive impairment/disorientation, dehydration/constipation, hypoxia, infection, immobility, pain, medication, nutrition, sensory impairment, and sleep. Additionally, examples of interventions that should be offered to all patients at risk of delirium include promoting daytime activities/

normal sleep-wake cycle, maintaining a quiet, well-lit environment, continuity of staff, minimizing excessive room changes, promoting sensorimotor orientation via hearing and visual aids, encouraging family member involvement, removing noxious stimuli, and minimizing unnecessary medical testing [12, 20, 30].

Orientation protocols allowing for the provision of clocks, calendars, and windows in patient rooms can help mitigate the confusion that may accompany being in an unfamiliar setting.

Communication with the patient should be done in a way that is empathic and straightforward, while avoiding directly confronting or arguing with the patient. Additionally, it is important to avoid any complex ideas or discussions which cannot be completely understood by the patient. Providers should involve the patient's family, to provide a reassuring presence both to help with the treatment process and to help with the transition back home post-discharge [28]. Involvement from family members should be encouraged and members of the treatment team should involve them in discussions and provide advice on how to talk to and monitor their family member so they can assist post-discharge [16].

All patients admitted to the hospital should have their baseline mental status assessed. Those with additional risk factors may warrant increased clinical monitoring. Patients with a decrease in cognitive functioning may warrant evaluation for delirium [16]. Additionally, even once a diagnosis of delirium has been established, frequent patient monitoring may act to prevent deterioration, monitor treatment course, and prevent complications.

There is currently no convincing evidence suggesting that pharmacologic interventions have an effect on mortality, ICU admission rates, rate of complications, or length of stay [15]. Thus, it follows that there are no FDA-approved medications for the treatment of delirium. However, there may be a role for pharmacologic intervention in regard to managing symptoms that may either be contributing to (e.g., pain) or resulting from (e.g., agitation, psychosis) the delirium itself. However, non-pharmacologic management remains the first-line therapy for agitation and involves a variety of verbal and non-verbal behavior management techniques designed to deescalate the situation.

The indications for pharmacological intervention in patients with delirium are severe agitation and anxiety causing significant distress to the patient resulting in the potential for harm to themselves or others, a lack of participation in care resulting in inability to carry out needed investigations or treatments, and persistent delirium despite best attempts at non-pharmacologic management [28]. Research has shown that in some patient populations, haloperidol or olanzapine can be used cautiously (lowest effective dose for less than 1 week). Risperidone (0.5–1 mg) and quetiapine (25–50 mg) are reasonable alternatives. Current guidelines recommend starting at the lowest dose and titrating up slowly to the lowest effective dose, with attempts to discontinue therapy as early as possible [15]. Note that benzodiazepines are used as first-line agents for delirium associated with alcohol or benzodiazepine withdrawal but are generally discouraged for other cases [20].

Prevention

About one-third of all delirium episodes are preventable [29]. Prevention of delirium is thought of in a similar vein as treatment. Non-pharmacologic multimodal therapy is regarded as the mainstay as treatment, but there is currently no role for routine pharmacologic prophylaxis, even in high-risk individuals. Examples of multimodal therapy for prevention that has been demonstrated to be cost-effective and realistic are the guidelines recommended by the National Institute for Health and Clinical Excellence (NICE) [29]. The guidelines are targeted at people 18 years of age or older in the setting of either hospitals or long-term residential care settings. There are 13 guidelines and most are similar to the risk factor modifications used in delirium treatment. The guidelines include early mobilization, orienting stimuli (calendars, clocks, etc.), therapeutic activities (reminiscing), encouragement of family visitation, assessment of hydration/nutrition status, asking about constipation, checking for hypoxia/optimizing oxygen saturation, checking for possible sources of infection, assessing for pain, carrying out a medication review, and addressing any reversible cause of sensory impairment [16, 27, 29].

Conclusion

As mentioned above, delirium is a neuropsychiatric syndrome that has been observed in many different clinical settings. Relative to its incidence and consequences, delirium appears to be a poorly understood and possibly neglected condition. Possibly due to its variable presentation, it is also consistently underdiagnosed [29]. Assessment for delirium should begin in all patients as soon as possible and be repeated in patients deemed at high risk for delirium development. Due to the ineffectiveness, and minimal options in regard to the treatment of delirium, the paradigm of management is shifting toward that of delirium prevention, of which multimodal therapies are considered the gold standard.

Psychosis

Psychosis can be broadly thought of as a disconnect between an individual's perception and reality. It can arise from psychiatric disorders (most commonly schizophrenia or other conditions in the schizophrenia spectrum, but may also occur in bipolar personality disorder or major depressive disorder with psychotic features), secondary medical conditions, or as a result of noxious insults or stimuli. Regardless of the etiology, symptoms of psychosis are highly distressing to the patient and are often accompanied by a substantial burden of disease to the greater community.

Schizophrenia, the most well-known primary psychiatric disorder causing psychosis, is one of the top 15 disorders causing the greatest number of years lived with disability (YLD) [31]. It is also associated with a massive cost, both to the person and the society. Schizophrenia is known to decrease both quality and quantity of life, with an average lifespan reduction of 20 years [32].

Early recognition and prompt treatment are crucial as duration of untreated psychosis (DUP) is an important modifiable risk factor. Due to the debilitating nature of psychosis, it is quite likely to be encountered within a hospital setting. Understanding how to identify and treat psychosis can better equip hospitalists to manage the illness and do their part in decreasing the burden of psychosis-related disorders on individuals and the healthcare system at large. This chapter aims to cover the epidemiology, clinical manifestations, workup, differential diagnosis, and management of psychosis within the context of hospital medicine.

Epidemiology

The lifetime prevalence of psychosis in the general population is approximately 3%, with 0.21% attributed to psychosis due to a secondary medical condition [33].

The incidence of psychosis worldwide is estimated at 50 per 100,000 individuals, whereas schizophrenia, the most commonly studied psychotic disorder, has an incidence of approximately 15 in 100,000 per year [31]. Furthermore, it is estimated that 13–23% of the population will experience symptoms of psychosis at some point in their lives, while 1–4% will meet criteria for diagnosis of a psychotic disorder [34].

Many primary psychiatric disorders have an established time course, requiring precise longitudinal monitoring for accurate diagnoses. Given that many cases of first-episode psychosis encountered in the emergency department or inpatient setting are often diagnosed retrospectively, the timeline of the illness can be difficult to determine. Many patients are given a diagnosis that is provisional or inaccurate.

Not only are psychotic episodes alarming during the current episode, but they can also indicate an insidious underlying condition that may cause repeated episodes. A study conducted in Suffolk County analyzed a group of 547 patients who had initially been admitted with a first-episode psychosis and were formally rediagnosed at 6 and 24-months post-discharge. At the 6-month follow-up, only 27.3% of those initially diagnosed with brief psychotic disorder (psychosis with duration of at least 1 day, but less than 1 month, with full return to premorbid functioning) still met diagnostic criteria. However, 91.7% of those initially diagnosed with schizophrenia retained their initial diagnosis [35]. The most common diagnosis at both the six-month and the 24-month follow-ups was schizophrenia (or other schizophrenia spectrum disorder, i.e., schizophreniform or schizoaffective). This lends credence to the idea of psychosis and psychiatric disorders as more of a relapsing remitting-type paradigm than that of a discrete incident.

Among all causes of psychosis, the distribution of the age of onset has not been well studied. However, with schizophrenia, age of onset is most typically 18–25 for men, 20–30 for women, and is rarely seen during childhood (prevalence of schizophrenia among 12 year olds or younger is 0.2–0.4 per 10,000) or after the age of 45 [34].

Risk factors for the development of psychosis in general are poorly understood but may include living in an urban area, immigration, genetics, and stressful life events.

Clinical Manifestations

As mentioned previously, psychosis can be generally thought of as a disconnect between an individual and reality; thus, it follows that a person experiencing symptoms of psychosis will have grossly impaired reality testing. Manifestations of psychosis may include hallucinations, delusions, and thought disorganization. Additionally, before the onset of psychosis, there is often a reported prodromal phase with premorbid signs and symptoms as well as possible neurocognitive impairments [36]. There is also increasing research implicating metabolic syndromes in the development of psychotic disorders [35].

Hallucinations are defined as having the apparent perception of a sensory stimuli without an external source. This is different from illusions which are a misinterpretation of an external stimuli. Hallucinations can occur with any of the five senses, with the most common being auditory, followed by visual, tactile, olfactory, and lastly gustatory. Auditory hallucinations are more commonly encountered in primary psychiatric disorders and may consist of either intelligible (i.e., spoken commands, ongoing narration of patients actions) or unintelligible sounds. Visual hallucinations are more commonly associated with psychosis due to secondary medical conditions, and they can range from misformed images and shapes to recognizable objects.

Delusions refer to a fixed false belief. However, this must take into account the patient's background as delusions must be incongruent with normal cultural or religious beliefs. Delusions may be generally classified as bizarre (non-believable) or nonbizarre (believable). Additionally, delusions may be defined by the specific type of delusion (e.g., persecutory, grandiose, delusions of reference, delusions of control). The content and severity of the delusions may vary based on the specific psychotic disorder. For example, delusions or hallucinations within the context of unipolar major depression with psychotic features may manifest as reinforcement of the patient's subjective feelings of guilt or worthlessness. Delusions may also occur alongside other psychotic symptoms (as in the case of schizophrenia) or may be a lone symptom (delusional disorder).

Thought disorganization refers to a disturbance in a person's ability to organize and express their thoughts in a sensical and logical way. It can be manifested by an inability to maintain a coherent conversation and can be observed in either written or spoken language [37]. While delusions and hallucinations may reflect an aberration in thought content, this is considered distinct from expression and organization of one's thoughts. Examples of thought disorder include tangentiality, clanging, circumstantiality, perseveration, and thought blocking.

It is reported that individuals who develop psychosis often have premorbid symptoms as well as a possible prodromal phase. Examples of premorbid symptoms include depression, neurocognitive impairment, and functional impairment. The prodromal phase occurs weeks to years before the onset of psychosis and may be accompanied by deteriorating function, subsyndromal psychosis, and the presence of negative symptoms. The prodromal phase is usually recognized retrospectively, but has important implications for the development of psychotic disorders. The prodromal phase may also be referred to as attenuated psychosis syndrome, or clinical high risk for psychosis (CHR-P). Symptoms of depression may be present during the prodromal phase or first episode of psychosis and if present are associated with a worse outcome. Additionally, neurocognitive impairments may also be prominent in the prodromal phase and may be manifested by detriments in memory, attention, processing speed, and executive function [32].

Metabolic abnormalities in association with psychotic disorders have long been thought to be the result of lifestyle choices or chronic antipsychotic treatments leading to an increased incidence of metabolic side effects. However, there is increasing evidence that metabolic abnormalities may be implicated during the prodromal phase and the first episode of psychosis in patients without prior exposure to antipsychotic medications. The association with metabolic syndrome among medication-naive patients implies that there may be an element of systemic disease.

Differential Diagnosis

In cases of acute psychosis etiology can be from primary psychiatric disorders and secondary due to general medical conditions. In general, organic causes must be evaluated and ruled out before considering psychosis a manifestation of a primary psychiatric disorder [38].

Primary psychiatric disorders known to cause acute psychosis include schizophrenia (and other schizophrenia spectrum disorders), mood disorders such as bipolar disorder and unipolar major depression with psychotic features, anxiety disorders such as post-traumatic stress disorder (PTSD) and obsessive compulsive disorder (OCD), autism, and other psychotic disorders such as brief psychotic disorders or attenuated psychosis syndrome.

Medical conditions that have been associated with psychosis include inflammatory, infectious, nutritional, autoimmune, neurological, and endocrine disorders. Additionally, especially in the case of chronic medical conditions, psychosis as a manifestation of delirium must also be considered. Depending on the etiology, these disorders may be uncovered via initial screening, or may need to be investigated further, based upon patient presentation. Regarding medications and substance abuse as a cause of psychosis, illicit substance use is the most frequent cause of acute psychosis. Known causative substances include cannabis, cocaine, amphetamines, benzodiazepines, and hallucinogens such as ketamine and phencyclidine (PCP) [37, 38].

Workup

Similar to that of delirium, the process of diagnostic evaluation will need to consist of an initial assessment, a thorough interview including a comprehensive mental status examination, as well as a preliminary medical workup. The goal is to rule out medical and/or organic causes before establishing a primary psychiatric diagnosis.

The idea behind the initial assessment is to determine the etiology of the condition causing psychotic symptoms. Additionally, a proper risk assessment is vital to ensure patient safety. Some components of this may include assessment of the patient for any thought of harm to self or others, as well as the ability of the patient to secure basic needs for themselves. These may factor into the setting or level of care in which the patient is treated. In both the initial risk assessment and the patient history, it is necessary to consider obtaining collateral from individuals known to the patient.

Noting the obvious challenges in taking the history of a patient experiencing acute psychosis, a detailed examination is important to guide diagnostic investigations and gain insight into the underlying etiology. In the case that the patient is unable or unwilling to participate in the interview, obtaining collateral information can be critical to understanding the situation.

Regarding the history of the presenting illness, there are some important factors to determine – symptom onset, both in rate and severity, duration, and nature of the symptoms. Additionally, it is important to determine if the patient is experiencing any concomitant mood symptoms, any thoughts of suicidal ideation or thoughts of harming self or others, or has experienced any recent traumatic stressors.

Important elements of the patient's psychiatric history that are important to consider include past psychiatric symptoms, diagnosis, or trials of medication or therapy. Additionally, in order to assess severity, it may be helpful to ask if there is history of being admitted or hospitalized, or if there is a history of harm caused to themselves or others. Lastly, it is important to inquire about familial history of psychiatric disorders.

Regarding past medical history, it is important to determine if the patient has any chronic medical conditions, especially those of neurocognitive or neurological domains. This is important both to aid in determining the underlying etiology and to screen for medical comorbidities prior to starting treatment. Additionally, acute insults such as traumatic injury, illness, or medication change should also be considered. It is important to thoroughly review all medications that the patient is taking (both prescribed and over the counter) and make a note of any medication changes or the presence of medications that may be causing/exacerbating symptoms. Similarly, it is important to inquire if the patient has a current or past history of substance use disorder, and if so any changes in the frequency of use.

Regarding psychosocial history, it is important to ask about any recent traumatic experiences or stressors as well as assess the patient's support network. Additionally, it is important to assess the patient's childhood/developmental history. Answers to these questions may give insight into the presence or absence of a prodromal phase as well as any possible neurocognitive deficits or functional impairment.

It is vitally important that a full and complete mental status examination be conducted. The mental status examination combines important elements of the history, alongside patient observation, and assessment of the patient's general appearance, mood, affect, speech, attention, and thought processes. Regarding dysfunction of thought, it is important to inquire about the presence of hallucinations and delusions. And as always, it is important to inquire about self-injurious thoughts or thoughts of harming others.

All patients being assessed for psychotic symptoms should receive a complete physical exam, including a neurological examination. Additionally, all patients experiencing an acute symptomatic psychosis (especially if it is their first episode) should receive laboratory investigations such as a complete blood count to rule out potential sources of infection, electrolytes to rule out possible metabolic/nutritional deficiencies, renal and liver panel to assess for organ dysfunction, thyroid stimulating hormone level, blood glucose level, blood phosphate and calcium, as well as a urinalysis and urine toxicology screen.

Additional workup if indicated may consist of HIV testing, screening for syphilis, hepatitis panel, copper studies, heavy metal screen, urine porphyrins, serum cortisol, serum folate/B12, sedimentation rate, antinuclear antibodies, and anti-N-methyl-D-aspartate receptor antibodies. Brain imaging may be indicated if a patient presents with focal neurologic deficit, unremitting headache, history of recent severe head trauma, or other features indicating a possible intracranial pathology. A lumbar puncture may be indicated to rule out inflammatory, paraneoplastic, or infectious central nervous system pathologies. An electroencephalogram (EEG) is not routinely indicated, but may be useful if a patient presents with suspected seizure disorder or unexplained change in level of arousal and awareness [38].

Management

Keeping in mind the impact that psychosis and/or psychotic disorders can have on both the individual and society, it is important for management to address safety, symptom control, and functionality. This is usually achieved through a variety of means including both pharmacological and nonpharmacological interventions.

The overall goal of psychosis management is to assure safety, strive to improve symptom control, and increase the degree of functional recovery.

As many episodes of psychosis present within a hospital setting, it is important for hospitalists to be aware of both the prevalence and the likelihood of repeat occurrences psychosis can have.

Regarding consulting psychiatric services, any patient with suspected initial presentation or recurrence of psychotic symptoms should be evaluated by a psychiatrist. This can take place in a number of different settings, including inpatient, emergency department, or even as an urgent outpatient evaluation. As mentioned previously, the decision upon which setting the treatment takes place in is part of the initial assessment and should be conducted in the least restrictive setting possible while being able to maintain the safety of the patient. This can be achieved on either a voluntary or involuntary basis, keeping in mind that this may be subject to local jurisdictions.

For the majority of cases of psychosis (even for those lacking a clear etiology), pharmacologic management with antipsychotic medications is recommended. The exceptions to this include suspected stimulant-induced psychosis or psychosis with catatonic features. Both situations should warrant administration of benzodiazepines instead of antipsychotics.

The efficacy of antipsychotic medications for acute symptomatic management of psychotic symptoms has been repeatedly well established [36]. While antipsychotic medications have been studied most extensively in the management of schizophrenia, they have demonstrated efficacy in a variety of psychiatric disorders including bipolar disorder, unipolar major depression with psychotic features (in conjunction with an antidepressant), and delirium with psychotic symptoms [39, 40].

Regarding selection of the individual antipsychotic agent, it is generally recommended when possible to use the newer second-generation antipsychotics in place of first-generation antipsychotics due to their more favorable side effect profile. Second-generation antipsychotics have less of an association with extrapyramidal (EPS) side effects when compared to their first-generation counterparts. Apart from the difference in EPS rates among side effect profiles, there has been a lack of convincing evidence demonstrating superior efficacy or adverse effects of one class of antipsychotics over the other. Given the lack of superiority of a single antipsychotic (with the exception of clozapine, which is not commonly recommended as a first-line treatment for psychosis), often times selection of an individual agent may be based on physician familiarity, patients comorbidities, and the side effects of the given medication. Patient factors or comorbidities to keep in mind when deciding upon a specific medication may include cardiovascular risk factors such as QT prolongation, metabolic syndrome, or orthostatic hypotension, advanced age (resulting in one being more sensitive to anticholinergic side effects of medications), and sexual dysfunction (a possible consequence of increased prolactin secretion).

Regarding initial dosing, it is recommended that medications be titrated up from the initial dose to the therapeutic as quickly as can be tolerated. However, if this is the patient's first episode of psychosis, or the patient is of older age, the patient may be more susceptible to the adverse effects of antipsychotic medications and as a result should be more slowly titrated and more closely monitored for adverse effects. The exact timeframe regarding titrations and dosages depends on the medication in question as well as the form in which it is administered. However, once the therapeutic dose is reached, patients should still be monitored for multiple days, before deciding whether to further increase the dosage. Studies have shown no additional benefit to raising dosages above the recommended range, and conversely at high dosages, the side effects of the antipsychotic medications may outweigh any benefits of increased dosage [41].

Follow-up monitoring is recommended on a weekly basis. After 3 months, if the patient is considered in remission, the follow-up monitoring can be switched to monthly [41].

Conclusion

It is approximated that one percent of the world's population is affected by psychotic illness. Symptoms of psychosis are associated with a massive burden to patients, their families, and the population at large. Early recognition of psychosis is important so as to decrease the duration of untreated psychosis experienced by the patient. Early use of antipsychotics and other interventions may improve both short-term symptomatic control and long-term prognosis.

Psychiatric conditions are difficult to treat in any setting, let alone in the hospital where many patients often have complicated comorbidities. Not only do they severely diminish the support system and development of patients but often affect the family and caregivers of the patient. Despite the obvious impact and the large amount of well-researched evidence, the healthcare system at large does not do all that it can to identify and effectively manage psychiatric conditions within the hospital. As discussed throughout the chapter, there are interventions that have been shown to be highly effective in the management of delirium. Implementing these simple, yet effective, interventions can significantly improve patients' quality of life, decrease long-term loss of function, decrease healthcare costs, and positively impact caregivers as well. The common barriers to implementing these initiatives include the lack of belief that they will make a difference, lack of awareness, and/or lack of structural incentives. As the prevalence of psychiatric disorders increases, it will be more and more important for hospital medicine doctors to be aware of how to work with their psychiatry colleagues to identify, treat, and prevent exacerbations of psychiatric disorders.

References

1. Hamer M, Stamatakis E, Steptoe A. Psychiatric hospital admissions, behavioral risk factors, and all-cause mortality the Scottish Health Survey. Arch Intern Med. 2008;168(22):2474–9. https://doi.org/10.1001/archinte.168.22.2474.
2. Hazlett SB, McCarthy ML, Londner MS, Onyike CU. Epidemiology of adult psychiatric visits to US emergency departments. Acad Emerg Med. 2004;11(2):193–5. https://doi.org/10.1197/j.aem.2003.09.014.

3. Siddiqi N, Harrison JK, Clegg A, Teale EA, Young J, Taylor J, Simpkins SA. Interventions for preventing deliriumin hospitalised non-ICU patients. Cochrane Database Syst Rev. 2016;3 https://doi.org/10.1002/14651858.CD005563.pub3.
4. Siddiqi N, House AO, Holmes JD. Occurrence and outcome of delirium in medical in-patients: a systematic literature review. Age Ageing. 2006;35(4):350–64. https://doi.org/10.1093/ageing/afl005.
5. Inouye SK, Westendorp RGJ, Saczynski JS. Delirium in elderly people. Lancet (London, England). 2014;383(9920):911–22. https://doi.org/10.1016/s0140-6736(13)60688-1.
6. Morandi A, Jackson JC, Ely EW. Delirium in the intensive care unit. Int Rev Psychiatry. 2009;21(1):43–58. https://doi.org/10.1080/09540260802675296.
7. Morandi A, Jackson JC. Delirium in the intensive care unit: a review. Neurol Clin. 2011;29(4):749. https://doi.org/10.1016/j.ncl.2011.08.004.
8. Dasgupta M, Dumbrell AC. Preoperative risk assessment for delirium after noncardiac surgery: a systematic review. J Am Geriatr Soc. 2006;54(10):1578–89. https://doi.org/10.1111/j.1532-5415.2006.00893.x.
9. Fok MC, Sepehry AA, Frisch L, Sztramko R, van der Burg BLS, Vochteloo AJH, Chan P. Do antipsychotics prevent postoperative delirium? A systematic review and meta-analysis. Int J Geriatr Psychiatry. 2015;30(4):333–44. https://doi.org/10.1002/gps.4240.
10. Lawlor PG, Gagnon B, Mancini IL, Pereira JL, Hanson J, Suarez-Almazor ME, Bruera ED. Occurrence, causes, and outcome of delirium in patients with advanced cancer – a prospective study. Arch Intern Med. 2000;160(6):786–94. https://doi.org/10.1001/archinte.160.6.786.
11. Kiely DK, Bergmann MA, Murphy KM, Jones RN, Orav EJ, Marcantonio ER. Delirium among newly admitted postacute facility patients: prevalence, symptoms, and severity. J Gerontol A Biol Sci Med Sci. 2003;58(5):441–5. https://doi.org/10.1093/gerona/58.5.M441.
12. Elie M, Rousseau F, Cole M, Primeau F, McCusker J, Bellavance F. Prevalence and detection of delirium in elderly emergency department patients. Can Med Assoc J. 2000;163(8):977–81.
13. Elie M, Cole MG, Primeau FJ, Bellavance F. Delirium risk factors in elderly hospitalized patients. J Gen Intern Med. 1998;13(3):204–12. https://doi.org/10.1046/j.1525-1497.1998.00047.x.
14. Fick DM, Agostini JV, Inouye SK. Delirium superimposed on dementia: a systematic review. J Am Geriatr Soc. 2002;50(10):1723–32. https://doi.org/10.1046/j.1532-5415.2002.50468.x.
15. Fiedler SM. An in-depth look into the management and treatment of delirium. In: Conrad K, editor. Clinical approaches to hospital medicine – advances, updates and controversies, vol. 1. Cham: Springer International Publishing; 2018.
16. Cerejeira J, Mukaetova-Ladinska EB. A clinical update on delirium: from early recognition to effective management. Nurs Res Pract. 2011, 2011; https://doi.org/10.1155/2011/875196.
17. Diagnostic and statistical manual of mental disorders : DSM-5 (2013). vol Accessed from https://nla.gov.au/nla.cat-vn6261708. American Psychiatric Association, Arlington.
18. Yurek DM, Hipkens SB, Hebert MA, Gash DM, Gerhardt GA. Age-related decline in striatal dopamine release and motoric function in Brown Norway Fischer 344 hybrid rats. Brain Res. 1998;791(1–2):246–56. https://doi.org/10.1016/s0006-8993(98)00110-3.
19. de Rooij SE, Schuurmans MJ, van der Mast RC, Levi M. Clinical subtypes of delirium and their relevance for daily clinical practice: a systematic review. Int J Geriatr Psychiatry. 2005;20(7):609–15. https://doi.org/10.1002/gps.1343.
20. Cortes-Beringola A, Vicent L, Martin-Asenjo R, Puerto E, Dominguez-Perez L, Maruri R, Moreno G, Vidan MT, Arribas F, Bueno H. Diagnosis, prevention, and management of delirium in the intensive cardiac care unit. Am Heart J. 2021;232:164–76. https://doi.org/10.1016/j.ahj.2020.11.011.
21. Lipowski ZJ. Delirium in the elderly patient. N Engl J Med. 1989;320(9):578–82.
22. Stagno D, Gibson C, Breitbart W. The delirium subtypes: a review of prevalence, phenomenology, pathophysiology, and treatment response. Palliat Support Care. 2004;2(2):171–9. https://doi.org/10.1017/s1478951504040234. PMID: 16594247.

23. Meagher D. Motor subtypes of delirium: past, present and future. Int Rev Psychiatry. 2009;21(1):59–73. https://doi.org/10.1080/09540260802675460.
24. Gupta AK, Saravay SM, Trzepacz PT, Chirayu P. Delirium motoric subtypes. Psychosomatics. 2005;46(2):158. https://doi.org/10.1007/s10725-005-5231-x.
25. Peterson JF, Pun BT, Dittus RS, Thomason JWW, Jackson JC, Shintani AK, Ely EW. Delirium and its motoric subtypes: a study of 614 critically ill patients. J Am Geriatr Soc. 2006;54(3):479–84. https://doi.org/10.1111/j.1532-5415.2005.00621.x.
26. Lam PT, Tse CY, Lee CH. Delirium in a palliative care unit. Prog Palliat Care. 2003;11(3):126–33. https://doi.org/10.1179/096992603235001393.
27. Sands MB, Dantoc BP, Hartshorn A, Ryan CJ, Lujic S. Single Question in Delirium (SQiD): testing its efficacy against psychiatrist interview, the confusion assessment method and the memorial delirium assessment scale. Palliat Med. 2010;24(6):561–5. https://doi.org/10.1177/0269216310371556.
28. Grover S, Avasthi A. Clinical practice guidelines for management of delirium in elderly. Indian J Psychiatry. 2018;60(7):329–40. https://doi.org/10.4103/0019-5545.224473.
29. Devlin JW, Skrobik Y, Gelinas C, Needham DM, Slooter AJC, Pandharipande PP, Watson PL, Weinhouse GL, Nunnally ME, Rochwerg B, Balas MC, van den Boogaard M, Bosma KJ, Brummel NE, Chanques G, Denehy L, Drouot X, Fraser GL, Harris JE, Joffe AM, Kho ME, Kress JP, Lanphere JA, McKinley S, Neufeld KJ, Pisani MA, Payen JF, Pun BT, Puntillo KA, Riker RR, Robinson BRH, Shehabi Y, Szumita PM, Winkelman C, Centofanti JE, Price C, Nikayin S, Misak CJ, Flood PD, Kiedrowski K, Alhazzani W. Clinical practice guidelines for the prevention and management of pain, agitation/sedation, delirium, immobility, and sleep disruption in adult patients in the ICU. Crit Care Med. 2018;46(9):E825–73. https://doi.org/10.1097/ccm.0000000000003299.
30. Flaherty JH, Yue JR, Rudolph JL. Dissecting delirium phenotypes, consequences, screening, diagnosis, prevention, treatment, and program implementation. Clin Geriatr Med. 2017;33(3):393. https://doi.org/10.1016/j.cger.2017.03.004.
31. Global, regional, and national incidence, prevalence, and years lived with disability for 328 diseases and injuries for 195 countries, 1990–2016: a systematic analysis for the global burden of disease study 2016. Lancet (London, England). 2017;390(10100):1211–59. https://doi.org/10.1016/s0140-6736(17)32154-2.
32. Correll CU, Galling B, Pawar A, Krivko A, Bonetto C, Ruggeri M, Craig TJ, Nordentoft M, Srihari VH, Guloksuz S, Hui CLM, Chen EYH, Valencia M, Juarez F, Robinson DG, Schooler NR, Brunette MF, Mueser KT, Rosenheck RA, Marcy P, Addington J, Estroff SE, Robinson J, Penn D, Severe JB, Kane JM. Comparison of early intervention services vs treatment as usual for early-phase psychosis a systematic review, meta-analysis, and meta-regression. JAMA Psychiat. 2018;75(6):555–65. https://doi.org/10.1001/jamapsychiatry.2018.0623.
33. Griswold KS, Del Regno PA, Berger RC. Recognition and differential diagnosis of psychosis in primary care. Am Fam Physician. 2015;91(12):856–63.
34. Olfson M, Lewis-Fernandez R, Weissman MM, Feder A, Gameroff MJ, Pilowsky D, Fuentes M. Psychotic symptoms in an urban general medicine practice. Am J Psychiatr. 2002;159(8):1412–9. https://doi.org/10.1176/appi.ajp.159.8.1412.
35. Schwartz JE, Fennig S, Tanenberg-Karant M, Carlson G, Craig T, Galambos N, Lavelle J, Bromet EJ. Congruence of diagnoses 2 years after a first-admission diagnosis of psychosis. Arch Gen Psychiatry. 2000;57(6):593–600. https://doi.org/10.1001/archpsyc.57.6.593.
36. Zammit S, Allebeck P, David AS, Dalman C, Hemmingsson T, Lundberg I, Lewis G. A longitudinal study of premorbid IQ score and risk of developing schizophrenia, bipolar disorder, severe depression, and other nonaffective psychoses. Arch Gen Psychiatry. 2004;61(4):354–60. https://doi.org/10.1001/archpsyc.61.4.354.
37. Rivkin PMD, Barta PMDPD thought disorder. Available via Unbound Medicine. https://www.hopkinsguides.com/hopkins/view/Johns_Hopkins_Psychiatry_Guide/787025/all/Thought_Disorder.

38. Preda A. Assessment of psychosis – differential diagnosis of symptoms | BMJ Best Practice. Br Med J. 2019; https://bestpractice.bmj.com/topics/en-gb/1066
39. Zhang JP, Gallego JA, Robinson DG, Malhotra AK, Kane JM, Correll CU. Efficacy and safety of individual second-generation vs. first-generation antipsychotics in first-episode psychosis: a systematic review and meta-analysis. Int J Neuropsychopharmacol. 2013;16(6):1205–18. https://doi.org/10.1017/s1461145712001277.
40. Yildiz A, Vieta E, Leucht S, Baldessarini RJ. Efficacy of antimanic treatments: meta-analysis of randomized, controlled trials. Neuropsychopharmacology. 2011;36(2):375–89. https://doi.org/10.1038/npp.2010.192.
41. Cooper SJ, Reynolds GP, Barnes TRE, England E, Haddad PM, Heald A, Holt RIG, Lingford-Hughes A, Osborn D, McGowan O, Patel MX, Paton C, Reid P, Shiers D, Smith J. BAP guidelines on the management of weight gain, metabolic disturbances and cardiovascular risk associated with psychosis and antipsychotic drug treatment. J Psychopharmacol. 2016;30(8):717–48. https://doi.org/10.1177/0269881116645254.

Chapter 10
Opioids: History, Pathophysiology, and Stewardship for Hospitalists

Marianne Maumus, Daniel Zumsteg, and Dileep Mandali

History and Evolution of the Opioid Epidemic in America

History is studied to understand the error of our ways. It is learned so as not to repeat the same mistakes leading us down on a path of failure. Had we paid closer attention to the initial use of opioids and their effects, we may have avoided battling one of the biggest epidemics in America.

The first opioid epidemic in America dates to more than 100 years ago, during the Civil War era. It was not called an epidemic, but rather attributed as "soldier's disease," cluing its unique distinguishment to those that fought in the Civil War. Physicians at the time coined the term "morphinism" to explain the liberal injection of morphine in the sick and in wounded soldiers leading to their dependency for years to come [1]. Morphine clinics increased in number to attend the wounds and long-term care of those injured, while opium, morphine's oral counterpart, began to be universally given in all cases of wounds, gangrene, diarrhea, and dysentery. Opium was even given for malaria in conjunction with quinine due to its analgesic and tranquilizing properties; it was praised as the one medicine "which the Creator himself seems to prescribe" [1]. By 1900, America had approximately 200,000 opioid addicts.

Given the strong, long-term dependency on morphine and opium, there was a race to create an alkaloid derivative that provided the same analgesic effects with significantly less addiction. In 1895, Bayer Corp in Germany commercialized an alkaloid derivative synthesized by British scientist C. R. Wright; it was advertised as being more potent than morphine and without the addictive side-effect drug. The group also believed that it would make a valuable contribution to medicine as a cough suppressant in those with severe lung disease. Their conviction of its potential "heroic" deeds led to the drug's name "heroin" [2]. Heroin was marketed heavily in America. However, it was ultimately proven ineffective as a cough suppressant and less potent in its analgesic effects than morphine. It also saw no therapeutic success in patients with advanced lung disease. Due to the absence of any legislation to restrict the production and consumerism of heroin, the question of addiction became a widespread public concern in America [2]. Heroin was readily available and accessible over the counter, and it could be sniffed, smoked, swallowed, and even injected due to its higher water solubility compared to morphine salts, facilitating its street use. Using the anti-German sentiment prevalent at the time, Congress successfully passed the Harrison Narcotics Tax Act in 1914, introducing federal narcotic controls and making heroin illegal in America [2].

Despite the Harrison Narcotics Tax Act, the use of heroin among Americans did not slow down. The global-scale World Wars allowed soldiers to easily access heroin in its highest purity outside of America; this resulted in the third opioid epidemic in America, right after the Vietnam War. Heroin was high in purity and very cheap at $6 in Vietnam (as opposed to 10% purity and $20 in America), and American soldiers often used it to get high and distract themselves from boredom, homesickness, and disturbed sleep [3]. After the Vietnam War, there was more regular use of narcotics and of heroin (as opposed to codeine), and more addiction to other drugs, particularly cannabis, due to persistent social stigma, high cost, and low purity of heroin in America. Post-Vietnam War, substance use disorder was rampant among 20% of the general population, and this compelled President Ronald Reagan to declare the "war on drugs" [4].

Opioid Epidemic: An American Cultural Phenomenon

The "war on drugs" failed to curb opioid use in America. This futile result can be attributed to lobbying for opioid use in a medical setting during the late twentieth and early twenty-first centuries. In 1986, Dr. Russell Protenoy and Dr. Kathleen Foley published a retrospective study of 38 patients with chronic pain, in favor of opioid use. Opioid maintenance therapy was begun in these patients (with age range of 25–82 years; without any history of substance abuse and malignancy) after many failed attempts of analgesia by surgical or medical means. They reported that in their study, 58% of patients reported either adequate or partial relief of pain, and 63% of patients reported notable enhancement in comfort [5]. They argued that their study corroborated the findings of three other studies at the time in favor of opioid use in a medical setting. They ultimately recommended that opioid maintenance therapy should be considered only after exhausting all reasonable attempts at pain control and that the patient's pain is a significant impediment to their function [5].

Using Drs. Portenoy and Foley's study and similar studies alike, Purdue Pharma aggressively marketed OxyContin in the 1990s, particularly for non-malignant chronic pain. It conducted more than 40 national conferences on pain management and recruited more than 5000 health professionals for its national speaker bureau, grossly influencing physicians' prescription practices and causing the Federation of State Medical Boards to release policies assuring that physicians would not face regulatory action for prescribing opioids [6]. Sophisticated marketing, by utilizing a database that monitored physicians' opioid prescription practices, the promise of lucrative bonuses to its sales representatives, and the use of a coupon program offering free limited 7- to 30-day supply to patients, catapulted liberal use of OxyContin, especially in territories where substance abuse was either rampant or on the rise. In 2001 alone, Purdue spent $200 million in marketing and promotions; between 1996 and 2001, its sales grew from $48 million to $1.1 billion. By 2004, OxyContin had become a leading drug of abuse due to its high availability [6].

In December 2001, the Joint Commission and the National Pharmaceutical Council, which is supported by the nation's major research-based biopharmaceutical companies, published a booklet entitled *Pain: Current Understanding of Assessment, Management, and Treatments*. It added further fuel to the opioid epidemic in the early twenty-first century – a time when deaths from opioid use were increasing with each passing year [7]. First, it stated that the "patient, not clinician, is the authority on the pain and that their self-report is the most reliable indicator of pain," persuading physicians to trust that their patients would report pain accurately. Second, it incorrectly argued that opioids are non-addictive, and though the addiction risk is unknown, it is thought to be quite minimal. Third, it adopted "pain'" as the fifth vital sign and it is just as important to assess as the other four vital signs in all patients. This became a standard practice for almost the first decade of the twenty-first century, which permitted the use of opioids to treat every kind of pain [7].

The liberal prescription of opioids is the driver behind the opioid epidemic becoming an American cultural phenomenon. Though they are useful for short-term or acute pain management, opioids are continuously prescribed for the management of chronic pain despite their ineffectiveness. In fact, higher pain scores are reported in chronic opioid users compared to non-opioid users; one of the common side effects in chronic opioid users is ironically hyperalgesia, an increased sensitivity and responsiveness to pain. Additionally, they report decreased quality of life and employment due to their debilitating addiction to opioids, and consequently, rely increasingly on disability and healthcare utilization [8]. For example, in Louisiana, opioid abuse costs the state approximately $296 million per year in healthcare cost, and from 2010 to 2016, the state has averaged around 122 opioid prescriptions per 100 persons. The opioid epidemic also has direct, synergistic effects on HIV and drug-related mortalities [9]. In 2016, around 64,000 people in the United States had died from drug overdose. This number exploded to 90,000 in 2020, of which 70,000 are from opioid overdose-related deaths [10]. This is more than car accident deaths and breast cancer deaths – causes that receive consistent national attention every year. As healthcare institutions become more attentive and cut back on opioid prescriptions, an increasing upward trend in heroin use has been observed, thereby highlighting that the opioid epidemic is not just a healthcare problem but rather a cultural problem that needs to be addressed aggressively by healthcare professionals, policy makers, and public health advocates.

Cardinal Features of the Opioid Epidemic

Over-prescription of opioid medications in the last 25 years is responsible for the progression of the opioid overdose epidemic, diversions of tablets in communities, and overutilization of healthcare resources. Opioid-dependent patients have complex psychiatric and medical illnesses, and most of them are also socially complex, lacking social support and frequently homeless. Opioids are known to topple neuroanatomical pathways that are responsible for Pavlovian learning, memory formation, judgment, and emotional control [11]. As a result, the impulsive (drug-seeking) behavior that may be seen in chronic opioid users is a drug-induced phenomenon, not a lack of moral character. Understanding the origins of chronic pain, withdrawal pain, and central sensitization is essential to treating these patients with evidence-based therapies and to tackle the features of the opioid epidemic: chronic pain, overutilization, substance use disorder, psychiatric illness, and diversion of tablets. A learning dive into the brain disease model of addiction, the pain matrix of a normal functioning brain, the effects of opioids on brain structures, and the neurophysiologic origins of central sensitization and central pain syndromes will serve as effective tools to gain such understanding.

The Brain Disease Model of Addiction

While it is debatable whether addiction and opioid dependence is a disease, or a normal response to the effect of opiates on brain tissue, the "Brain Disease Model of Addiction" serves as a great place to start learning the effects of opioids on the brain. The areas involved are noted in Fig. 10.1. The brain disease model of addiction as outlined was derived from years of neuropsychopharmacology research. Pavlovian learning, a type of learning that occurs due to the subject's instinctive responses, is driven by the ventral tegmental area and the nucleus accumbens, i.e., the learning and pleasure centers of the brain, respectively. Given the intertwined connection, a pleasure signal entices to repeat action to stimulate remembrance [12]. The signal begins with a dopamine flash in these two areas when a person learns something new, and this is followed by a weak dopamine signal sent to the prefrontal cortex.

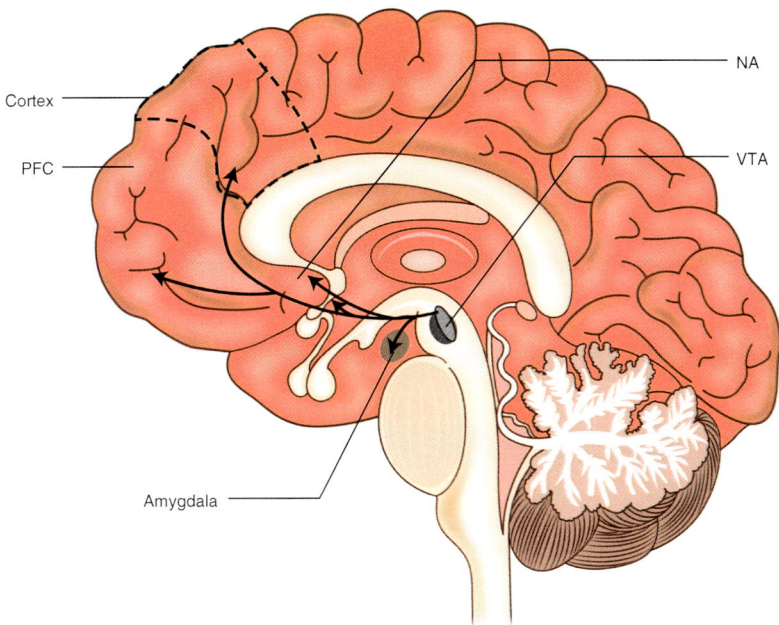

Fig. 10.1 Brain disease model of addiction. PFC prefrontal cortex, NA nucleus accumbens, VTA ventral tegmental area

The prefrontal cortex then begins to make connections with cortical nerve fibers to create memory and feedback loops to the emotional center of the brain, the amygdala. The amygdala does not fully mature until the age of 24, and without prefrontal control, it tips the balance of behavior toward impulsive actions [11, 12].

Opioid use induces euphoria, through a dopamine "blast" instead of a healthy pleasurable "flash" in the ventral tegmental area and nucleus accumbens. As a result of overstimulation, the brain undergoes several adaptive changes, intracellularly and within the synapse, in order to reduce the effects of dopamine; this causes an increasing requirement of opioid dose to achieve the same effect [11, 12]. The adaptive response in the prefrontal cortex is recession of affected neuron dendrites, which consequently impairs memory formation and disconnects control over the amygdala. This causes an individual to lose their impulse control and their ability to progress academically and intellectually, putting them at a risk for progressive psychiatric disorders [11, 12].

Hypofrontality has been observed in the prefrontal cortex as well as in the regions of anterior cingulate and ventral orbital cortex in addicted individuals. The development of enduring neuroplasticity was observed through neuroimaging with functional MRI scans and direct visualization of reduced prefrontal cortical measures of blood flow, metabolism, and striatal levels of dopamine D2 receptors. The capacity for biologically relevant stimuli to activate the prefrontal cortex is impaired in patients with prolonged opioid use; however, drug-associated stimuli continue to markedly activate the prefrontal cortex [11]. The role of dopamine transitions from promoting new learning to enabling the use of learned information to execute adaptive behavioral response. Behavior evolves from a declarative process into a habitual behavior utilizing working memory circuits, which lead to automatic behaviors that lack conscious control and cause compulsive relapse [11]. The ability of prefrontal, declarative circuit to intrude and disrupt drug-seeking habit is also impaired. Over time, adaptive changes that occur early in disease progression promote behaviors toward addiction but can resolve with abstinence; however, later in the disease, habit circuitry is fully formed [11].

Addiction is a progression of brain pathology, and lack of behavioral control is a pharmacologically induced phenomenon. There is a hierarchy of events, a 3-tiered progression, that occurs with repeated exposure over time. Addiction progresses from intracellular changes to changes in function and anatomy of neural circuits, establishment of permanent unconscious behaviors and drug-related memories, and loss of unconscious control from conscious dependence [11]. Given that neuroplasticity leads to permanent drug-associated memories, addiction should be recognized as a chronic relapsing disease, not as an acute episodic illness.

The Pain Matrix

As seen in Fig. 10.2, the pain pathway involves the parts of the brain that control and modulate sensory input from the dorsolateral spinothalamic tract of the spinal cord. It consists of a constellation of brain regions, a multi-tiered hierarchical neural network, and the pattern or neural activation created by the sensory input that represents the *pain signature* of the experience. The stream of input is continuous, and the brain interprets it, gives it meaning, and then reflects it back to the original source [12].

First, the nociceptive input arrives to the thalamus. Second, perceptual-attentional areas of the cortex interpret it; this is known as *conscious modulation* and is shown in Fig. 10.3. Third, the nociceptive input is reflected into reappraisal-emotional areas so that importance can be assigned to the information; this is known as *unconscious modulation* and is shown in Fig. 10.4. After the sensory input is filtered through these three regions, *descending modulation* of the pain signature occurs. The signal first enters the periaqueductal gray zone, where a high concentration of opioid receptors either inhibits or facilitates the pain signature in order to tone down or increase the response. The altered signature enters the rostral ventral medulla, which contains "on" cells and "off" cells, before traveling back to the dorsal horn and then to the original source. These midbrain structures are analogous to "volume

Pain matrix: nociceptive input arrives

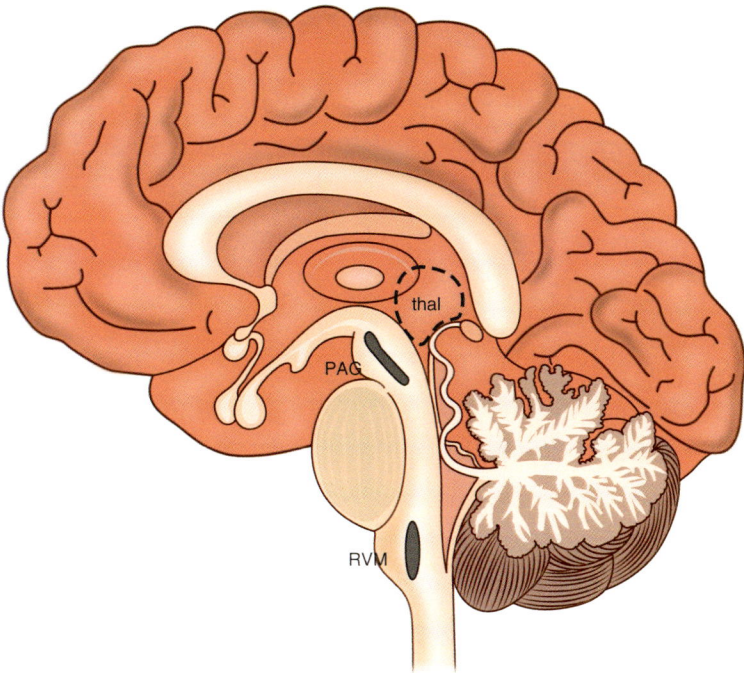

Fig. 10.2 Nociceptive input arrives

control" and "on/off switch" for pain; the pain signature deintensifies with time and distraction before it is reflected back to the original source.

Opioids inhibit the reflection of the pain signature at the levels of periaqueductal gray zone and rostral ventral medulla, where the function of "on" cells is blocked. In addition, opioids cause release of cytokines, interleukins, and glutamate from microglial cells, thereby intensifying neuroinflammation and leading to cell dysfunction and death in these areas [13]. Opioids are also known to disrupt the function of glial cells in the dorsal horn of spinal cord, causing spontaneous neuronal firing and leading to hyperalgesia and chronic pain. The pain associated with neuroinflammation is known as *central sensitization* [13].

Opioids also intensify the pleasure signal through stimulation of the ventral tegmental and nucleus accumbens areas [11]. When the effect of opioids begins to wear off, the rostral ventral medulla and the periaqueductal gray zone relieve the signal and the pleasure signal also disappears; the patient's perception of pain gets worse. This triggers intense fear and avoidance behaviors in patients that clinically manifest as *pain catastrophizing* behavior; it is the behavior focused on the

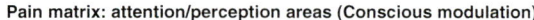

Pain matrix: attention/perception areas (Conscious modulation)

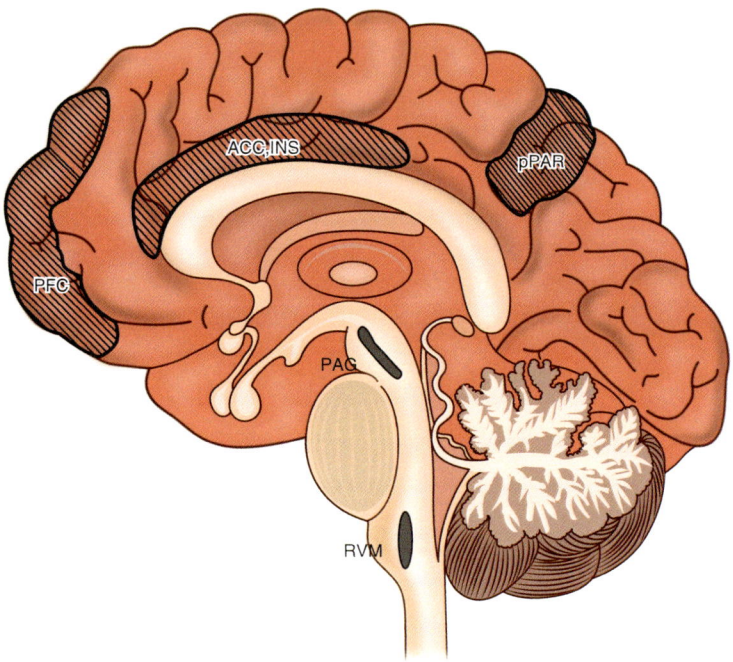

Fig. 10.3 Attention/perception areas (conscious modulation)

anticipation of the worst possible outcome, with increased attention to pain and associated symptoms [14]. The repeated use of opioids progresses maladaptive neuroplastic changes seen in the addiction pathway over time, inhibiting prefrontal cortex control over both the amygdala and the periaqueductal gray zone, strengthening habit circuity, and ultimately leading to highly emotional patients in constant pain.

Shared Neural Networks

The pain matrix and learning reward system share overlapping neural networks, mainly between the medial prefrontal cortex and nucleus accumbens. Prefrontal brain regions are involved in nociceptive inhibition and in the transition from declarative memories to habitual working memory circuits. The periaqueductal gray zone is located right next to the ventral tegmental area and receives input from the prefrontal cortex, insula, and other important structures. Because of the proximity of these regions to one another, the systems of human learning, pleasure, and pain are intimately connected. This is necessary since learning to avoid painful events deters risky behavior and stimulates the seeking of healthy, safe environments as well as cooperation within human communities.

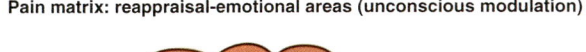

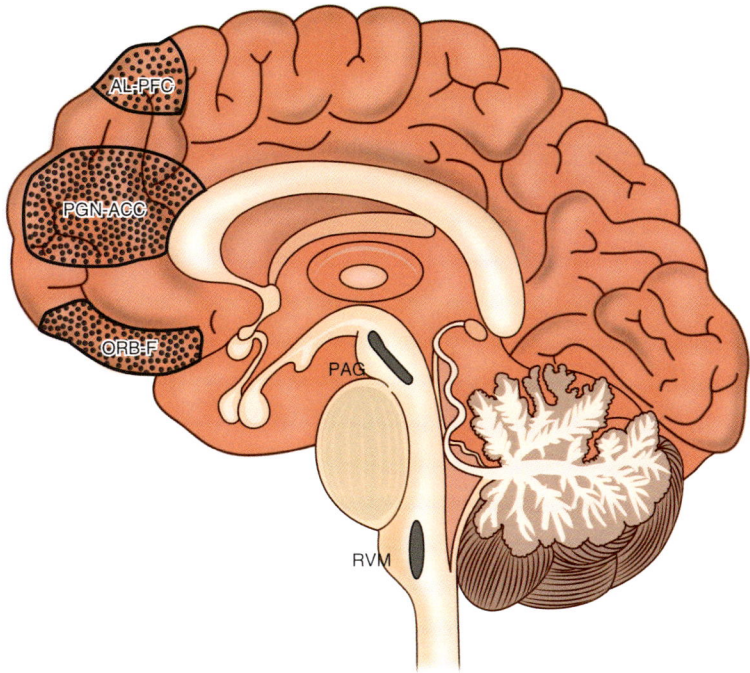

Fig. 10.4 Reappraisal-emotional areas (unconscious modulation). PAG periaqueductal gray zone, RVM rostral ventral medulla, thal thalamus ACC, INS anterior cingulate cortex, insula, pPAR posterior parietal lobe, PFC prefrontal cortex, AL-PFC anterior lateral prefrontal cortex, PGN-ACC perigenual anterior cingulate cortex, ORB-F orbital frontal lobe

On the other hand, chronic pain and psychiatric disorders also share neural mechanisms, and their relationship is bidirectional. For example, chronic pain leads to depression, and depression leads to chronic pain. In the opioid epidemic context, chronic pain leads to substance use disorders, and substance use disorders, including cannabis use, lead to chronic pain [14]. Additionally, suicide risk factors have increased prevalence among patients with chronic pain. Patients with personality disorders and neuroticism (negative thoughts) have increased sensitivity to pain, greater disability, and a lower quality of life, further signifying the shared neural networks between chronic pain and psychiatric disorders [14].

A third condition – addiction – is also intimately intertwined with chronic pain and psychiatric disorders within the brain. With prolonged, persistent use of opioids, acute pain progresses to chronic pain, eventually resulting in conscious opioid dependence and then finally to unconscious addiction. The prefrontal cortex dysfunction coupled with prolonged fear of withdrawal leads to chronic anxiety and the development of personality disorders. Due to the intertwined connection among chronic pain, psychiatric disorders, and addiction, these ultimately cannot be separated in clinical practice; they must be considered as the same disease process and treated together.

Chronic Pain, Central Pain Syndromes, Hyperalgesia, and Withdrawal Pain

Chronic pain is pain lasting for more than 3 months. It is not the same disease as acute pain. It has association with fear and avoidance behaviors, so psychosocial issues come under scrutiny. It also has a different pathophysiology than acute pain and, therefore, it needs a multimodal approach [15]. Chronic pain can impact many body systems: gastrointestinal, psychological, endocrine, and sleep. Its presence implies that neuroinflammation and neuroplastic changes in the brain have begun to develop. Its pathophysiology may include central pain syndromes, central sensitization of the periaqueductal gray zone and rostral ventral medulla of the midbrain, or a failure of descending modulation of glial cells in the dorsal horn of the spinal cord (complex regional pain syndrome). It may also be peripheral in origin, as in peripheral neuropathy or osteoarthritis [15].

Some examples of central pain syndromes include phantom limb pain, pain associated with Parkinson's disease, pain associated with spinal cord injury, and multiple sclerosis. This form of pain arises when the brain constructs painful reality within unconscious brain structures as the pain signature is born and persists from direct insult to nerve tissue. Microglial cells activate and induce neuroinflammation with the release of cytokines, interleukins, and glutamate, which ultimately lead to mental dysfunction and depression as a result of cell death. Opioid use fails to provide relief and can actually potentiate the central pain [13].

Complex regional pain syndrome is due to failure of descending modulation of signal by glial cells in the dorsal horn of the spinal cord. These cases require a multimodal treatment approach, as the perception of pain is real to the patient. Although the pain signature arises from a peripheral nerve, it is amplified at the level of spinal cord. As noted in its name, this form of pain syndrome is complex, difficult to treat, and requires a referral to a chronic pain specialist [13].

Opioids are often the go-to treatment to treat pain. However, not all pain can be treated with them. The opioid-induced hyperalgesia is an important cause of pain and is often overlooked. It is also greatly associated with fear and avoidance behavior and with pain catastrophizing. Opioid-induced hyperalgesia was first reported in the medical literature in 1870 and has persistently been noted since. It is characterized by increased sensitization to painful stimuli after exposure to opioids and often mimics the patient's original pain condition [15]. Opioid-induced hyperalgesia may have both a central and a spinal origin. Central sensitization in opioid-induced hyperalgesia is caused by neuroinflammation in the midbrain structures. Function of glial cells is also disrupted, where the mitigation of the pain signal in the dorsal horn of the spinal cord is compromised [15]. Opioid-induced hyperalgesia needs to be considered when a patient fails to resolve their pain with opioid use. A thorough history of pain, opioid use, and psychiatric issues is critical to the formation of a treatment plan for a patient who has a history of opioid use.

Pain from opioid withdrawal is also chronic, cyclical, associated with anxiety, and often unrecognized. It has a similar pathophysiology to opioid-induced hyperalgesia and should be considered when opioid therapy fails [15]. Opioids turn off the natural endogenous opioid system in the brain, and it may take 3–5 days to recover after the opioid is discontinued. The pain perception of central sensitization can take 1 month to resolve [13]. Due to the pharmacologic effects of opioids, the withdrawal pain can be greater than the original painful event. As the opioids wear off, the midbrain structures release the pain signature and the pleasure signal in the nucleus accumbens also diminishes, enhancing pain perception. As a result, objective monitoring of the patient's functional status (rather than use of a subjective pain scale) is crucial to dictate the pace of the weaning process. Opioids also induce fear and anxiety, which amplify pain perception, so patients typically are very emotional and expressive when they present with withdrawal [15]. During this sensitive period, a patient will need reassurance, motivational interviewing, and guidance to overcome their withdrawal. They may respond well to dialog about the central origins of their pain and reaffirmation that their pain perception is real, although their physical condition is stable. A useful analogy that a patients may understand is when one moves their hand from a cold bath to a warm one, the temperature may initially feel very hot but will stabilize in time. Many patients are willing to endure this sensitive, suffering period, if the goal is independence from pharmacotherapy and improved quality of life. Additionally, distraction is a known treatment method that can assist with this endeavor [13].

Opioid Stewardship for Hospitalists

The rest of this chapter will discuss the common risks, such as respiratory depression and behavioral disturbances, involved with opioid use, the special complications of opioid use, the characteristics that put an individual at a greater risk, and the management necessary to mitigate these risks. This lays down the clinical foundation for opioid stewardship for hospitalists and provides guidance on the multimodal approach to treat opioid dependency and withdrawal.

Table 10.1 Risk factors and monitoring of respiratory suppression

Respiratory suppression risk factors and monitoring	
Risk factors	Monitoring
Renal and pulmonary conditions Neurologic or psychiatric conditions Higher dose First 24 hours of opioid therapy Prolonged surgery Polypharmacy Substance use disorder	Capnography Telemetry Naloxone reversal orders Neurological checks periodically Quick weaning protocols

Understanding Opioid Risk

Respiratory Depression

Respiratory depression is a very well-known side effect associated with opioid medication. However, as noted in Table 10.1, there are risk factors that make certain patient populations more likely to experience opioid-induced respiratory depression (OIRD) [16]. OIRD is due to the decreased respiratory drive and reduced supraglottic airway tone induced by opioids. If left untreated, OIRD may be fatal.

Risk Factors

Risk factors for OIRD include patient characteristics, certain comorbidities, and iatrogenic risks. Presence of one or more of these risk factors should prompt the hospitalist to institute an appropriate monitoring system to assess and, if necessary, reverse opioid toxicity.

Patients who are female, greater than 60 years of age, or less than 24 hours postsurgery are at an increased risk of OIRD. Orthopedic, transplant, and general surgery patients are particularly at high risk for OIRD, as are patients with an American Society of Anesthesia (ASA) score of 3–4 prior to their surgery. As an example, a patient with a remote history of a myocardial infarction (MI) or cerebral vascular accident (CVA) would likely have an ASA score of 3, while a patient with a recent MI or CVA would have an ASA score of 4 [17]. Patients who are opioid dependent at baseline are also at increased risk.

Patients with underlying renal disease, liver disease, neurologic disease (e.g., stroke, dementia), pulmonary disease (including chronic obstructive pulmonary disease), or cardiac disease (including coronary artery disease, congestive heart failure, and arrhythmias) are at an increased risk for OIRD. Diagnosed or suspected obstructive sleep apnea, obesity, and diabetes mellitus are also comorbidities associated with OIRD.

Finally, iatrogenic factors associated with OIRD include concomitant use of sedatives, multiple prescribers, multiple routes of administration, and excessive doses.

Management

Management of opioid patients at high risk for respiratory suppression includes monitoring for changes in clinical picture, as well as the placement of naloxone reversal orders. High-risk patients should be treated in a step-down unit, where capnography and telemetry are available. For these patients, as well as patients at lower risk for OIRD, periodic neurologic checks and alternative treatment modalities for pain should be considered. Finally, protocols for the rapid weaning of opioids should be in place for all patients at risk of OIRD.

Behavioral Disturbances

The neuropathological effects of opioids, as discussed previously, generate behavior in patients that is disruptive or counter-productive to the goals of care, or perhaps to the point of endangering the safety of hospital staff.

Risk Factors

Perhaps unsurprisingly, patients with a history of substance use disorder (SUD), persistent refusal to take medication-assisted therapy (MAT), and opioid dependence are at an increased risk of behavioral disturbances in the hospital setting. Patients who demonstrate poor frontal lobe function, refusal of self-care, or self-mutilation behaviors are also at risk for behavioral disturbances.

An adversarial relationship with the healthcare system, such as a history of verbal abuse of staff or non-adherence to medical or psychiatric care, is predictive of behavioral disturbances.

Similarly, patients with recurrent administrations to the same hospital, with frequent short stays at multiple hospitals (so-called "hospital shopping"), or who have been terminated from a practice in the past are more likely to cause behavioral disturbances.

Behavioral management is a very delicate task that can make or break the therapeutic relationship between the patient and hospital staff. Addressing behavioral disturbances compassionately requires clear communication to the patient and among the staff to ensure that therapeutic goals can be met while also maintaining the safety and well-being of all parties.

Table 10.2 Behavioral disturbances risk factors and monitoring

Risk factors	Monitoring
History of SUD/opioid dependence	Proactive violence prevention strategies
Persistent non-adherence to medical care	De-escalation
History of engaging in verbal abuse	Joint rounding with nursing and security
Evidence of poor frontal lobe function	Collate patients
Persistent refusal for self-care	Communicate risk to nursing
Self-mutilation	Create and utilize long-term care plans
Persistent refusal to take MAT	Develop a multi-disciplinary care team
Recurrent admissions to the hospital/hospital shopping	Steer patients into treatment programs
Receipt of a seek care elsewhere policy	

Management

As noted in Table 10.2, strategies for management of behavioral disturbances may be divided into those that directly involve the patient and those which inform the structure and coordination of the hospital care team.

For a patient with a history of behavioral disturbances, the most effective approaches are preventative in nature. These may include creation of a long-term care plan with the patient, and counselling to steer patients into treatment programs. Long-term care plans create a point of consensus and mutual understanding that reduces the discontinuity between patient and staff about routine medical care, such as blood draws or neurological checks.

A multi-disciplinary team consisting of psychiatry, medicine, pharmacy, and infectious disease staff allows for a consistent and holistic approach to patient care that minimizes the perception or actual presence of conflicting medical recommendations. Similarly, communication among nursing and physician teams regarding the patient's risk of behavioral disturbances ensures that all members of the care team are prepared when interacting with that patient. This is especially important if there are particular triggers for a patient's outbursts. Finally, all staff should be trained in verbal de-escalation strategies so that they respond to a patient's behavior appropriately.

At an administrative level, joint rounding, which is rounding within a team framework, with hospital security and representatives from the patient provider relations department may reduce risk to healthcare workers. Ensuring effective and adequate communication is key to proper medical care and well-being of all caregivers. The collation of patients at risk of behavioral disturbances to a designated set of beds on the hospital floor can allow for the centralization of properly trained staff and resources. Furthermore, these strategies reduce the impact of behavioral disturbances on all other patients on that floor.

> **Key Points**
> - OIRD is a serious and potentially fatal complication of opioid use.
>   - Postsurgical patients and chronically ill patients are at high risk of OIRD.
>   - Monitoring, multimodal therapies, early mobilization prevent respiratory depression.
> - Behavioral disturbances disrupt patient care and can pose a threat to staff.
>   - De-escalation training is recommended for all staff.
>   - Foster patient buy-in to treatment plans.
>   - Joint rounding and care team communication reduce risk of violence.

Stewardship and Acute Pain

The emergency department is often the first port of call for many patients seeking treatment for pain and, therefore, a critical point for opioid stewardship.

Acute vs Chronic Pain

Acute pain management begins with the decision to treat with opioid or non-opioid therapy. Multimodal pain management including acute nerve blocks should be the mainstay therapy whenever possible. In the event that opioid therapy is indicated, the Centers for Disease Control (CDC) recommends using the lowest effective dose with the shortest duration of treatment [18]. Ideally, a treatment plan should be established with the patient to ascertain the goals of opioid therapy as well as risks and benefits.

Once the decision to utilize opioid therapy for acute pain has been made, physicians should assess opioid risk. This can be accomplished by checking the prescription monitoring program, performing a pain, psychiatry, and drug history, and performing a urine drug screen. When considering which opioid medication to prescribe, short-acting opioids should be preferred. Finally, a comprehensive review of the patient's medications should be undertaken to avoid co-prescribing opioids with benzodiazepines or other sedatives.

Chronic pain has a different pathophysiology than acute pain. Although there is significant overlap between the two, chronic pain is associated with fear, avoidance behaviors, and additional psychosocial factors such as substance use disorder and dependency. Patients who are expected to be admitted to the hospital for a short period of time and are otherwise stable, without any signs of substance use disorder and dependency, on a chronic pain regimen should be kept on their long-term medicine regimen and discharged to follow-up with the provider who prescribes their opioid medications.

During the course of hospitalization, complications and side effects of opioids, such as hyperalgesia, gastroparesis, and nausea, should be anticipated and addressed. Hospitalization is an opportunity to screen patients for these complications. If present, the patient's medications should be discontinued, as ongoing use will lead to debilitation, adverse outcomes, and readmission. The patient will need other options for pain management. If weaning of opioids is not possible, then palliative care consultation is warranted. Care should be taken to avoid making a patient opioid-dependent, including weaning and education on the risks of long-term opioid use.

American College of Emergency Physicians Opioid Recommendations [19]

Several questions need to be considered before prescribing opioids in the emergency department:

- In adult patients experiencing an acute painful condition, do the benefits of prescribing a short course of opioids on discharge from the emergency department outweigh the potential harms?
  - Preferentially prescribe nonopioid analgesic therapies (nonpharmacologic and pharmacologic) rather than opioids as the initial treatment of acute pain in patients discharged from the emergency department.
  - For cases in which opioid medications are deemed necessary, prescribe the lowest effective dose of a short-acting opioid for the shortest time indicated.
- In adult patients with an acute exacerbation of noncancer chronic pain, do the benefits of prescribing a short course of opioids on discharge from the emergency department outweigh the potential harms?
  - Do not routinely prescribe opioids to treat an acute exacerbation of noncancer chronic pain for patients discharged from the emergency department. Nonopioid analgesic therapies (nonpharmacologic and pharmacologic) should be used preferentially.
  - For cases in which opioid medications are deemed appropriate, prescribe the lowest indicated dose of a short-acting opioid for the shortest time that is feasible.
- In adult patients with an acute episode of pain being discharged from the emergency department, do the harms of a short concomitant course of opioids and muscle relaxants/sedative-hypnotics outweigh the benefits?
  - Do not routinely prescribe, or knowingly cause to be co-prescribed, a simultaneous course of opioids and benzodiazepines (as well as other muscle relaxants/sedative-hypnotics) for treatment of an acute episode of pain in patients discharged from the emergency department.

- In adult patients experiencing opioid withdrawal, is emergency department-administered buprenorphine as effective for the management of opioid withdrawal compared with alternative management strategies?
  - When possible, treat opioid withdrawal in the emergency department with buprenorphine or methadone as a more effective option compared with nonopioid-based management strategies such as the combination of α2-adrenergic agonists and antiemetics.
  - Preferentially treat opioid withdrawal in the emergency department with buprenorphine rather than methadone.
- As per the US Substance Abuse and Mental Health Services Administration recommendations, physicians should prescribe naloxone to at-risk patients such as the following [20]:
  - Discharged from the emergency department following opioid intoxication or poisoning
  - Taking high doses of opioids or undergoing chronic pain management
  - Receiving rotating opioid medication regimens
  - Having legitimate need for analgesia combined with history of substance abuse
  - Using extended release/long-acting opioid preparations
  - Completing mandatory opioid detoxification or abstinence programs
  - Recent release from incarceration and past abuser of opioids

Key Points
- Avoid prescribing opioids in the emergency department whenever possible.
- ACEP guidelines apply to hospitals for treatment of acute pain.
- Prescribe naloxone in the emergency department and hospital.
- Prescribe two doses due to short-acting effect.
- Distribute to patient, family, caretakers.

Special Complications of Opioids

Unique to opioids is the development of pain sensitization and catastrophizing of pain. Hyperalgesia due to opioid use should be suspected in patients for whom opioids paradoxically make the patient's pain worse. For hospitalists, this syndrome is often seen in postoperative settings and cannot be treated with additional opioids. In fact, treatment entails removing the opioid. A short-term prescription for antiseizure medication for neuropathy may reduce the hyperactivity and reduce symptoms of pain and emotionality. Recognition of opioid-induced hyperalgesia is important because any delay in treatment leads to unnecessary suffering of the patient.

Opioid-withdrawal hypersensitivity is an allodynia-like sensation of pain in the patient's typical location which flares when the dosage of opioids is reduced. This hypersensitivity lasts approximately 24–72 hours after a change in dosing and is associated with a spike in the patient's anxiety and catastrophizing about the nature of their pain.

Multimodal Therapy

Multimodal therapy is the synergistic utilization of non-opioid analgesics to address pain, as an alternative to opioids [21]. Multimodal therapy comprises both general (i.e., systemic medications) and regional (i.e., field blocks and neuraxial blocks) approaches to pain management. Unless contraindicated, patients should receive an around-the-clock regimen of non-steroidal anti-inflammatory drugs (NSAIDs), COX-2 inhibitors (COXIBs), or acetaminophen. The choice of medication, dose, route, and duration of therapy should be individualized, and dosing regimens should be administered to optimize efficacy while minimizing the risk of adverse events. When appropriate, or prior to a surgical procedure, regional blockade with local anesthetic should be considered [22].

Classes of Multimodal Therapy

Each class of medication used in the context of multimodal therapy is briefly discussed below.

NSAID use decreases opioid consumption and provides superior analgesia when combined with opioids [23, 24]. These drugs are considered first-line medications for mild-to-moderate pain. Adverse effects include gastric bleeding, colonic or diverticular bleeding, and renal impairment [25, 26]. COXIBS have a lower risk of bleeding compared with traditional NSAIDs but have an increased risk for cardiovascular events [27].

Acetaminophen is a non-opioid antipyretic analgesic without anti-inflammatory activity [28]. It has an incompletely understood mechanism of action, but studies show a synergistic effect with NSAIDs [29]. Acetaminophen is recommended to be administered using a dosing schedule. Both PO and IV routes of administration are equally efficacious for moderate-to-severe pain, but IV administration is recommended when oral medications are contraindicated, e.g., nausea and vomiting [30].

Tramadol is a weak opioid agonist which acts on the μ-opioid receptor. It also acts as a selective serotonin reuptake inhibitor (SSRI) and serotonin-norepinephrine reuptake inhibitor (SNRI) [31]. Tramadol is a cytochrome p450 (CYP450) substrate and may cause interactions with other medications that are processed via the

CYP450 system [32]. Because of the SSRI capacity of tramadol, it should be used with caution on patients who take other SSRI medications to prevent serotonin syndrome. Presently, evidence does not support the concept that tramadol is less addictive than other opioid medications [33].

N-methyl-D-aspartate (NMDA) receptor antagonists include drugs like ketamine, magnesium, methadone, and dexamethasone [34, 35]. The NMDA receptor is associated with central sensitization of nociceptive signals and is therefore an important target in the treatment of chronic and postoperative pain. Ketamine is particularly versatile, with intranasal administration as a safe and efficacious alternative to intranasal fentanyl [36].

Anticonvulsant agents such as gabanoids, gabapentin, and pregabalin are neuromodulators that reduce excitability of pre-synaptic calcium-gated channels. This class of therapy promotes opioid cessation after surgery, but has no effect on postoperative pain [37]. However, gabanoids are effective first-line agents for neuropathic pain [38]. Of note, evidence suggests that diversion and abuse of gabanoids occur in approximately 1% of the general population and at higher rates among patients with opioid use disorder [39].

Fixed-dose combinations of opioid and non-opioid medications are an important element in multimodal therapy that decrease pill burden on patients by combining NSAID medications with small doses of opioids [40]. Common drug pairings include oxycodone/ibuprofen, hydrocodone/ibuprofen, and hydrocodone/acetaminophen, which decreases the liver toxicity associated with acetaminophen [41].

Regional anesthesia is an effective option to reduce or eliminate the need for opioids. Administration is via continuous local infiltration in patients requiring prolonged analgesia, and benefits include a reduction in hospital resource utilization, decreased nausea and vomiting, and an improvement in patient satisfaction [42]. Additional medications added to the regional anesthetic can provide additional benefit to patients. Anti-inflammatory medications, such as COX-2 inhibitors and steroids, or motor and sensory blocks such as liposomal bupivacaine may be used when indicated [43].

Field blocks are a non-specific subset of regional anesthesia, in which local anesthetic is administered into fascial planes. A single injection may last hours but requires ultrasound-guidance and a larger volume of anesthetic compared to peripheral nerve blocks [44].

Key Points
- There are multiple methods to address acute and chronic pain in patients.
- Opioids are often inferior to other analgesic agents such as NSAIDs.
- Appropriate combinations of two or more methods can be safe and effective.
- Be aware of drug-drug interactions and potential complications.

Compassionate Withdrawal of Opiates

Overview

The most effective strategy for the treatment of opioid use disorder is that of prevention. Early weaning of opioid medication and transition to multimodal therapy after acute pain are paramount to opioid stewardship. Failing to wean a patient from their opioid medications prior to discharge is one of the biggest mistakes a hospitalist can make. For patients who are already taking opioids, the decision to taper or completely stop opioids should be made when there is evidence of complications, dependence, or substance use disorder. Doing so in a compassionate manner requires making a correct diagnosis and understanding the complications of opioid withdrawal. Strategies to address the psychological components of a patient's pain are often as important as the medication regimens themselves. Peer recovery coaches, nurses, case managers, therapists, clinical psychologists, inpatient and chronic pain specialists, addiction medicine specialists, and hospitalists should all be capable of recognizing complications, performing motivational interviews and bedside cognitive behavioral therapies to help guide the patient's progress through opioid withdrawal.

Empathic Strategies

Validation and reassurance should be used frequently when withdrawing patients from opioids. The sensation of worsening pain may be temporary, but the pain itself is very real, and dismissing patient complaints of pain can negatively affect the physician-patient relationship. All patients should be given the time and space to express themselves and feel respected by the care team. The role of the clinician is often that of a coach, helping to redirect the patient's attention away from the immediate pain of withdrawal and toward their future state.

Coping strategies are also helpful for many patients during this time, and mind-body therapies have some evidence for a decrease in opioid-treated pain [45]. Meditation, hypnosis, relaxation, guided imagery, therapeutic suggestion, and cognitive behavioral therapy are all options to discuss with patients. A variety of strategies not only gives the patient agency in deciding the approach to their treatment, but it also avoids the tendency for patient to succumb to treatment nihilism should the first approaches prove unsuccessful. If all else fails, simply walking the halls of the unit can offer a change of scenery, however brief, that can precipitate a change in focus away from the patient's current sensation of withdrawal. Early mobility in a safe environment builds confidence, documents functional status, and prepares a patient for a safe discharge.

Providing patients with education materials is another helpful strategy during the withdrawal of opioids. Understanding the pain pathways and how pain is generated can help reinforce validation and reassurance. Furthermore, tying the education materials into the pain-reducing strategies currently being used by the patient can improve the patient's buy-in to the clinical plan. Finally, documenting the education provided to the patient can ensure that the next provider who sees the patient does not make assumptions about what the patient does or does not know about their condition. This helps the patient to feel that they are being seen, heard, and understood by their care team.

Suggested Stepwise Withdrawal

The first step in withdrawing prescription opioids from a patient is to establish a provider-patient relationship. Buy-in to the care plan from both the patient and their family is critical to a successful withdrawal. The provider should also document reasoning for withdrawal recommendation, including patient behavior, as well as a complete medical and surgical evaluation.

Once the patient and family agree with the care team regarding the recommendation to withdraw opioids, the next step is education. Handouts may be useful to allow all parties to consider the decision, as well as to formulate any questions or concerns about the process. A discussion about the anticipated symptoms is warranted, especially the concept of hyperalgesia, i.e., the increased sensation of pain is not indicative of new pathology. Nursing staff, caretakers, and family should all be informed of the decision to withdraw opioids, as discussed previously.

Once withdrawal is initiated, the transition period should involve close monitoring for new issues and treatment of symptoms as they arise. Chronic pain and withdrawal hypersensitivity pain should be treated with non-opioid alternatives, as discussed previously. Non-pharmacologic approaches such as physical and occupational therapy, as well as cognitive behavioral therapy and ongoing education about the neurologic effects of opioids, should be utilized where appropriate.

Documentation of symptom progression is an important component in managing the withdrawal period. Functional status of patients and any occurrence of aberrant behaviors should be recorded and addressed. As patients withdrawing from opioids have a higher risk of leaving against medical advice (AMA), decision-making capacity assessments should be documented daily and before the AMA discharge. Additionally, hydration and electrolyte status should be monitored, especially in patients with ongoing diarrhea or vomiting due to the withdrawal.

Timeline of Withdrawal

Clinicians should be aware that while acute physical withdrawal lasts between 3 and 5 days, physical withdrawal symptoms can last for up to 3 months, and psychological dependence lasts years. Patients need close monitoring in the period after withdrawal to screen for relapse and ensure adequate psychosocial support. Over 90% of patients go through opioid withdrawal relapse within a month [46]. Removing any habit may take numerous attempts before success is attained.

With regard to the trajectory of medications, benzodiazepines should be weaned first to eliminate the risk of seizures. Opioids may be weaned by 25% every other day and more if tolerated. The tapering of medications for central sensitization should begin at least 1 month after cessation to give time for neural activity to calm down. They may be tapered slowly according to the patient's symptoms. All patients should be supported with naloxone, given the risk of death from relapse.

> **Key Points**
> - Withdrawal of opioids should be conducted in a stepwise fashion, with buy-in from patient and family followed by education, monitoring, and treatment of symptoms.
> - Risk of overdose and death is highest in the post-hospital period – all patients should be supported with naloxone.

Opioid Use Disorder: Diagnosis and Treatment Strategies

The correct diagnosis of opioid use disorder is only the first step of treatment. The DSM-5 classification of opioid use disorder is outlined in Table 10.3. It is also important to communicate this diagnosis to other providers, nursing staff, and insurance companies to ensure appropriate care for each patient.

OUD encompasses both opioid dependence and the more severe opioid use disorder. Dependence is associated with either physiologic or psychologic withdrawal. In contrast, opioid use disorder is characterized by compulsive drug-seeking behavior, dysfunction, and the persistent use of opioids despite adverse consequences.

Patients with OUD are often hospitalized due to the presence of new complications secondary to drug use. For these patients, the decision to wean, educate, and discontinue opioids versus the commencement of medication assisted therapy is crucial. Opioid risk assessment tools can be helpful to differentiate between acute and chronic pain and between iatrogenic opioid dependency and substance use disorder.

When considering opioid withdrawal, medications are recommended over abrupt cessation ("quitting cold-turkey"). Tapering schedules for opioid withdrawal usually last between 6 and 10 days, depending on the patient's individual need. For iatrogenic opioid dependence, a gradual taper of the patient's prescription can be undertaken. For patients with substance use disorder, a long-term approach is needed. Medication-assisted therapy may include methadone, buprenorphine, or extended-release naloxone. For the management of side effects, clonidine,

Table 10.3 DSM-5 opioid use disorder (OUD) [46]

Opiate use AND the recurrence within 12 months of ≥2 of the following:
Continued use despite worsening physical or psychological health
Continued use leading to social and interpersonal consequences
Decreased social or recreational activities
Difficulty fulfilling professional duties at school or work
Excessive time to obtain opioids or recover from taking them
More taken than intended
Presence of cravings
Withdrawal
Inability to decrease amount used
Development of tolerance
Use despite physically dangerous settings

loperamide, ondansetron, acetaminophen, and NSAIDs are appropriate [46]. The help of an addiction medicine specialists is indicated.

Patients should also be counseled on the risks of relapse and overdose, especially following discharge from the hospital, as a loss of tolerance to their usual dose of opioids can result in fatal respiratory depression if that dose is resumed. A best practice is to include a prescription of naloxone at the time of discharge. Medications that reduce the sensation of craving and thus the risk of relapse are discussed in detail below.

Medication-Assisted Therapy (MAT)

Overview

Patients with iatrogenic opioid dependence deserve a trial of abstinence (with naloxone), especially if they do not have an underlying psychiatric or attachment disorder. However, for patients with longstanding opioid use disorder, MAT has been shown to be highly effective. Chief among the benefits of MAT such as buprenorphine/naloxone is the lower rate of overdose, the decreased risk of abuse or diversion, and the increased retention of patients in treatment programs where, ideally, the psychosocial factors may also be addressed.

Importantly, if a patient is admitted to the hospital and is already on MAT, it is appropriate to continue their medication regimen throughout their stay. Whenever possible, confirm with the prescribing provider the patient's dosage schedule and active status of treatment.

Medications of MAT

Methadone is an orally administered long-acting full agonist at the mu-opioid receptor, appropriate for use in medically supervised withdrawal and maintenance of abstinence from opioids [47]. Due to the duration of occupation of the opioid receptor, methadone reduces cravings and withdrawal symptoms for an extended period of time. Additionally, methadone's occupation of the opioid receptor blunts the effects of additional opioids. Methadone is classified as a Schedule II controlled substance and, therefore, administration is limited to the acute inpatient setting and certified outpatient clinics [48].

Buprenorphine is a partial agonist at the mu-opioid receptor, weaker than full agonists such as methadone. For this reason, buprenorphine has a lower potential for misuse than other opioids [46]. By occupying the opioid receptor, buprenorphine reduces the symptoms associated with physiological dependence on opioids, such as cravings and withdrawal. Suboxone is a common formulation of buprenorphine and naloxone, which precipitates withdrawal when injected but not when taken orally. Buprenorphine is classified as a Schedule III controlled substance, which requires a waiver for physicians to prescribe, as discussed below [48].

Unlike methadone and buprenorphine, naltrexone is a competitive antagonist at the mu-opioid receptor. Its chief utility is to prevent relapse in patients who have completed medically supervised withdrawal and are no longer taking opioids. Because it binds and antagonizes the opioid receptor, naltrexone blunts both the sedative and euphoric effects of opioids but may precipitate withdrawal in patients who have unmetabolized opioids still in their system. Because it is not a controlled substance, naltrexone does not have the prescribing restrictions of other drugs used in MAT.

Barriers to MAT

Like any therapy, MAT does have its downsides. Chief among these is the need for patients to secure follow-up after their discharge from the hospital. This is compounded by the relative lack of providers with the X-license necessary to prescribe MAT. Recent announcements suggest that X-licenses may not be required for physicians in the future, but as of this writing, this is hypothetical [49].

Discharge disposition is also often a barrier, since many long-term acute care facilities and nursing homes are reluctant to take patients on MAT, due to the stereotype of opioid patients as "difficult." Paradoxically, patients receiving closer clinical attention at such facilities would be less likely to have unmet medical needs, be more adherent with enhanced supervision, and have improved outcomes and behaviors. Achieving adherence in a supervised setting is more likely to improve long-term care arrangement in the outpatient drug treatment program.

Among clinicians, there is a lack of education about the efficacy and elements of MAT, leading to a perception of a high risk involved in its use. Providers have medical legal concerns about complex laws restricting the use of medications, stigmatize and treat substance use disorders. Stemming perhaps in part from this lack of understanding, providers can be reluctant to assume the kind of partnership with their patients that is a necessary component of effective MAT [50].

In addition to individual-level stigma, access to MAT in the United States is often accompanied by structural-level stigma that negatively impacts utilization and retention in MAT programs. This is best characterized by patterns of restricted access to MAT services and low tolerance of patient noncompliance [51]. For example, MAT is not commonly provided in correctional facilities [47]. In the community setting, MAT is often administered by specialty clinics physically and ideologically separate from clinics, which treat other forms of chronic illness that are more easily treated in a primary care setting.

Further commentary on the racial and socioeconomic barriers to MAT is beyond the scope of this chapter. Clinicians should be mindful of the conditions that patients are likely to face in their communities once discharged.

Initiation of Buprenorphine

As mentioned previously, buprenorphine is a partial agonist at the mu-opioid receptor commonly used for MAT. Initiation of buprenorphine can increase the risk of precipitating acute withdrawal in patients who take opioids. It is recommended that buprenorphine be started only after current opioid medications are stopped and mild to moderate symptoms of withdrawal begin, as measured using a validated tool like the Clinical Opioid Withdrawal Scale (COWS) [52].

A typical starting dose is 2–4 mg by mouth once or twice a day, though this should be titrated up in increments of 2–4 mg until symptoms are managed for 24 hours [53]. An average daily dose of buprenorphine is 8 mg but can be as high as 16–24 mg [54]. Psychosocial treatment, such as motivational interviewing and bedside CBT, is an important adjunct to initiation of buprenorphine, as patients may benefit from the coping strategies as they adjust to a new medication regimen.

As mentioned previously, the transition of care from hospital to outpatient setting can be difficult and potentially dangerous. Ensuring the patient's seamless transition to an outpatient provider of MAT is the responsibility of the hospitalist. Once in the outpatient setting, the decision to taper off of buprenorphine may be considered. Should the patient desire tapering and eventual discontinuation of MAT, the process should be done slowly with close monitoring for symptoms of withdrawal. This is because patients are at the highest risk of mortality in the first month after discontinuation of treatment [55].

References

1. Courtwright DT. Opiate addiction as a consequence of the civil war. Civ War Hist. 1978;24(2):101–11. https://doi.org/10.1353/cwh.1978.0039.
2. Sneader W. The discovery of heroin. Lancet. 1998;352(9141):1697–9. https://doi.org/10.1016/S0140-6736(98)07115-3.
3. Robins LN, Davis DH, Nurco DN. How permanent was Vietnam drug addiction? Am J Public Health. 1974;64(Suppl 12):38–43. https://doi.org/10.2105/ajph.64.12_suppl.38.
4. Hall W, Weier M. Lee Robins' studies of heroin use among US Vietnam veterans. Addiction. 2017;112(1):176–80. https://doi.org/10.1111/add.13584.
5. Portenoy RK, Foley KM. Chronic use of opioid analgesics in non-malignant pain: report of 38 cases. Pain. 1986;25(2):171–86. https://doi.org/10.1016/0304-3959(86)90091-6.
6. Van Zee A. The promotion and marketing of oxycontin: commercial triumph, public health tragedy. Am J Public Health. 2009;99(2):221–7. https://doi.org/10.2105/AJPH.2007.131714.
7. Scalpel S. The joint commission deserves some blame for the opioid crisis. Mo Med. 2016;113(6):449.
8. Quinlan J, Cox F. Acute pain management in patients with drug dependence syndrome. Pain Rep. 2017;2(4):e611. https://doi.org/10.1097/PR9.0000000000000611.
9. Louisiana Commission on Preventing Opioid Abuse. The opioid epidemic: evidence based strategies legislative report. 2017. Retrieved from: https://ldh.la.gov/assets/docs/BehavioralHealth/Opioids/LCPOAFinalReportPkg20170331.pdf.
10. Baumgartner JC, Radley DC. The Drug overdose mortality toll in 2020 and near-term actions for addressing it. The Commonwealth Fund. 2021. Retrieved from: https://www.commonwealthfund.org/blog/2021/drug-overdose-toll-2020-and-near-term-actions-addressing-it.
11. Kalivas PW, O'Brien C. Drug addiction as a pathology of staged neuroplasticity. Neuropsychopharmacology. 2008;33(1):166–80. https://doi.org/10.1038/sj.npp.1301564.
12. Volkow ND, Koob GF, McLellan AT. Neurobiologic advances from the brain disease model of addiction. N Engl J Med. 2016;374(4):363–71. https://doi.org/10.1056/NEJMra1511480.
13. Schwartzman RJ, Grothusen J, Kiefer TR, Rohr P. Neuropathic central pain: epidemiology, etiology, and treatment options. Arch Neurol. 2001;58(10):1547–50. https://doi.org/10.1001/archneur.58.10.1547.
14. Hooten WM. Chronic pain and mental health disorders: shared neural mechanisms, epidemiology, and treatment. Mayo Clin Proc. 2016;91(7):955–70. https://doi.org/10.1016/j.mayocp.2016.04.029.
15. Lee M, Silverman SM, Hansen H, Patel VB, Manchikanti L. A comprehensive review of opioid-induced hyperalgesia. Pain Physician. 2011;14(2):145–61.
16. Gupta K, Prasad A, Nagappa M, Wong J, Abrahamyan L, Chung FF. Risk factors for opioid-induced respiratory depression and failure to rescue: a review. Curr Opin Anaesthesiol. 2018;31(1):110–9.
17. Saklad M. Grading of patients for surgical procedures. Anesthesiology. 1941;2(3):281–4. https://doi.org/10.1097/00000542-194105000-00004.
18. Dowell D, Haegerich TM, Chou R. CDC guideline for prescribing opioids for chronic pain – United States. MMWR Recomm Rep. 2016;65(1):1–49. https://doi.org/10.15585/mmwr.rr6501e1.
19. Cantrill SV, Brown MD, Carlisle RJ, Delaney KA, Hays DP, Nelson LS, O'Connor RE, Papa A, Sporer KA, Todd KH, Whitson RR, American College of Emergency Physicians Opioid Guideline Writing P. Clinical policy: critical issues in the prescribing of opioids for adult patients in the emergency department. Ann Emerg Med. 2012;60(4):499–525. https://doi.org/10.1016/j.annemergmed.2012.06.013.
20. Substance Abuse and Mental Health Services Administration. Opioid overdose prevention TOOLKIT. 2018. Retrieved from: https://store.samhsa.gov/sites/default/files/d7/priv/sma18-4742.pdf.

21. Wardhan R, Chelly J. Recent advances in acute pain management: understanding the mechanisms of acute pain, the prescription of opioids, and the role of multimodal pain therapy. F1000Res. 2017;6:2065. https://doi.org/10.12688/f1000research.12286.1.
22. American Society of Anesthesiologists Task Force on Acute Pain M. Practice guidelines for acute pain management in the perioperative setting: an updated report by the American Society of Anesthesiologists Task Force on acute pain management. Anesthesiology. 2012;116(2):248–73. https://doi.org/10.1097/ALN.0b013e31823c1030.
23. Maund E, McDaid C, Rice S, Wright K, Jenkins B, Woolacott N. Paracetamol and selective and non-selective non-steroidal anti-inflammatory drugs for the reduction in morphine-related side-effects after major surgery: a systematic review. Br J Anaesth. 2011;106(3):292–7. https://doi.org/10.1093/bja/aeq406.
24. Wong I, St John-Green C, Walker SM. Opioid-sparing effects of perioperative paracetamol and nonsteroidal anti-inflammatory drugs (NSAIDs) in children. Paediatr Anaesth. 2013;23(6):475–95. https://doi.org/10.1111/pan.12163.
25. Varrassi G, Pergolizzi JV, Dowling P, Paladini A. Ibuprofen safety at the Golden anniversary: are all NSAIDs the same? A narrative review. Adv Ther. 2020;37(1):61–82. https://doi.org/10.1007/s12325-019-01144-9.
26. Castellsague J, Riera-Guardia N, Calingaert B, Varas-Lorenzo C, Fourrier-Reglat A, Nicotra F, Sturkenboom M, Perez-Gutthann S, Safety of Non-Steroidal Anti-Inflammatory Drugs P. Individual NSAIDs and upper gastrointestinal complications: a systematic review and meta-analysis of observational studies (the SOS project). Drug Saf. 2012;35(12):1127–46.
27. Masso Gonzalez EL, Patrignani P, Tacconelli S, Garcia Rodriguez LA. Variability among nonsteroidal antiinflammatory drugs in risk of upper gastrointestinal bleeding. Arthritis Rheum. 2010;62(6):1592–601. https://doi.org/10.1002/art.27412.
28. Ennis ZN, Dideriksen D, Vaegter HB, Handberg G, Pottegard A. Acetaminophen for chronic pain: a systematic review on efficacy. Basic Clin Pharmacol Toxicol. 2016;118(3):184–9. https://doi.org/10.1111/bcpt.12527.
29. Ong CK, Seymour RA, Lirk P, Merry AF. Combining paracetamol (acetaminophen) with nonsteroidal antiinflammatory drugs: a qualitative systematic review of analgesic efficacy for acute postoperative pain. Anesth Analg. 2010;110(4):1170–9. https://doi.org/10.1213/ANE.0b013e3181cf9281.
30. Jibril F, Sharaby S, Mohamed A, Wilby KJ. Intravenous versus oral acetaminophen for pain: systematic review of current evidence to support clinical decision-making. Can J Hosp Pharm. 2015;68(3):238–47. https://doi.org/10.4212/cjhp.v68i3.1458.
31. Duehmke RM, Derry S, Wiffen PJ, Bell RF, Aldington D, Moore RA. Tramadol for neuropathic pain in adults. Cochrane Database Syst Rev. 2017;6:CD003726. https://doi.org/10.1002/14651858.CD003726.pub4.
32. Lassen D, Damkier P, Brosen K. The pharmacogenetics of tramadol. Clin Pharmacokinet. 2015;54(8):825–36. https://doi.org/10.1007/s40262-015-0268-0.
33. Shah K, Stout B, Caskey H. Tramadol for the management of opioid withdrawal: a systematic review of randomized clinical trials. Cureus. 2020;12(7):e9128. https://doi.org/10.7759/cureus.9128.
34. Jones JL, Mateus CF, Malcolm RJ, Brady KT, Back SE. Efficacy of ketamine in the treatment of substance use disorders: a systematic review. Front Psych. 2018;9:277. https://doi.org/10.3389/fpsyt.2018.00277.
35. Shin HJ, Na HS, Do SH. Magnesium and pain. Nutrients. 2020;12(8):2184. https://doi.org/10.3390/nu12082184.
36. Kamp J, Van Velzen M, Olofsen E, Boon M, Dahan A, Niesters M. Pharmacokinetic and pharmacodynamic considerations for NMDA-receptor antagonist ketamine in the treatment of chronic neuropathic pain: an update of the most recent literature. Expert Opin Drug Metab Toxicol. 2019;15(12):1033–41. https://doi.org/10.1080/17425255.2019.1689958.
37. Hah J, Mackey SC, Schmidt P, McCue R, Humphreys K, Trafton J, Efron B, Clay D, Sharifzadeh Y, Ruchelli G, Goodman S, Huddleston J, Maloney WJ, Dirbas FM, Shrager J,

Costouros JG, Curtin C, Carroll I. Effect of perioperative gabapentin on postoperative pain resolution and opioid cessation in a mixed surgical cohort: a randomized clinical trial. JAMA Surg. 2018;153(4):303–11. https://doi.org/10.1001/jamasurg.2017.4915.
38. Finnerup NB, Attal N, Haroutounian S, McNicol E, Baron R, Dworkin RH, Gilron I, Haanpaa M, Hansson P, Jensen TS, Kamerman PR, Lund K, Moore A, Raja SN, Rice AS, Rowbotham M, Sena E, Siddall P, Smith BH, Wallace M. Pharmacotherapy for neuropathic pain in adults: a systematic review and meta-analysis. Lancet Neurol. 2015;14(2):162–73. https://doi.org/10.1016/S1474-4422(14)70251-0.
39. Evoy KE, Morrison MD, Saklad SR. Abuse and misuse of pregabalin and gabapentin. Drugs. 2017;77(4):403–26. https://doi.org/10.1007/s40265-017-0700-x.
40. Oldfield V, Perry CM. Oxycodone/ibuprofen combination tablet: a review of its use in the management of acute pain. Drugs. 2005;65(16):2337–54. https://doi.org/10.2165/00003495-200565160-00011.
41. Derry S, Derry CJ, Moore RA (2013) Single dose oral ibuprofen plus oxycodone for acute postoperative pain in adults. Cochrane Database Syst Rev (6):CD010289. https://doi.org/10.1002/14651858.CD010289.pub2.
42. Kandarian BS, Elkassabany NM, Tamboli M, Mariano ER. Updates on multimodal analgesia and regional anesthesia for total knee arthroplasty patients. Best Pract Res Clin Anaesthesiol. 2019;33(1):111–23. https://doi.org/10.1016/j.bpa.2019.02.004.
43. Emelife PI, Eng MR, Menard BL, Myers AS, Cornett EM, Urman RD, Kaye AD. Adjunct medications for peripheral and neuraxial anesthesia. Best Pract Res Clin Anaesthesiol. 2018;32(2):83–99. https://doi.org/10.1016/j.bpa.2018.06.011.
44. Williams L, Iteld L. Moving toward opioid-free breast surgery: regional blocks and a novel technique. Clin Plast Surg. 2021;48(1):123–30. https://doi.org/10.1016/j.cps.2020.09.003.
45. Garland EL, Brintz CE, Hanley AW, Roseen EJ, Atchley RM, Gaylord SA, Faurot KR, Yaffe J, Fiander M, Keefe FJ. Mind-body therapies for opioid-treated pain: a systematic review and meta-analysis. JAMA Intern Med. 2020;180(1):91–105. https://doi.org/10.1001/jamainternmed.2019.4917.
46. Dydyk AM, Jain NK, Gupta M. Opioid use disorder. In: StatPearls. Treasure Island. 2021.
47. Moore KE, Roberts W, Reid HH, Smith KMZ, Oberleitner LMS, McKee SA. Effectiveness of medication assisted treatment for opioid use in prison and jail settings: a meta-analysis and systematic review. J Subst Abus Treat. 2019;99:32–43. https://doi.org/10.1016/j.jsat.2018.12.003.
48. Preuss CV, Kalava A, King KC. Prescription of controlled substances: benefits and risks. In: StatPearls. Treasure Island. 2021.
49. D'Onofrio G, Melnick ER, Hawk KF. Improve access to care for opioid use disorder: a call to eliminate the X-waiver requirement now. Ann Emerg Med. 2021;78(2):220–2. https://doi.org/10.1016/j.annemergmed.2021.03.023.
50. Madden EF. Intervention stigma: how medication-assisted treatment marginalizes patients and providers. Soc Sci Med. 2019;232:324–31. https://doi.org/10.1016/j.socscimed.2019.05.027.
51. McElrath K. Medication-assisted treatment for opioid addiction in the United States: critique and commentary. Subst Use Misuse. 2018;53(2):334–43. https://doi.org/10.1080/10826084.2017.1342662.
52. Wesson DR, Ling W. The Clinical Opiate Withdrawal Scale (COWS). J Psychoactive Drugs. 2003;35(2):253–9. https://doi.org/10.1080/02791072.2003.10400007.
53. Cisewski DH, Santos C, Koyfman A, Long B. Approach to buprenorphine use for opioid withdrawal treatment in the emergency setting. Am J Emerg Med. 2019;37(1):143–50. https://doi.org/10.1016/j.ajem.2018.10.013.
54. Kapuganti A, Turner T, Thomas CJ. Evaluation of buprenorphine/naloxone dose and use of sedating supportive medication on treatment outcomes in veterans with opioid use disorder. Ment Health Clin. 2017;7(6):271–5. https://doi.org/10.9740/mhc.2017.11.271.
55. National Academies of Sciences E, Medicine, Health, Medicine D, Board on Health Sciences P, Committee on Pain M, et al. In: Phillips JK, Ford MA, Bonnie RJ, editors. Pain management and the opioid epidemic: balancing societal and individual benefits and risks of prescription opioid use. Washington, D.C., 2017. https://doi.org/10.17226/24781.

Chapter 11
Overview, Updates, and New Topics in Perioperative Care

Lakshmi N. Prasad Ravipati and Marisa Doran

Introduction

Perioperative care encompasses the care of a patient before, during, and after undergoing a surgical procedure. The aim of this chapter is to discuss the components of perioperative care, the methods for risk assessment of predictable complications and outcomes, and optimization of patient's chronic medical conditions. Furthermore, this chapter will discuss updates in newer topics, such as the role of prehabilitation and new challenges faced with the current COVID-19 pandemic.

The utilization of perioperative care within a healthcare system holds a critical role not only at the individual patient level but also at the scale of the hospital system. Proper perioperative care has the ability to improve patient outcomes through preoperative counseling, education, optimizing patient's chronic conditions, improved operating room efficiency through avoidance of same day surgery cancellations, shorter length of hospital stays, improved communication among different providers, appropriate documentation of patient's comorbidities, successful coordination of postoperative care, improvement in long-term health outcomes, reduction in in-hospital mortality and reduced costs for healthcare systems [1].

L. N. Prasad Ravipati (✉)
Perioperative Care Center, Ochsner Health, New Orleans, LA, USA
e-mail: lravipati@ochsner.org

M. Doran
University of Queensland-Ochsner Clinical School, New Orleans, LA, USA

© The Author(s), under exclusive license to Springer Nature Switzerland AG 2022
K. Conrad (ed.), *Clinical Approaches to Hospital Medicine*,
https://doi.org/10.1007/978-3-030-95164-1_11

What Is Perioperative Care?

The Role of the Medical Team in Perioperative Care

Perioperative care traditionally involved the surgical team performing the procedure, the anesthesiologist performing an evaluation. Therefore, a lot of patients expect to see the Anesthesiologist during the preoperative assessment. Now, there is a greater movement toward a multifaceted and multidisciplinary approach in perioperative care. The perioperative assessment includes the evaluation by the primary care provider (Internist/Family medicine doctor), or relevant subspecialists such as a Cardiologist or Pulmonologist, along with other ancillary staff. The ancillary care team may include dietitians, physical therapists, occupational therapists, mental health therapists, smoking cessation specialists, and social workers who assist in the risk assessment and risk modification of patients prior to undergoing surgery [2]. There is an emphasis on prehabilitation that focuses on improving functional health through addressing physical unfitness, malnutrition, and cognitive assessment to avoid postoperative debility and improve recovery [3].

The risk assessment process involves collecting information about surgical and anesthetic factors in conjunction with patient factors. This includes anesthesia type, the extent and duration of the surgical procedure. Patient factors range from demographic information like age, lifestyle, ability to perform physical activities, availability of support from family, and friends to help with recovery and other comorbidities. The goal is to understand how each of these factors interact such that predictable possible complications are avoided, risk is minimized, and the recovery is optimized. This allows for the patient, their family, care givers, and the operating team to make an informed medical decision.

The Preoperative Clinic Medical Evaluation, Assessment, and Plan

During the preoperative clinic visit, it is important to understand that the structure and goal is like that of an Internal/Family medicine clinic visit, but with specific emphasis on the patient's chronic preexisting medical conditions and the goal of optimizing the patient for surgery. Our current population is aging, and older patient groups are becoming increasingly more burdened by multiple comorbid health conditions [4]. Young, healthy individuals require surgeries less often.

The surgical problem for the patient can be from almost any system, including but not limited to Orthopedic, Urological, Gynecological, ENT, abdominal, thoracic, head and neck, spine, plastic, breast, ophthalmic, or cardiovascular. After obtaining the immediate history that led up to the patient's need for surgery, the review of systems extends beyond the focus of the surgical problem to be addressed, tactically focusing on the presence of any risk factors for surgery. At this point, it is essential to emphasize the importance of documentation of the visit. The preoperative clinic note plays a very important role. It should not be overlooked as a routine history and physical but rather considered an effective tool of communication between the different members of the perioperative care team, in addition to appropriately documenting the patient's comorbidities. It has the interest of patient safety at the core. The preoperative medical evaluation/consultation note serves to document all the chronic medical conditions that the patient has, as a problem list in the electronic health record, such that the true state of the patient's health is being reflected. This helps not only with the care of the patient but also with hospital reimbursement.

When taking a patient history, it is important to have a routine, such as a checklist or template so that important aspects of patient's health are not missed. The review of systems, although comprehensive, can be tailored to obtain a focused history of relevant factors of perioperative care. The following can serve as an outline for the review of systems, as it will be broken down into specific body systems with conditions to focus on, along with risk factors and risk assessment tools.

Perioperative Cardiac Disease and Risk Assessment

Relevant aspects of the patient's history for cardiac evaluation include any preexisting heart disease such as coronary artery disease (CAD), heart failure, valvular disease, arrhythmias, renal disease, and diabetes mellitus. The presence of cerebrovascular disease can be concerning for related vascular disease like CAD or peripheral arterial disease. The assessment must also determine the stability of the known cardiac conditions or if there are any new acute cardiac conditions, like that of unstable coronary artery syndromes or decompensated heart failure. There is importance in performing a thorough cardiovascular examination. Greater cardiac risk is associated with high-risk surgeries, such as vascular, intraperitoneal, and intrathoracic procedures. The functional status of the patient is also important to assess. This can be done by asking about the patient's physical activity.

Risk assessment models for noncardiac surgery patients include the Revised Cardiac Risk Index (RCRI) [5], American College of Surgeons National Surgical Quality Improvement risk (ACS-NSQUIP), and the Myocardial Infarction and Risk calculator (MICA NSQUIP) database risk model [6]. The RCRI includes six factors: high-risk surgery, history of ischemic heart disease (IHD), history of congestive heart failure (CHF), history of cerebrovascular disease, preoperative treatment with insulin, and preoperative serum creatinine >2.0 mg/dL. Recommendations include utilizing the RCRI in conjunction with MICA-NSQUIP because they provide complementary prognostics [7].

Pulmonary Disease, Risk Assessment, and Complications

Thorough evaluation of pulmonary risk factors can help identify patients at risk of postoperative complications. Risk factors include older age, dependent functional status, American Society of Anesthesiologist (ASA) class >2, chronic obstructive pulmonary disease (COPD), pulmonary hypertension, and heart failure. Screening for sleep apnea can be done by STOPBANG questions-assessing for loud snoring, tiredness, observed apnea, high blood pressure, BMI >35, age > 50 years, neck circumference > 40 cm, and male gender [8]. Pulse oximetry, chest radiographs, pulmonary function tests, and exercise testing may be helpful to determine the severity of known pulmonary conditions. Closer proximity of surgical site to the lung, as in upper abdominal procedures, longer procedures, and use of general anesthesia over regional anesthesia also increase risk. Possible postoperative complications include atelectasis, bronchospasm, pneumonia, pulmonary edema, pulmonary embolism, aspiration, postoperative respiratory failure requiring ventilatory support, and exacerbation or worsening of preexisting lung conditions such as sleep apnea or COPD. The route of surgical approach is also an important consideration now that there are advances in laparoscopic and robotic-assisted procedures. The decision for approach may consider cosmetic outcomes, type of surgery, and the patient's medical and surgical history. For example, laparoscopic approach in patients with COPD has been shown to have less postoperative complications and shorter length of hospital stay [9].

Pulmonary risk prediction tools include the Assess Respiratory Risk in Surgical Patients in CANET (ARISCAT) risk index [10], Arozullah respiratory failure index, and the Gupta calculators for postoperative respiratory failure and pneumonia [10, 11].

To improve pulmonary status in the perioperative period, several measures can be suggested to the patient. Prior to surgery, patients with relevant conditions are counseled on tobacco cessation, scheduled use of inhaler treatment and inhaler technique reinforcement, optimizing medical management for COPD based on disease severity with long-acting beta-agonists, inhaled corticosteroid use, long-acting muscarinic antagonists, inspiratory muscle training, increasing physical activity, use of mucolytic/expectorant treatment, and weight loss, in relevant patients. The physician may also work with the surgeon on the surgical approach, i.e., if laparoscopic, advise that low head position and abdominal insufflation may be a risk factor in patients with lung disease. In the postoperative period, it is beneficial to minimize the use of sedating medications such as opioids or benzodiazepines. Anesthesiologists can consider use of a regional block to reduce the need for systemic opioid treatment, use opioid sparing analgesia, avoid diaphragmatic splinting in upper abdominal procedures through adequate pain control, avoid use of excessive FiO2 as it can reduce the hypoxic respiratory drive in patients with hypoxic hypercapnic respiratory failure, and consider empirical treatment with CPAP if there is a high index of suspicion for sleep apnea. The surgical team may consult respiratory therapy and physical therapy and encourage deep breathing exercises, early ambulation, incentive spirometer use, oral care, and rest with head of bed elevated [12]. This is in addition to having the patient in a monitored care area so that hemodynamic and respiratory status can be closely monitored.

Renal Disease, Risk Assessment, and Complications

The patient's history of kidney disease is an important aspect of the perioperative renal risk assessment. Not only is preexisting renal disease a risk factor for acute kidney injury in the perioperative period, but the history of chronic renal insufficiency or end stage renal disease-requires additional attention. Acute kidney injury (AKI), defined as a rapid loss of renal function, is normally identified in the postoperative period by an increase in serum creatinine from the patient's baseline and decreased urine output. Risk factors for AKI in the surgical setting include high-risk surgeries such as transplant, abdominal aortic surgery, emergency surgery, cardiac valve surgery [13], preexisting chronic kidney disease, diabetes mellitus, congestive heart failure, peripheral vascular disease, and postoperative hypotension. Measures to reduce the risk of AKI include utilizing minimally invasive surgical techniques [14], optimizing volume status, ensuring renal perfusion through maintenance of adequate hemodynamic status, and avoiding nephrotoxic medications. These include, but are not limited to, nonsteroidal anti-inflammatory agents (NSAIDs), radio contrast agents, aminoglycosides, and amphotericin.

Patients with chronic kidney disease have a significant risk of perioperative complications with high morbidity and mortality. Complications include hyperkalemia, infections, arrhythmias, and bleeding [15]. There are also special considerations for patients on hemodialysis or peritoneal dialysis. Surgery should be scheduled such that it follows the hemodialysis day, or the hemodialysis regimen is adjusted such that it is scheduled the day before surgery. It is beneficial for the patient to be at their dry weight prior to surgery and the dialysis prescription to allow for serum electrolytes to be as close to normal as possible. For peritoneal dialysis patients, it is recommended that additional dialysis is done in the 48–72 hours prior to surgery [16]. There is also a benefit in aiming for peritoneal dialysis patients to be at their dry weight prior to surgery, as fluids are typically given for treatment of postoperative hypotension that is likely caused by anesthetic agents. The decision to restart peritoneal dialysis will depend on type of surgery and the surgeon's preference, with possible interval hemodialysis [17]. There are no specific guidelines on the continuation of angiotensin converting enzyme (ACE) inhibitors and angiotensin receptor blockers. There is some research that recommends withholding those medications on the morning of surgery for reduction in risk of hypotension [18].

Postoperative urinary retention is a common problem for some. It can lead to bladder overdistention, urinary tract infections, and catheterizations [19]. Urinary retention is more common in older or male patients, in patients with benign prostatic hyperplasia, and in preexisting neurological conditions such as multiple sclerosis or cerebral palsy. Medications that may predispose to urinary retention include opioids, anticholinergic agents, and sympathomimetics. The score risk for postoperative urinary retention can be calculated based on surgery length, congestive heart failure, low BMI, diabetes mellitus, and beta-blocker use [20]. The decision for timing of removal of urinary catheterization remains controversial. Earlier removal places patients at risk of urinary retention that requires re-catheterization [21]. However, longer catheterization places patients at risk of catheter-associated urinary tract infections. It is advised that select patients with risk factors for postoperative urinary retention receive alpha-1a antagonists to avoid re-catheterization.

Liver Disease and Risk Assessment

The risk of morbidity and mortality is increased in patients with chronic liver disease that undergo surgery. Tools for calculation of risk in surgical patients with liver disease include the model of end-stage liver disease (MELD) score [22], Child-Turcotte-Pugh score, and the Mayo risk score. The inputs for calculation of Mayo risk score include age, ASA score as either compensated or decompensated liver disease, bilirubin, creatinine, INR, and the etiology of cirrhosis (alcohol, cholestatic, viral or other). The outputs are probability of mortality at 7 days, 30 days, 90 days, 1 year, and 5 years. There is observation that the use of the Mayo risk score may overestimate surgical risk in liver disease patients [23]. The VOCAL-Penn model has improved postoperative mortality prediction in cirrhotic patients compared to the risk assessment models. VOCAL-Penn variables include the age, total bilirubin, surgery category, emergency surgery indication, preoperative albumin, platelet count, and presence of obesity and fatty liver disease. This prediction tool gives postoperative predicted mortality at 30, 90, and 180 days [24].

Neurological and Musculoskeletal Disease: Delirium, Frailty, and Functional Status

Delirium is a common neurological complication that can occur in the postoperative period. Delirium is associated with prolonged hospital stay and increased mortality. It is more common in older patients and in those with a history of dementia. Other important aspects of the patient's medical history to elicit include prior episodes of delirium or confusion, reduced mobility, chronic opioid use, and chronic benzodiazepine use. Measures to avoid delirium in the postoperative period include minimization or avoidance, if possible, of certain medications. This includes benzodiazepines, anticholinergics, antihistamines such as Benadryl, and opioid medications. Opioids should be used in the lowest possible doses and for the shortest duration possible. The use of multimodal analgesia is also beneficial to reduce opioid use. Other measures include maintaining a normal sleep/wake cycle by keeping window shades open during the day and closed at night, and the use of a clock and calendar in the room for orientation. It is also important to encourage the presence of family members to assist with reorientation of the patient and to alert medical staff should there be deviations from baseline mental status. Smaller changes in mentation are more easily detected by family members. Assessment and preventative measures are the current best methods, along with measures to return the patient to their normal daily routine [25].

Frailty is considered a risk factor for perioperative delirium but also a risk for surgical complications. Frailty describes a patient's decrease in physical function and can involve malnutrition, loss of muscle mass, or inflammation depending on the individual patient's clinical picture. There are different tools that can be used to assess a patient's frailty, with the Clinical Frailty Scale supported with strong evidence [26]. The Clinical Frailty Scale includes 9 points ranging from very fit to terminally ill [27]. Other methods for assessing frailty can include evaluation of functional status. This can include a Timed Up and Go and examining ambulation and transfers [28]. Identifying patients with reduced functional status and frailty is important, as these patients are more likely to have postoperative complications such as further functional decline and increased morbidity and mortality. Identification of such individuals can provide insight into the necessity for a prehabilitation program [29]. These programs include physical therapy and nutrition and have been shown to reduce lengths of hospital stay and readmission rates [30].

Hematological Conditions and Anticoagulation

Patients with a history of atrial fibrillation, artificial heart valves, or a history of thrombosis likely take oral anticoagulation therapy. With surgery, this then places them at risk of excessive bleeding with continuing anticoagulation that must be balanced with their risk of thromboembolic complications, when withholding anticoagulation for surgery. For patients on vitamin K antagonists, e.g., warfarin, it is common to instruct patients to discontinue the medication 5–7 days before surgery and is most often safe to resume the evening or morning after surgery. Some patients deemed to be at a higher risk when withholding anticoagulation for surgery may use low-molecular-weight heparin (LMWH) or unfractionated heparin as bridging therapy prior to surgery. There is, however, no consensus between a difference of risk of thromboembolic complications in either treatment strategy.

Use of direct oral anticoagulants (DOACs) is a far newer anticoagulation therapy. General recommendation is to discontinue use 1 day prior to surgery with a low bleeding risk and 2 days prior to surgery with a high bleeding risk, with resumption after 24 hours and 48–72 hours, respectively. It is important to note whether the patient has renal dysfunction, as this can affect clearance of the medication. The use of perioperative laboratory testing for DOAC levels is not standard. There is not a clear interpretation and standardization guideline of the laboratory results and no consensus on the utility of the results [31]. For reversal of direct factor Xa inhibitors, e.g., rivaroxaban and apixaban, the FDA has approved the use of andexanet alfa but only in adults with life threatening or uncontrolled bleeding. It has yet to be studied in other contexts [32]. Idarucizumab is an FDA-approved specific reversal agent for, dabigatran, a direct thrombin inhibitor [33].

Management of anticoagulation prior to surgery may deviate from the above procedures in patients with other underlying hypercoagulable states. Patients with antiphospholipid syndrome are at increased risk of thrombosis [34]. In patients with high therapeutic INR targets on warfarin, it is recommended to discontinue treatment 7 days prior to surgery and start bridging therapy with either unfractionated heparin or LMWH. LMWH can be used up to 24 hours prior to surgery. Unfractionated heparin can be administered up to 4–6 hours before surgery [34]. An individualized plan should be determined and communicated with each member of the team, the provider managing anticoagulation, and, most importantly, the patient. This is another instance of the importance of clear and thorough documentation.

Anemia and thrombocytopenia may be encountered in the preoperative assessment; screening for low hemoglobin is not typically recommended but should be performed based on the clinical context. Although various transfusion guidelines exist, the current threshold for red blood cell transfusion is a hemoglobin level of 6–8 g/dL, and typically not performed when >10 g/dL [35]. Platelet count thresholds may differ depending on the type of procedure to be performed. Platelet count threshold is typically $>20 \times 10^9/l$ in venous central lines, $>40 \times 10^9$ in lumbar puncture, $>80 \times 10^9$ for insertion or removal of epidural catheter, $>50 \times 10^9$ in major surgery, $>100 \times 10^9$ in neurosurgery or ophthalmic surgery, and $> 50 \times 10^9$ in percutaneous liver biopsy. If the platelet count drops below that threshold, platelet transfusion may be indicated [36].

Endocrine: Steroid Use and Diabetes Mellitus

Encountering a patient with a history of long-term glucocorticoid therapy is not uncommon. This chronic therapy places them at risk of an insufficient adrenal response during stress or surgery. Therefore, some patients may require a stress dose of steroids. There is no strict set of guidelines to follow, but current best treatment includes an individualized approach. Most patients are kept on their current baseline dosage of steroid therapy and will not require a high-dose corticosteroid [37]. More research into this area is needed.

For patients with a history of diabetes mellitus (DM), there are multiple aspects that need to be considered. CAD is more common in this population, and there should be focus on assessing blood glucose control and presence of diabetic complications. DM is associated with higher risk of 6-month postoperative mortality, major complications, ICU admission, mechanical ventilation, and longer length of stay. Furthermore, higher hemoglobin A1c (HbA1c) is associated with poorer surgical outcomes [38]. Achieving a HbA1c < 8.5% is typically considered acceptable prior to surgery, although long-term goal is <7% to indicate adequate glycemic control. Perioperative glucose control is another important aspect to manage to reduce risk of perioperative complications. It is important to ask patients about their insulin regimen and whether the patient is using an insulin pump, as this requires different management. Although insulin pumps can be used during the perioperative period, there needs to be consideration for the fasting state that patients require prior to surgery. If possible, it is best to minimize time fasted by scheduling elective surgeries in diabetic patients early in the morning. Prior to surgery, these patients require a basal assessment which will establish whether they have a stable blood glucose concentration in the fasting state. The optimal target for blood sugar has some controversy, overall. It differs for minor and major procedures and in the critically ill patient. Working with an endocrinologist is highly recommended [39]. Patients that have been unable to achieve glucose control on metformin alone may also be taking sodium glucose cotransporter 2 (SGLT2) inhibitors. This medication should be stopped 3 days prior to surgery due to risk of euglycemic diabetic ketoacidosis [40].

Connective Tissue Disorders

A history of connective tissue disease is another important aspect of perioperative care. Connective tissue disorders include a broad array of systems and are relevant to discuss here because of these patient's frequent need for orthopedic surgery. Patients are at an increased risk for cardiac and pulmonary complications and require evaluation of other risk factors [41]. For example, patients with rheumatoid arthritis are at risk of cervical spine involvement; therefore, screening with flexion and extension radiographs of the cervical spine to assess atlantoaxial instability is recommended. In patients with systemic lupus erythematosus (SLE) and antiphospholipid syndrome, use of anticoagulation prophylaxis should be considered.

Surgical Site Infections

The surgical site is important to consider in the context of avoidance of infection and optimization of wound healing. Risk factors for poor wound healing include a history of peripheral arterial disease, venous insufficiency, prior infection, radiation, presence of prostheses, diabetes mellitus, obesity, sickle cell disease, tobacco use, and malnutrition, most which have been discussed above. Surgical site infection prevention includes use of intravenous prophylactic antibiotics within 1 hour before incision, glucose control, and maintenance of normothermia. Other strategies include preoperative bathing with an antimicrobial body wash and compliance of healthcare personnel with handwashing throughout patient interactions [42].

Medication Review

Obtaining an accurate medication history is a key part of the perioperative assessment. Best possible medication history includes patients bringing in each of the medications they take, inclusive of over-the-counter vitamins and supplements. The involvement of a pharmacist at this stage has also proven to be helpful [43]. As discussed in prior sections, focus on anticoagulants and antiplatelet agents is essential. It is also important to consider medications that a patient has been taking over a long period of time. Complications can occur with abrupt cessation of a medication for surgery [44]. The continuation of beta-blockers in the perioperative period needs careful consideration. In general, if a patient is taking a beta-blocker, it should be continued in the perioperative period.

The patient's substance use history is an important aspect of the preoperative evaluation. This includes alcohol and tobacco. Risky alcohol intake, which is approximately 2–3 standard drinks per day, is linked to postoperative complications such as increased overall morbidity, general infections, wound complications, and pulmonary complications [45]. Tools for assessing alcohol misuse include the Alcohol Use Disorders Identification Test Consumption (AUDIT-C) and the CAGE questionnaire [46, 47]. Abstinence from alcohol is recommended for 4–8 weeks prior to surgery, as even short-term avoidance is associated with decreased risk postoperatively [45]. Smoking, in addition to pulmonary complications, also places the patient at risk of surgical anastomoses, nonunion, wound complications, and delayed fracture healing. Patients are recommended to quit smoking 8 weeks prior to surgery [48]. It is important to recommend for any patient that is currently using tobacco to quit, although most patients are already aware of the risks of smoking. Suggested methods to help patients quit smoking include referral to a smoking cessation service, use of nicotine replacement therapy (NRT), behavioral support, and advice from many members of the perioperative care team [48]. For patients that refuse overall cessation, even discussion about short-term abstinence or reduction in frequency of smoking is beneficial and could lead to cessation later [48].

Laboratory Investigations

Following a focused history and physical examination, the next step during the perioperative assessment is to decide if further investigations are necessary prior to surgery. This is a critical decision, as ordering more tests increases the possibility of an abnormal results, requiring potential further testing or intervention. This can lead to healthcare expenditure beyond what is necessary. In general, for patients with American Society of Anesthesiology Score of I or II and undergoing low-risk procedures, there is no need for laboratory testing if there is not a change in their clinical condition [49]. A one-size-fits-all, capture-all approach is not appropriate in this situation. Be prudent.

ERAS Protocols and Perioperative Surgical Home

Enhanced recovery after surgery (ERAS) protocols are developed pathways used in multidisciplinary teams to reduce the patient's surgical stress response, maximize physiologic function, and aid recovery. ERAS has benefits in reducing length of hospital stays without an increase in readmission [50], morbidity, or mortality. This overall has positive financial implications [51].

The Perioperative Surgical Home (PSH) is a system that aims to incorporate each stage of the surgical experience smoothly without discontinuity of care. This is especially useful in managing patients with opioid tolerance. Strategies for managing opioid-tolerant patients begin in the preoperative period and throughout the postoperative period. This includes the use of multimodal analgesia regimens such as perineural catheters and addition of NSAIDs [52].

COVID-19

Undergoing surgery during the current setting of the COVID-19 pandemic is not without risk. There is a possibility of increased mortality following surgery, as well as possible risk of contracting COVID in the hospital setting [53]. It is therefore necessary for all surgical patients to obtain COVID testing prior to surgery, in addition to undergoing screening based on exposure risk and prevalence of infection in the community [54]. The decision to undergo surgery can be considered in the context of the urgency of the procedure and explained to the patient for informed consent [55]. The management of COVID-19 in perioperative care is constantly being influenced by new research and implementation of new hospital policies. There are still many unknowns remaining.

Advanced Care Planning and Informed Consent

The discussion with the patient and their family about the risks of undergoing surgery and the importance of gaining consent should not be overlooked. With any surgical procedure, there is a risk of complication and death. There is a distinct difference between informed consent and "clearance" for surgery. Individual patients with different comorbidities and different reasons for undergoing surgery may have different views of their risk of surgery. It is the job of the perioperative medicine team to explain to the patient these factors, such that they can weigh up for themselves whether they are willing to undergo surgery based on the risk assessment. Especially in high-risk surgeries, it is important to have a discussion of advanced care planning (ACP). This includes the patient's goals and values, what they prefer for treatment, and who will be their surrogate decision-maker [56]. Difficult discussions such as these are better suited prior to surgery when there is less likely to be a conflict of emotions.

Conclusion

This chapter discussed the role of perioperative medical, subspecialist, and ancillary evaluations for patients planning to undergo surgery. Each major system from cardiac and pulmonary through to endocrine, etc. was discussed from obtaining past medical history, assessing disease severity, and the methods of risk assessment. Apart from focusing only on risk assessment of medical complications, efforts should be put in to optimize the patient's chronic medical conditions. If a determination is made that the patient is at risk of a postoperative complication, this should be documented in the chart, along with suggested measures to reduce the risk of that complication. This serves to guide the multiple other members of the patient care team to work together toward prevention of predictable complications. Utilizing a thorough and systematic approach and embracing the nature of teamwork is key in this increasingly complex field of medicine. We discussed risk assessment for Cardiac Disease; Pulmonary Disease; Renal Disease; liver disease, Neurological and Musculoskeletal Disease: Delirium, Frailty, and Functional Status; Hematological Conditions; Endocrine: Steroid Use and Diabetes Mellitus; Connective Tissue Disorders; Surgical Site Infections; Medication Review; Laboratory Investigations; COVID-19; ERAS Protocols and Perioperative Surgical Home; and Advanced Care Planning and informed consent. The methods for improved assessment of patients may constantly be in development and changing, but the goal is the same: optimization of the patient prior to surgery.

References

1. Blitz JDMD, Mabry CMD. Designing and running a preoperative clinic. Anesthesiol Clin. 2018;36(4):479–91. https://doi.org/10.1016/j.anclin.2018.07.001.
2. Carli F, Baldini G, Feldman LS. Redesigning the preoperative clinic: from risk stratification to risk modification. JAMA Surg. 2020. https://doi.org/10.1001/jamasurg.2020.5550.
3. Carli F. Prehabilitation for the anesthesiologist. Anesthesiology. 2020;133(3):645–52. https://doi.org/10.1097/ALN.0000000000003331.
4. Ofori-Asenso R, Chin KL, Curtis AJ, Zomer E, Zoungas S, Liew D. Recent patterns of multimorbidity among older adults in high-income countries. Popul Health Manag. 2019;22(2):127–37. https://doi.org/10.1089/pop.2018.0069.
5. Lee TH, Marcantonio ER, Ludwig LE, Pedan A, Goldman L, Mangione CM, Thomas EJ, Polanczyk CA, Cook EF, Sugarbaker DJ, Donaldson MC, Poss R, Ho KKL. Derivation and prospective validation of a simple index for prediction of cardiac risk of major noncardiac surgery. Circulation. 1999;100(10):1043–9. https://doi.org/10.1161/01.CIR.100.10.1043.
6. Bilimoria KY, Liu Y, Paruch JL, Zhou L, Kmiecik TE, Ko CY, Cohen ME. Development and evaluation of the universal ACS NSQIP surgical risk calculator: a decision aide and informed consent tool for patients and surgeons. J Am Coll Surg. 2013;217(5):833–842.e833. https://doi.org/10.1016/j.jamcollsurg.2013.07.385.
7. Mureddu GF. Current multivariate risk scores in patients undergoing non-cardiac surgery. Monaldi Arch Chest Dis. 2017;87(2):848. https://doi.org/10.4081/monaldi.2017.848.
8. Chung FM, Abdullah HRM, Liao PMD. STOP-Bang Questionnaire. Chest. 2016;149(3):631–8. https://doi.org/10.1378/chest.15-0903.

9. Singh S, Merchant AM. A propensity score-matched analysis of laparoscopic versus open surgery in patients with COPD. J Investig Surg. 2021;34(1):70–9. https://doi.org/10.1080/08941939.2019.1581307.
10. Gupta S, Fernandes R, Rao J, Dhanpal R. Perioperative risk factors for pulmonary complications after non-cardiac surgery. J Anaesthesiol Clin Pharmacol. 2020;36(1):88–93. https://doi.org/10.4103/joacp.JOACP_54_19.
11. Gupta HMD, Gupta PKMD, Fang XP, Miller WJMS, Cemaj SMD, Forse RAMDP, Morrow LEMDF. Development and validation of a risk calculator predicting postoperative respiratory failure. Chest. 2011;140(5):1207–15. https://doi.org/10.1378/chest.11-0466.
12. Cassidy MR, Rosenkranz P, McCabe K, Rosen JE, McAneny D. I COUGH: reducing postoperative pulmonary complications with a multidisciplinary patient care program. JAMA Surg. 2013;148(8):740–5. https://doi.org/10.1001/jamasurg.2013.358.
13. Grayson AD, Khater M, Jackson M, Fox MA. Valvular heart operation is an independent risk factor for acute renal failure. Ann Thorac Surg. 2003;75(6):1829–35. https://doi.org/10.1016/S0003-4975(03)00166-8.
14. Cheng D, Martin J, Shennib H, Dunning J, Muneretto C, Schueler S, Von Segesser L, Sergeant P, Turina M. Endovascular aortic repair versus open surgical repair for descending thoracic aortic disease: a systematic review and meta-analysis of comparative studies. J Am Coll Cardiol. 2010;55(10):986–1001. https://doi.org/10.1016/j.jacc.2009.11.047.
15. Kellerman PS. Perioperative care of the renal patient. Arch Intern Med. 1994;154(15):1674–88. https://doi.org/10.1001/archinte.154.15.1674.
16. Kleinpeter MA, Krane NK. Perioperative management of peritoneal dialysis patients: review of abdominal surgery. Adv Perit Dial. 2006;22:119–23.
17. Lew SQ. Peritoneal dialysis immediately after abdominal surgery. Perit Dial Int. 2018;38(1):5–8. https://doi.org/10.3747/pdi.2017.00089.
18. Vaquero Roncero LM, Sánchez Poveda D, Valdunciel García JJ, Sánchez Barrado ME, Calvo Vecino JM. Perioperative use of angiotensin-converting-enzyme inhibitors and angiotensin receptor antagonists. J Clin Anesth. 2017;40:91–8. https://doi.org/10.1016/j.jclinane.2017.04.018.
19. Baldini G, Bagry H, Aprikian A, Carli F. Postoperative urinary retention : anesthetic and perioperative considerations. Anesthesiology. 2009;110(5):1139–57. https://doi.org/10.1097/ALN.0b013e31819f7aea.
20. Medairos R, Berger G, Prebay Z, Foss H, Liu J, Tarima S, O'Connor R. MP10-04 post-operative urinary retention (pour) score – can incomplete bladder emptying after surgery be predicted? J Urol. 2019;201(Supplement 4):e118. https://doi.org/10.1097/01.JU.0000555148.66465.04.
21. Tam V, Lutfi W, Morgan K, Vasan R, Scaife R, Mahler B, Medich DS, Celebrezze JP, Watson AR, Holder-Murray J. Impact of enhanced recovery pathways and early urinary catheter removal on post-operative urinary retention. Am J Surg. 2020;220(5):1264–9. https://doi.org/10.1016/j.amjsurg.2020.06.057.
22. Teh SH, Nagorney DM, Stevens SR, Offord KP, Therneau TM, Plevak DJ, Talwalkar JA, Kim WR, Kamath PS. Risk factors for mortality after surgery in patients with cirrhosis. Gastroenterology. 2007;132(4):1261–9. https://doi.org/10.1053/j.gastro.2007.01.040.
23. Kim SY, Yim HJ, Park SM, Kim JH, Jung SW, Kim JH, Seo YS, Yeon JE, Lee HS, Lee SW, Um SH, Byun KS, Choi JH, Ryu HS. Validation of a Mayo post-operative mortality risk prediction model in Korean cirrhotic patients. Liver Int. 2011;31(2):222–8. https://doi.org/10.1111/j.1478-3231.2010.02419.x.
24. Mahmud N, Fricker Z, Hubbard RA, Ioannou GN, Lewis JD, Taddei TH, Rothstein KD, Serper M, Goldberg DS, Kaplan DE. Risk prediction models for post-operative mortality in patients with cirrhosis. Hepatology. 2021;73(1):204–18. https://doi.org/10.1002/hep.31558.
25. Jin Z, Hu J, Ma D. Postoperative delirium: perioperative assessment, risk reduction, and management. Br J Anaesth. 2020;125(4):492–504. https://doi.org/10.1016/j.bja.2020.06.063.
26. Aucoin SD, Hao M, Sohi R, Shaw J, Bentov I, Walker D, McIsaac DI. Accuracy and feasibility of clinically applied frailty instruments before surgery: a systematic review and meta-analysis. Anesthesiology. 2020;133(1):78–95. https://doi.org/10.1097/ALN.0000000000003257.

27. Rockwood K, Song X, MacKnight C, Bergman H, Hogan DB, McDowell I, Mitnitski A. A global clinical measure of fitness and frailty in elderly people. CMAJ. 2005;173(5):489–95. https://doi.org/10.1503/cmaj.050051.
28. Greene BR, Doheny EP, O'Halloran A, Anne Kenny R. Frailty status can be accurately assessed using inertial sensors and the TUG test. Age Ageing. 2014;43(3):406–11. https://doi.org/10.1093/ageing/aft176.
29. Debes C, Aissou M, Beaussier M. Prehabilitation. Preparing patients for surgery to improve functional recovery and reduce postoperative morbidity. Ann Fr Anesth Reanim. 2014;33(1):33–40. https://doi.org/10.1016/j.annfar.2013.12.012.
30. Santa Mina D, Scheede-Bergdahl C, Gillis C, Carli F. Optimization of surgical outcomes with prehabilitation. Appl Physiol Nutr Metab. 2015;40(9):966–9. https://doi.org/10.1139/apnm-2015-0084.
31. Shaw JR, Kaplovitch E, Douketis J. Periprocedural management of oral anticoagulation. Med Clin North Am. 2020;104(4):709–26. https://doi.org/10.1016/j.mcna.2020.02.005.
32. Favresse J, Hardy M, van Dievoet MA, Sennesael AL, Douxfils J, Samama CM, Vornicu O, Dincq AS, Lessire S, Mullier F. Andexanet alfa for the reversal of factor Xa inhibitors. Expert Opin Biol Ther. 2019;19(5):387–97. https://doi.org/10.1080/14712598.2019.1599355.
33. Reilly PAP, van Ryn JP, Grottke OMDP, Glund SP, Stangier JP. Idarucizumab, a specific reversal agent for dabigatran: mode of action, pharmacokinetics and pharmacodynamics, and safety and efficacy in phase 1 subjects. Am J Med. 2016;129(11):S64–72. https://doi.org/10.1016/j.amjmed.2016.06.007.
34. Kim JW, Kim TW, Ryu KH, Park SG, Jeong CY, Park DH. Anaesthetic considerations for patients with antiphospholipid syndrome undergoing non-cardiac surgery. J Int Med Res. 2020;48(1):300060519896889. https://doi.org/10.1177/0300060519896889.
35. Fusaro MV, Nielsen ND, Nielsen A, Fontaine MJ, Hess JR, Reed RM, DeLisle S, Netzer G. Restrictive versus liberal red blood cell transfusion strategy after hip surgery: a decision model analysis of healthcare costs. Transfusion. 2017;57(2):357–66. https://doi.org/10.1111/trf.13936.
36. Estcourt LJ, Birchall J, Allard S, Bassey SJ, Hersey P, Kerr JP, Mumford AD, Stanworth SJ, Tinegate H. Guidelines for the use of platelet transfusions. Br J Haematol. 2017;176(3):365–94. https://doi.org/10.1111/bjh.14423.
37. Chilkoti G, Singh A, Mohta M, Saxena A. Perioperative "stress dose" of corticosteroid: pharmacological and clinical perspective. J Anaesthesiol Clin Pharmacol. 2019;35(2):147–52. https://doi.org/10.4103/joacp.JOACP_242_17.
38. Yong PH, Weinberg L, Torkamani N, Churilov L, Robbins RJ, Ma R, Bellomo R, Lam QT, Burns JD, Hart GK, Lew JF, Mårtensson J, Story D, Motley AN, Johnson D, Zajac JD, Ekinci EI. The presence of diabetes and higher HbA1cAre independently associated with adverse outcomes after surgery. Diabetes Care. 2018;41(6):1172–9. https://doi.org/10.2337/dc17-2304.
39. Partridge H, Perkins B, Mathieu S, Nicholls A, Adeniji K. Clinical recommendations in the management of the patient with type 1 diabetes on insulin pump therapy in the perioperative period: a primer for the anaesthetist. Br J Anaesth. 2016;116(1):18–26. https://doi.org/10.1093/bja/aev347.
40. American Diabetes A. 15. Diabetes care in the Hospital: standards of medical care in diabetes-2020. Diabetes Care. 2020;43(Suppl 1):S193–202. https://doi.org/10.2337/dc20-S015.
41. Goodman SM, Goodman SM, Figgie MP, Figgie MP, MacKenzie CR, MacKenzie CR. Perioperative management of patients with connective tissue disease. HSS J. 2011;7(1):72–9. https://doi.org/10.1007/s11420-010-9180-1.
42. Bashaw MADNPRN, Keister KJPRNCNE. Perioperative strategies for surgical site infection prevention. AORN J. 2019;109(1):68–78. https://doi.org/10.1002/aorn.12451.
43. Renaudin A, Leguelinel-Blache G, Choukroun C, Lefauconnier A, Boisson C, Kinowski J-M, Cuvillon P, Richard H. Impact of a preoperative pharmaceutical consultation in scheduled orthopedic surgery on admission: a prospective observational study. BMC Health Serv Res. 2020;20(1):747. https://doi.org/10.1186/s12913-020-05623-6.

44. Castanheira L, Fresco P, Macedo AF. Guidelines for the management of chronic medication in the perioperative period: systematic review and formal consensus. J Clin Pharm Ther. 2011;36(4):446–67. https://doi.org/10.1111/j.1365-2710.2010.01202.x.
45. Fernandez AC, Claborn KR, Borsari B. A systematic review of behavioural interventions to reduce preoperative alcohol use: review preoperative alcohol use. Drug Alcohol Rev. 2015;34(5):508–20. https://doi.org/10.1111/dar.12285.
46. Higgins-Biddle JC, Babor TF. A review of the alcohol use disorders identification test (AUDIT), AUDIT-C, and USAUDIT for screening in the United States: past issues and future directions. Am J Drug Alcohol Abuse. 2018;44(6):578–86. https://doi.org/10.1080/00952990.2018.1456545.
47. Bradley KA, DeBenedetti AF, Volk RJ, Williams EC, Frank D, Kivlahan DR. AUDIT-C as a brief screen for alcohol misuse in primary care. Alcohol Clin Exp Res. 2007;31(7):1208–17. https://doi.org/10.1111/j.1530-0277.2007.00403.x.
48. Aveyard P, Dautzenberg B. Temporary abstinence from smoking prior to surgery reduces harm to smokers. Int J Clin Pract. 2010;64(3):285–8. https://doi.org/10.1111/j.1742-1241.2009.02300.x.
49. Edwards AFMD, Forest DJMD. Preoperative laboratory testing. Anesthesiol Clin. 2018;36(4):493–507. https://doi.org/10.1016/j.anclin.2018.07.002.
50. Paton F, Chambers D, Wilson P, Eastwood A, Craig D, Fox D, Jayne D, McGinnes E. Effectiveness and implementation of enhanced recovery after surgery programmes: a rapid evidence synthesis. BMJ Open. 2014;4(7):e005015. https://doi.org/10.1136/bmjopen-2014-005015.
51. Pickens RC, Cochran AR, Lyman WB, King L, Iannitti DA, Martinie JB, Baker EH, Ocuin LM, Riggs SB, Davis BR, Matthews BD, Vrochides D. Impact of multidisciplinary audit of enhanced recovery after surgery (ERAS)® programs at a single institution. World J Surg. 2021;45(1):23–32. https://doi.org/10.1007/s00268-020-05765-y.
52. Wenzel JTMD, Schwenk ESMD, Baratta JLMD, Viscusi ERMD. Managing opioid-tolerant patients in the perioperative surgical home. Anesthesiol Clin. 2016;34(2):287–301. https://doi.org/10.1016/j.anclin.2016.01.005.
53. Brown WA, Moore EM, Watters DA. Mortality of patients with COVID-19 who undergo an elective or emergency surgical procedure: a systematic review and meta-analysis. ANZ J Surg. 2020. https://doi.org/10.1111/ans.16500.
54. Anesthesiologists ASo. ASA and APSF statement on perioperative testing for the COVID-19 Virus. 2020. https://www.asahq.org/about-asa/newsroom/news-releases/2020/12/asa-and-apsf-statement-on-perioperative-testing-for-the-covid-19-virus.
55. Wainstein AJA, Drummond-Lage AP, Ribeiro R, Castro Ribeiro HS, Pinheiro RN, Baiocchi G, Sousa Fernandes PH, Anghinoni M, Laporte GA, Coelho Junior MJ, Dall'Inha VN, Oliveira AF. Risks of COVID-19 for surgical cancer patients: the importance of the informed consent process. J Surg Oncol. 2020;122(4):608–10. https://doi.org/10.1002/jso.26065.
56. Tang VL, Dillon EC, Yang Y, Tai-Seale M, Boscardin J, Kata A, Sudore RL. Advance care planning in older adults with multiple chronic conditions undergoing high-risk surgery. JAMA Surg. 2018;154(3):261–4. https://doi.org/10.1001/jamasurg.2018.4647.

Chapter 12
Virtual Hospital Medicine

Charit Fares and Margaret Malone

Background

Telemedicine is a rapidly expanding field in today's climate of advancing technology, combined with increasing demand for contactless communication in the context of the novel coronavirus disease 2019 (COVID-19). Much has been written on the role of telemedicine in outpatient medical settings, with its ability to reach both rural areas without access to specialists and people at risk of contracting COVID-19. However, the pandemic has additionally introduced a previously less-considered purpose for telemedicine, which is the use of remote technology for inpatient medicine with the goal of reducing infection risk and conserving personal protective equipment (PPE).

Inpatient telehealth already exists in several contexts. Perhaps the most prolific is its use for pediatric patients in community or rural hospitals that do not have pediatric specialists available for consults on-site [1]. It is also used for critical care consults at such hospitals [2].

Telemedicine can be utilized in cases of stroke in remote areas as well; by virtually consulting an expert in stroke medicine, the essential time to administration of tissue plasminogen activator (tPA) can be decreased, especially in rural communities [3].

Virtual hospital medicine (VHM) extends to other specialist consults from rural hospitals, including in ophthalmology (in addition to specially trained technologists

C. Fares (✉)
Hospital Medicine, Ochsner Health, New Orleans, LA, USA
e-mail: charit.fares@ochsner.org

M. Malone
The University of Queensland-Ochsner Clinical School, New Orleans, LA, USA

© The Author(s), under exclusive license to Springer Nature Switzerland AG 2022
K. Conrad (ed.), *Clinical Approaches to Hospital Medicine*,
https://doi.org/10.1007/978-3-030-95164-1_12

to assist) [4]. In psychiatry, some smaller hospitals use a virtual consult/liaison service [5], while medical/surgical units in Pittsburgh have also piloted virtual consults [6]. Allergists may be consulted virtually in cases of severe allergy requiring specialist management [7]. Telemedicine has also been used for complex issues in intensive care units (ICU) since at least 2002 [8], although acceptance of this use by healthcare personnel varies according to a 2018 survey of ICU nurses [9].

The above examples refer to specialist consults, but uses for the specific role of "telehospitalist" are also increasing. Need has been identified for a nighttime telehospitalist who can consult from home in areas that are not able to sustain an on-site hospitalist 24 hours per day [10]. In addition, the Veterans Health Administration (VHA) has produced a pilot program that allows telehospitalists to provide care for patients that live too far to realistically commute to a physical hospital [11].

The COVID-19 pandemic brought new uses for the technology of telemedicine and accelerated other uses that were already in development. In the setting of a pandemic, reducing the number of providers circulating through each patient's room is essential to limiting the spread of the disease. Dermatology [12] and infectious disease [13] consults moved to largely virtual applications, as many cases in these specialties can be effectively diagnosed via photographs and laboratory results. Inpatient diabetes management has also accelerated its use of virtual medicine [14].

Virtual Hospital Medicine at Ochsner Health

The Ochsner Health System, in New Orleans, LA, was one of the first hospitals in the nation to establish a telehospitalist program in the context of COVID-19. Louisiana was one of the earliest- and hardest-hit states during the pandemic; in March through May of 2020, the state had the highest deaths per capita in the United States and among the highest in the world [15]. This unprecedented situation called for major rethinking of how healthcare was delivered, bearing in mind infection control, a huge patient census, and the need to conserve PPE. Our VHM program was a solution to these problems, allowing virtual hospitalists to manage many patients at once from a remote headquarters without the need to enter each room individually.

We used existing hardware where possible to increase the speed and financial expediency of deploying the new program. Since telepsychiatry and teleneurology programs already existed within the Ochsner system, we were able to adapt their telemedicine carts for hospitalists. These were wheeled tables equipped with desktop computers, microphones, and a high resolution camera that could be operated remotely. Due to the large number of cases, it was also necessary to order iPad tablets on poles that could be left in each room so that the provider could "visit" multiple times per day. One Ochsner campus had installed VHM hardware in its rooms a few years prior to the pandemic; this was invaluable, as the hardwired equipment provided much better sound and video quality than the tablets and did not rely on battery power.

Patients most appropriate for the program were those recovering from COVID-19 who still required inpatient care but were no longer in critical condition. These patients had to meet criteria to be eligible for VHM and were transferred back to in-person care if their condition again became critical. At first, nurses assisted the telehospitalists by performing basic exams and bringing tablets into each room. However, eventually a new role of "telepresenter," a staff member at each hospital dedicated specifically to this task, allowed offloading of some of this burden from nurses.

As with any new program, we faced a number of challenges with implementing Ochsner's new VHM system. Hardware was one difficulty; communication was more difficult with tablets due to inferior sound and video quality. Tablets and carts also raised infection control concerns as they required sanitization when being moved between rooms. Hardwired rooms were best as the hospitalist could check the room first, then "drop in" on a dedicated screen near the television in the room. However, installing equipment in rooms for this purpose was expensive, and stakeholder and physician buy-in was another challenge we faced in the early days of the program. We had several myths and misconceptions to work through, including that virtual medicine provided a lower quality evaluation, or the fear that VHM would replace hospitalists. However, we were eventually able to show that this method was safe, reliable, and not inferior to an inpatient visit. Patients reported satisfaction with the experience as well.

As adoption of VHM increased systemwide, the culture began to change. Our team made site visits and remained in constant contact with all levels of leadership and key stakeholders in the process. We listened to and incorporated feedback from both leadership and from our virtual medicine providers, which was invaluable. In addition, "telemedicine champions" at each site were able to promote VHM usage, which was useful to advocate for the program. As a result of these efforts, several more campuses invested in hardwiring their rooms for VHM.

We have learned several important lessons from this process that may benefit other, similar programs:

1. Stakeholder engagement is key; the earlier, the better.
2. Close communication with multidisciplinary teams of nurses, physicians, allied health, and hospital leadership is essential to assess the efficacy of the program and make necessary changes.
3. Similarly, remaining open to feedback at all levels is significant both for improvement and for buy-in from leaders and stakeholders.
4. While the COVID-19 pandemic required lightning speed setup, it is still important to be systematic when launching a new program. Taking on too much at one time can prove to be deleterious and eventually lead to a negative perception of the program, so it was incumbent on us to understand our own limitations.

5. VHM programs should be honest about the limitations of virtual medicine; it is not appropriate for all patients, and does not exist to replace inpatient providers. Rather, the program is designed to augment the current model of care.
6. Having a leader who is appreciative of the team and is available for contact creates a culture of trust and engagement.
7. VHM is a unique skill set separate from hospital care. Providers who staff VHM programs should already have at least a year of inpatient experience before taking on virtual care.

Other Programs

Two similar programs in hard-hit states were created at the same time as the one at Ochsner. One was within several hospitals associated with Stanford University in California [16], and the other was in Westchester, NY [17]. Both of these programs were also created rapidly, so they also adapted preexisting hardware and software for speed of deployment. Both augmented existing hardware with iPad tablets on carts. At Stanford, like Ochsner, emphasis was placed on the need for teamwork. The Stanford team found that "field service workers," similar to Ochsner's "telemedicine champions," were invaluable for troubleshooting problems as they arose. Stanford also found that rooms hardwired for VHM were optimal [16]. In Westchester, a preexisting tele-ICU program was adapted that relied on tablets. After trying several methods, the hospital placed one tablet outside and one within each room, so that any healthcare personnel, including nursing and allied health, could utilize VHM. Like Ochsner, the Westchester team found that key stakeholders should be alerted early in the process, and multidisciplinary groups must be involved at every step [17].

Conclusion

The unprecedented COVID-19 pandemic created a need for rapid deployment of large-scale, effective telehospitalist programs. Ochsner Health was one of the first to develop such a program, using available hardware and tablets. Like its peers, the team at Ochsner found that early stakeholder engagement, multidisciplinary teamwork, and dedicated staff members were essential to success. Virtual medicine is here to stay; defining its role in healthcare and educating providers about its use will be essential in the future.

Key Points

1. Early stakeholder engagement is essential
2. Close communication with multidisciplinary teams of nurses, physicians, allied health, and hospital leadership is essential to assess the efficacy of the program and make necessary changes.
3. Remaining open to feedback at all levels is significant both for improvement and for buy-in from leaders and stakeholders.
4. While the COVID-19 pandemic required a rapid deployment, it is still important to be systematic when launching a new program.
5. VHM programs should be honest about the limitations of virtual medicine; it is not appropriate for all patients, and does not exist to replace inpatient providers. Rather, the program is designed to augment the current model of care.

References

1. Burke BL Jr, Hall RW, Section On Telehealth C. Telemedicine: pediatric applications. Pediatrics. 2015;136(1):e293–308. https://doi.org/10.1542/peds.2015-1517.
2. Berrens ZJ, Gosdin CH, Brady PW, Tegtmeyer K. Efficacy and safety of pediatric critical care physician telemedicine involvement in rapid response team and code response in a satellite facility. Pediatr Crit Care Med. 2019;20(2):172–7. https://doi.org/10.1097/pcc.0000000000001796.
3. Witrick B, Zhang D, Switzer JA, Hess DC, Shi L. The association between stroke mortality and time of admission and participation in a telestroke network. J Stroke Cerebrovasc Dis. 2020;29(2):104480. https://doi.org/10.1016/j.jstrokecerebrovasdis.2019.104480.
4. Woodward MA, Bavinger JC, Amin S, Blachley TS, Musch DC, Lee PP, Newman-Casey PA. Telemedicine for ophthalmic consultation services: use of a portable device and layering information for graders. J Telemed Telecare. 2017;23(2):365–70. https://doi.org/10.1177/1357633x16634544.
5. Arevian AC, Jeffrey J, Young AS, Ong MK. Opportunities for flexible, on-demand care delivery through telemedicine. Psychiatr Serv. 2018;69(1):5–8. https://doi.org/10.1176/appi.ps.201600589.
6. Graziane JA, Gopalan P, Cahalane J. Telepsychiatry consultation for medical and surgical inpatient units. Psychosomatics. 2018;59(1):62–6. https://doi.org/10.1016/j.psym.2017.08.008.
7. Portnoy JM, Pandya A, Waller M, Elliott T. Telemedicine and emerging technologies for health care in allergy/immunology. J Allergy Clin Immunol. 2020;145(2):445–54. https://doi.org/10.1016/j.jaci.2019.12.903.
8. Kahn JM, Cicero BD, Wallace DJ, Iwashyna TJ. Adoption of ICU telemedicine in the United States. Crit Care Med. 2014;42(2):362–8. https://doi.org/10.1097/CCM.0b013e3182a6419f.
9. Canfield C, Galvin S. Bedside nurse acceptance of intensive care unit telemedicine presence. Crit Care Nurse. 2018;38(6):e1–4. https://doi.org/10.4037/ccn2018926.
10. Sanders RB, Simpson KN, Kazley AS, Giarrizzi DP. New hospital telemedicine services: potential market for a nighttime telehospitalist service. Telemed J E Health. 2014;20(10):902–8. https://doi.org/10.1089/tmj.2013.0344.
11. Gutierrez J, Moeckli J, Holcombe A, O'Shea AM, Bailey G, Rewerts K, Hagiwara M, Sullivan S, Simon M, Kaboli P. Implementing a telehospitalist program between veterans health administration hospitals: outcomes, acceptance, and barriers to implementation. J Hosp Med. 2021;16(3):156–63. https://doi.org/10.12788/jhm.3570.

12. Trinidad J, Kroshinsky D, Kaffenberger BH, Rojek NW. Telemedicine for inpatient dermatology consultations in response to the COVID-19 pandemic. J Am Acad Dermatol. 2020;83(1):e69–71. https://doi.org/10.1016/j.jaad.2020.04.096.
13. Monkowski D, Rhodes LV, Templer S, Kromer S, Hartner J, Pianucci K, Kincaid H. A retrospective cohort study to assess the impact of an inpatient infectious disease telemedicine consultation service on hospital and patient outcomes. Clin Infect Dis. 2020;70(5):763–70. https://doi.org/10.1093/cid/ciz293.
14. Jones MS, Goley AL, Alexander BE, Keller SB, Caldwell MM, Buse JB. Inpatient transition to virtual care during COVID-19 pandemic. Diabetes Technol Ther. 2020;22(6):444–8. https://doi.org/10.1089/dia.2020.0206.
15. Louisiana T. COVID-19 deaths by U.S. County per 1000 residents. https://public.flourish.studio/visualisation/1627392/. 2020. Accessed Aug 13 2021.
16. Vilendrer S, Patel B, Chadwick W, Hwa M, Asch S, Pageler N, Ramdeo R, Sliba-Gustafsson EA, Strong P, Sharp C. Rapid deployment of inpatient telemedicine in response to COVID-19 Across three health systems. J Am Med Inform Assoc. 2020;27(7):1102–9. https://doi.org/10.1093/jamia/ocaa077.
17. Becker CD, Forman L, Gollapudi L, Nevins B, Scurlock C. Rapid implementation and adaptation of a telehospitalist service to coordinate and optimize care for COVID-19 patients. Telemed J E Health. 2021;27(4):388–96. https://doi.org/10.1089/tmj.2020.0232.

Chapter 13
Palliative Care for Hospitalists

Susan Nelson and Megha Koduri

What Is Palliative Care?

Palliative care is a medical specialty that provides medical care to individuals living with serious illness. Palliative care has evolved over the past several decades from exclusively providing end-of-life care to serving patients with life-limiting medical conditions by providing supportive, comprehensive care throughout their journey. Specialist palliative care services use an interdisciplinary approach to provide holistic care for both chronically and acutely unwell patients by aiming to reduce the burden of their symptoms and improve their quality of life. The palliative care team consists of a variety of healthcare workers, including physicians, nurses, spiritual leaders, social workers, and other individuals vital to the patient's care.

Palliative care services can and should be sought at all stages of severe illness and are typically provided alongside medically curative treatment. The role of consult palliative care teams can broadly be broken down into four domains:

1. Pain and symptom assessment and management.
2. Communication between patients, their families, and the healthcare teams involved in the patient's care.
3. Provision of support to patients, families, and healthcare teams involved.
4. Hospice care services.

S. Nelson (✉)
Ochsner Health, New Orleans, LA, USA
e-mail: susan.nelson@ochsner.org

M. Koduri
The University of Queensland School of Medicine, Ochsner Clinical School, New Orleans, LA, USA

As a point of clarification, palliative medicine has often been incorrectly used interchangeably with hospice care. Hospice care, often referred to as end-of-life care, aims at providing comfort focused treatment for patients with a prognosis of fewer than 6 months to live or patients whose health is demonstrably declining. Hospice is palliative medicine at the end of life.

Pain and Symptom Management Since the COVID-19 Pandemic

The rapid, global spread of the COVID-19 virus led to an international pandemic that has caused a rapid rise in the utilization of healthcare services and a surge in demand for palliative care [1]. Specialist palliative care services employ a multidisciplinary approach to care for both chronically and acutely unwell patients, often with multiple comorbidities, as well as both social and medical complications in care. Such populations are most at risk of experiencing severe illness in the context of COVID-19 [2]. Novel strategies have emerged as specialist palliative care services have struggled to meet both the increased medical needs of hospitalized patients and the additional difficulties that the isolation of infected individuals poses to both the patients and their families [1, 3]. As discussed later in this chapter, the development of COVID-specific communication materials has aided the ability of clinicians, regardless of specialty, to lead conversations that palliative care specialists would typically conduct. The current pandemic has necessitated educational interventions that expand the pool of nonspecialist palliative care providers during these times [2, 4].

The Waikato Specialist Palliative Care Service in New Zealand developed a Palliative Care Pack containing information sheets with specific recommendations for nonspecialist palliative care clinicians to aid in the medical management of dyspnea, respiratory secretions, delirium, and patients with preexisting renal failure [2]. In another paper, Blinderman et al. discuss a three-part preliminary palliative care educational resource that also includes recommendations for symptom management, in addition to the VitalTalk communication resource (discussed below), and institution-specific palliative care resources at New York Presbyterian (NYP) Hospital [1]. In contrast to the "Palliative Care Pack" approach, the NYP resources were disseminated in the form of both reading materials and Zoom teaching sessions. The Center to Advance Palliative Care (CAPC) has also developed a curriculum for clinicians from all specialties to train non-palliative care specialists in core skills [5]. Course topics include pain management, communication skills, symptom management, and preventing crisis through patient care [5]. As an additional benefit, this online course also counts for continuing education credits for clinicians seeking to fulfill those requirements [5].

The "upskilling of non-specialist palliative care clinicians" [2] via the production and dissemination of educational resources both encourages inter-team collaboration and aims to address the acute need for palliative care services during this pandemic.

Table 13.1 SPIKES model for delivering bad news

S – Setting	Arrange for an appropriate, private location Clearly introduce yourself and your role in the patient's care Rehearse the conversation mentally, and be prepared with the medical facts
P – Perception	Determine the patient's perception of their medical condition
I – Invitation	Inquire as to how much information the patient wants to hear
K – Knowledge	Provide information in simple, direct language
E – Empathize	Expect and respond to patient's emotions
S – Summarize	Summarize the relevant clinical information, reiterate patient wishes, make a plan of action

Table 13.2 Ask-tell-ask model for delivering bad news

Ask	Ask the patient to describe their understanding of their medical course
Tell	Tell the patients necessary information in clear, simple, and direct language
Ask	Ask the patient to describe their understanding of the information you provided them

Table 13.3 NURSE mnemonic for statements of verbal empathy

N: Name	Name the emotion being expressed "It sounds like you are upset"
U: Understand	Acknowledge and legitimize the intensity of the emotion and the patient/family's experience "I cannot imagine what you are going through at this time."
R: Respect	Respect the patient/family's experience and praise their efforts "You have been handling your treatments tremendously."
S: Support	Ensure the patient/family knows who is available to support them/reiterate your role in supporting them "I will do everything I can to ensure you are receiving the best care."
E: Explore	Further the empathetic connection by allowing for the opportunity to more information to be obtained and explored. "Would you mind telling me more about that?"

Communication

Palliative medicine clinicians commonly lead difficult conversations regarding deteriorating health, goals of care, and end-of-life discussions. Multiple conversations are often necessary for both patients and their families to comprehend difficult news. Such discussions should include the patient, relevant clinicians and members of the patient's care team, and any family members the patient would like to involve. Several models have been developed to guide healthcare providers in leading these challenging discussions: "SPIKES model for delivering bad news," "ask-tell-ask model for delivering bad news," and "nurse mnemonic for statements of verbal empathy" (Tables 13.1, 13.2, and 13.3).

Six principles that should guide these conversations are:

1. *Scheduling the meeting:* To ensure that everybody attending the meeting is as prepared as possible, meetings should be planned in advance [6]. Clinicians and other members of the healthcare team who will be present should discuss the patient's case and their individual roles in the discussion ahead of time.
2. *Acknowledging the patient:* The meeting should begin with a clear explanation of the meeting's purpose and an introduction from each individual of the patient's care team. The patient's current understanding of their illness and how much they wish to learn about their medical condition should be assessed.
3. *Providing information:* Clinicians should provide information in accordance with how much the patient wishes to know. Clinicians should explain the patient's condition in simple terms, avoiding the use of medical jargon [7].
4. *Expect and respond to emotion*: Clinicians should expect a range of emotion from patients and their families in such difficult conversations. Expressing empathy both verbally and nonverbally, such as through touch, facial expression, and nodding, can be appropriate responses. The NURSE mnemonic for statements of verbal empathy (Table 13.3) may provide some guidance for clinicians.
5. *Discussing transitions of care and goals of care:* If patients are willing to discuss goals of care, clinicians should ask questions to elicit the concerns and values of the patient, while providing a realistic perspective about the patient's prognosis. Should the patient prefer to defer this conversation to a later date, plans for further discussion should be made.
6. *Debrief:* The healthcare team should take time to reflect on the meeting, the patient, and their own emotions following this discussion.

In lieu of the COVID-19 pandemic, clinicians outside of palliative care specialty services and primary hospitalist teams have had to lead difficult conversations regarding end-of-life expectations, resource rationing, and goals of care. The development of COVID-19 specific communication resources, as noted in Tables 13.4, 13.5, 13.6, and 13.7, continues to serve as an adjunct to existing road maps for common palliative care-related conversations. In addition to providing mnemonics for initiating such discussions, the "VitalTalk COVID Ready Communication Playbook" provides quick scripted answers for commonly asked questions with regard to topics such as COVID screening, triaging, and counseling [8]. The Social Worker Hospice and Palliative Care Network has also provided a document to guide clinicians on how to best communicate with families facing undesired outcomes of COVID-19 [9]. (Place Tables 13.4, 13.5, 13.6, and 13.7 here, below paragraph.)

Telemedicine in Palliative Care

Though the field of palliative care medicine has grown immensely in larger hospitals over the past few years, access to palliative care medicine is a continued struggle in many remote and rural communities [10, 11]. An aging American population and an

Table 13.4 CALMER mnemonic for COVID-19 contingency and crisis planning: discussions regarding preferences and goals of care conversations [8]

C – *Check-in*	Assess where they are at emotionally "How are you handling all of this?"
A – *Ask* about COVID	Listen to them "What's been on your mind regarding COVID and your situation?"
L – *Lay* out issues	"This is something I would like us to be prepared or" "Is there anything you would like us to know about you and your care if you get COVID/if you become very ill from COVID?"
M – *Motivate* them to choose a proxy and talk about what matters	"If your health were to take a turn for the worse, what you discuss now can assist your family/loved ones""Who would you like to make decisions for you in the event that you were unable to speak?" (Ideally list two people) "We are living through unprecedented times, what matters most to you about your life and your healthcare?" Make a recommendation if possible, "Based on what we've discussed, I would recommend [the following]. How do you feel about that?"
E – Expect emotion	*Expect and acknowledge their emotion*
R – Record the discussion	Document the discussion to assist the patient and your colleagues in the future "Thank you for having this very helpful conversation with me. I'll note what you have said in your cart."

Table 13.5 SHARE mnemonic for COVID-19 contingency and crisis planning: discussions regarding resource allocation [8]

S – *Show* the guideline	"This is the guideline that our hospital/institution/area is adhering to for patients with this condition" Tip: begin with the section most relevant your current conversation
H – *Headline* what this means for the patient's care	"So for you/your loved one, this means that we will …" "What we will not do is …" Tip: initiate this portion with what you *will* do first
A – *Affirm* the care that you will provide	"We will be doing …" "We hope that you will recover with this care plan."
R – *Respond* to emotion	"I can see that you are scared"
E – *Emphasize* that the same rules apply to everyone	"We are living through challenging times and we are doing our best to allocate our resources fairly. Every patient in this hospital/institution/region is being treated according to this same set of rules. You are not being singled out."

increase in patients living with chronic illness place a larger burden on palliative medicine each year, regardless of geographic region [12]. Telemedicine can generally be defined "as the use of telecommunications technologies to provide medical information and services" [13]. Over the past two decades, this has come to mean providing medical care via telephone or, more recently, video communication services, when clinically appropriate. This technology was initially employed to facilitate the delivery of specialist medical care to medically underserved areas and has since led to a fewer urgent care and emergency room visits and increased elderly and homebound patient satisfaction [14].

Table 13.6 LOVE mnemonic for the last family call [8]

L - *Lead* the way forward	Introduce yourself "This is a very difficult situation for most people.""I am here to walk you through it if you would like,"
O – *Offer* the four things that matter to most people	"So we have the chance to make this time memorable, here are five things you might want to say if any of them seem right for you." 1. Please forgive me 2. I forgive you 3. Thank you 4. I love you 5. Goodbye "Do any of those sound good to you?"
V - *Validate* what they want to say	"I think that sounds lovely" "If my loved one said that to me, I would feel so loved." "I think your loved one can hear you even if they can't respond."
E – *Expect* emotion	"I can see that you two were close" "Can you stay on the line for just another minute? I'd like to check in with you just to see how you're doing/handling this."

Few quantitative studies have been conducted to measure the effectiveness of telehealth specifically in the field of palliative care. Though the majority of existing knowledge regarding the role of telemedicine in this field is qualitative in nature, it is apparent that the benefits of telemedicine are vast. Studies conducted in the United Kingdom have shown that telemedicine visits allowed palliative care specialists to provide symptom assessment and consultation and lead goals of care and end-of-life discussions to remote nursing homes [15]. Palliative care specialists were also able to provide "off hours" care to minimize unnecessary emergency room visits and hospital admissions [15, 16].

Chronic severe illness, such as advanced cancer, often hinders patient's ability to attend routine appointments leading to multiple emergency department visits and hospital admissions that may be mitigated by facilitating access to symptom management services. A small study in advanced cancer patients showed that access to palliative care telemedicine services functioned as a helpful adjuvant to in-person assistance, leading to fewer emergency department visits and increased confidence in family members' ability to care for these patients [17].

Another study assessing the quality of telehealth compared to standard in person visits in the care of 900 patients with Parkinson's disease resulted in 85 percent of visits rated as "satisfactory" or above. Additionally, via telehealth, clinicians were able to allow for longer appointment times in this study [18].

Telemedicine may also have a role in supporting self-management in patients suffering from cancer and other chronic illnesses by allowing physicians to remotely monitor patient's fluid intake/output and vitals. Such "remote patient monitoring" may prevent emergency department visits by facilitating personal/family intervention for conditions that may be managed at home, such as dehydration [14].

Table 13.7 SWHPN's seven tips for communicating with families of patients facing undesired outcomes due to COVID-19 [9]

1. Setting	If in person, find a quiet place to talk. If using virtual communication, encourage family to find a quiet place to have the discussion if possible
2. "Stay grounded"	Remember the importance of this conversation and do your best to remain calm
3. "Listen to the family's concerns"	"This is a very challenging situation for most people, how can I best help you at this time?" Do not make assumptions regarding how the family is interpreting the situation Note that "terminal extubation" may cause a sense of relief for some family members, which can unveil feelings of guilt which may be expressed as anger
4. "No bandwagons allowed"	Listen empathetically to the family's reaction Do not join in on placing blame Acknowledge that these are difficult times and we are living through an extraordinary situation Do not trivialize the family's reactions
5. Active listening	Employing active listening techniques, such as reflecting on feelings and summarizing thoughts can be helpful Keep reflections brief Allow space for the family's reactions
6. Explore family's cultural and religious views	If appropriate and desired by the patient or family, you may seek a spiritual counselor

7. Provide information	Provide honest information that is relevant to the current situation. This may include:
	    Explaining the visitor's policy
	    Discussing measures that can help minimize family's risk of exposure
	    Reassuring that the staff will minimize their loved one's suffering as much as possible
	    If appropriate, discussing the parameters of the patient's death and disease

Many palliative care services opted to increase the use of telemedicine in the midst of the COVID-19 pandemic with the intention of minimizing the spread of the virus in particularly vulnerable populations. This allowed patients with palliative care needs to remain with their loved ones while efficiently establishing goals of care for these patients in the event that they experience acute illness from COVID-19 [1]. The employment of telemedicine has also allowed for out-of-state palliative care physicians to relieve the workload of overburdened hospitals, primarily by leading goals of care conversations with patients and their families.

Pitfalls of telemedicine include an inability to visualize the patient if the visit is conducted via audio communication (telephone call), general connectivity and video quality problems, and difficulty directing a primarily elderly population to appropriately use the necessary technology [14]. Telehealth is least useful in very ill, elderly patient populations, in whom the challenge of navigating new technology outweighs the benefits. As this population most often requires in-person assessments for changes in their medical condition, palliative care via telemedicine has not been studied in these populations [19].

In summary, it is apparent that palliative care telemedicine is most beneficial for remotely conducting important family and goals of care discussions, remotely providing symptom assessment, and remotely monitoring patients with chronic illnesses. However, very elderly patients and patients whose condition has deteriorated to a point that significantly hinders their ability to interact with technology are least likely to benefit from these remote services.

Virtual Reality in Palliative Care

Virtual reality (VR), also referred to as augmented reality, is the use of technology such as computers and other multimedia devices to create a simulated environment that can be shockingly realistic. Studies investigating the role of VR in palliative care have employed stand-alone audiovisual headsets to create a 360° simulated environment.

A preliminary, prospective, multicenter study conducted in japan used Google Earth VR® software to provide terminal cancer patients with virtual travel experiences lasting 30 minutes per session [20]. These virtual experiences provided a relative benefit to most patient's mental health, most notably with regard to improving symptoms of depression and anxiety [20]. The majority of patients with life-limiting illness enrolled in a pilot study investigating the benefit of 30-minute virtual reality sessions reported that they would recommend VR to other individuals living with terminal illness [21]. Of note, however, neither of these studies revealed a statistically significant improvement in measured patient symptoms, such as shortness of breath, fatigue, nausea, or pain.

The patients most likely to benefit from VR are patients at the end of their life who are unable to die at home. Particularly in the current context of the COVID-19 pandemic, the necessary isolation of infected individuals has resulted in hundreds of thousands of patients dying in hospitals, isolated from their loved ones. While many patients have been using video conferencing technologies to spend their last moments with their loved ones, VR can provide an alternative setting, in which the patient can be virtually transported to various locations across the globe, and peaceful scenery/settings can be set up to provide a simulated escape from the hospital room [22]. VR can also be used to record patients during their final days, creating "hologram-like projections" for their loved ones to cherish [22]. As VR technology continues to grow, it is likely that upcoming advancements may allow for virtual, "real-time interaction" to simulate the presence of loved ones around the patient in their final hours [22].

Music Therapy in Palliative Care

Music therapy is a recognized allied health profession wherein board certified music therapists employ music as an intervention to accomplish an array of goals. Within palliative care, music therapy is gaining popularity as a complimentary treatment to improve a patient's quality of life by relieving psychological distress and facilitating communication [23]. Music therapists use singing, song writing, lyrical analysis, guided meditations with music and imagery, and music therapy relaxation, among other techniques to address each patient's specific needs.

Music therapy has been proven to produce a statically significant improvement in both observer-rated and self-reported perception of pain, mood, and patient anxiety [24, 25]. Graphic analysis of patients treated with vocal improvisation therapy indicated significantly decreased discomfort behaviors with music therapy, and the playing of spiritual music has been proven to enhance the spiritual well-being of terminally ill patients [26, 27]. Phase III randomized trials of music therapy as an intervention for improving the quality of life in palliative care patients are currently underway [28].

Though more quantitative studies are needed to empirically evaluate the benefits of music therapy in palliative care patient populations, qualitative studies have shown that music therapy can be helpful in addressing social isolation, depression, anxiety, distressing emotions, neurological impairments, spiritual needs, as well as physical symptoms such as pain and shortness of breath [12]. With this qualitative success of music therapy in improving quality of life, music therapists are increasingly sought out as a valuable addition to palliative care teams in their endeavor to provide holistic patient care [29].

Key Points
- *Involve palliative care services early!* Palliative care medicine is more than just hospice! When possible, involve the palliative care services as a part of the multidisciplinary team for patients with severe illnesses.
- *Be proactive about your own learning!* The recent pandemic has necessitated the provision of certain palliative care services by non-palliative care specialists. Resources such as the CAPC (https://www.capc.org/) provide courses for all clinicians to acquaint themselves with palliative care topics. (Many CAPC courses require membership.)
- *Do not to shy away from difficult conversations!* Following the "six principles to guide difficult conversations" and employing the various mnemonics presented above in this chapter can facilitate the success of these conversations. As an additional resource, the CAPC also offers an online course on communication skills to further support your training and confidence.
- *Do bring up goals of care early in a patient's care!* Understanding the patient's wishes is a critical component of providing good, comprehensive patient care.
- *Keep an eye out for what's to come in palliative care medicine!* Research and technology advance our understanding and ability to deliver palliative care medicine every day. Inventions like virtual reality may be changing the landscape of providing palliative care in the near future. Keep an eye out for these interesting new advancements!

References

1. Blinderman CD, Adelman R, Kumaraiah D, Pan CX, Palathra BC, Kaley K, Trongone N, Spillane K. A comprehensive approach to palliative care during the coronavirus pandemic. J Palliat Med. 2020; https://doi.org/10.1089/jpm.2020.0481.
2. Ferguson L, Barham D. Palliative care pandemic pack: a specialist palliative care service response to planning the COVID-19 pandemic. J Pain Symptom Manag. 2020;60:e18–20. https://doi.org/10.1016/j.jpainsymman.2020.03.026.
3. Wallace CL, Wladkowski SP, Gibson A, White P. Grief during the COVID-19 pandemic: considerations for palliative care providers. J Pain Symptom Manag. 2020;60:e70–6. https://doi.org/10.1016/j.jpainsymman.2020.04.012.
4. Powell VD, Silveira MJ. What should palliative care's response be to the COVID-19 pandemic? J Pain Symptom Manag. 2020;60:e1–3. https://doi.org/10.1016/j.jpainsymman.2020.03.013.
5. Communication and Symptom Management. https://www.capc.org/toolkits/training-all-clinicians-in-essential-communication-and-symptom-management-skills/. Accessed 21 Feb 2021.
6. Smith RC, Hoppe RB. The patient's story: integrating the patient- and physician-centered approaches to interviewing. Ann Intern Med. 1991;115:470–7. https://doi.org/10.7326/0003-4819-115-6-470.
7. Chapman K, Abraham C, Jenkins V, Fallowfield L. Lay understanding of terms used in cancer consultations. Psychooncology. 2003;12:557–66. https://doi.org/10.1002/pon.673.
8. COVID Ready Communication Playbook. In: VitalTalk. https://www.vitaltalk.org/guides/covid-19-communication-skills/. Accessed 20 Feb 2021.
9. Working with Families Facing Undesired Outcomes During the COVID-19 Crisis. https://www.swhpn.org/index.php?option=com_dailyplanetblog&view=entry&year=2020&month=03&day=19&id=35:working-with-families-facing-undesired-outcomes-during-the-covid-19-crisis. Accessed 20 Feb 2021.
10. Burge FI, Lawson BJ, Johnston GM, Grunfeld E. A population-based study of age inequalities in access to palliative care among cancer patients. Med Care. 2008;46:1203–11. https://doi.org/10.1097/MLR.0b013e31817d931d.
11. Morrison RS, Augustin R, Souvanna P, Meier DE. America's care of serious illness: a state-by-state report card on access to palliative care in our Nation's hospitals. J Palliat Med. 2011;14:1094–6. https://doi.org/10.1089/jpm.2011.9634.
12. Kelley AS. Epidemiology of care for patients with serious illness. J Palliat Med. 2013;16:730–3. https://doi.org/10.1089/jpm.2013.9498.
13. Perednia DA, Allen A. Telemedicine technology and clinical applications. JAMA. 1995;273:483–8. https://doi.org/10.1001/jama.1995.03520300057037.
14. Worster B, Swartz K. Telemedicine and palliative care: an increasing role in supportive oncology. Curr Oncol Rep. 2017;19:37. https://doi.org/10.1007/s11912-017-0600-y.
15. Kidd L, Cayless S, Johnston B, Wengstrom Y. Telehealth in palliative care in the UK: a review of the evidence. J Telemed Telecare. 2010;16:394–402. https://doi.org/10.1258/jtt.2010.091108.
16. Lloyd-Williams M. Out-of-hours palliative care advice line. Br J Gen Pract. 2001;51:677.
17. Hennemann-Krause L, Lopes AJ, Araújo JA, Petersen EM, Nunes RA. The assessment of telemedicine to support outpatient palliative care in advanced cancer. Palliat Support Care. 2015;13:1025–30. https://doi.org/10.1017/S147895151400100X.
18. Achey M, Beck C, Beran D, Boyd C, Schmidt P, Willis A, Riggare S, Simone R, Biglan K, Dorsey E, Aldred J, Ayan J, Bull M, Carter J, Duderstadt K, Dunlop B, Galifianakis N, Hickey P, Hunter C, Zadikoff C. A randomized controlled trial of telemedicine for Parkinson's disease (Connect. Parkinson) in the United States: Interim assessment of investigator and participant experiences. 2015. pp. S64.
19. Bensink M, Hailey D, Wootton R. A systematic review of successes and failures in home telehealth: preliminary results. J Telemed Telecare. 2006;12:8–16. https://doi.org/10.1258/135763306779380174.

20. Niki K, Okamoto Y, Maeda I, Mori I, Ishii R, Matsuda Y, Takagi T, Uejima E. A novel palliative care approach using virtual reality for improving various symptoms of terminal cancer patients: a preliminary prospective, multicenter study. J Palliat Med. 2019;22:702–7. https://doi.org/10.1089/jpm.2018.0527.
21. Virtual reality use for symptom management in palliative care: a pilot study to assess user perceptions - PubMed. https://pubmed-ncbi-nlm-nih-gov.ezproxy.library.uq.edu.au/31895637/. Accessed 21 Feb 2021.
22. Wang SSY, Teo WZW, Teo WZY, Chai YW. Virtual reality as a bridge in palliative care during COVID-19. J Palliat Med. 2020;23:756. https://doi.org/10.1089/jpm.2020.0212.
23. Hilliard RE. Music therapy in hospice and palliative care: a review of the empirical data. Evid Based Complement Alternat Med. 2005;2:173–8. https://doi.org/10.1093/ecam/neh076.
24. Gallagher LM, Steele AL. Developing and using a computerized database for music therapy in palliative medicine. J Palliat Care. 2001;17:147–54.
25. Krout RE. The effects of single-session music therapy interventions on the observed and self-reported levels of pain control, physical comfort, and relaxation of hospice patients. Am J Hosp Palliat Care. 2001;18:383–90. https://doi.org/10.1177/104990910101800607.
26. Batzner KW. The effects of therapist vocal improvisation on discomfort behaviors of in-patient hospice clients. PhD Thesis, University of Kansas, Music and Dance. 2003.
27. Wlodarczyk N. The effect of music therapy on the spirituality of persons in an in-patient hospice unit as measured by self-report. J Music Ther. 2007;44:113–22. https://doi.org/10.1093/jmt/44.2.113.
28. McConnell T, Graham-Wisener L, Regan J, McKeown M, Kirkwood J, Hughes N, Clarke M, Leitch J, McGrillen K, Porter S. Evaluation of the effectiveness of music therapy in improving the quality of life of palliative care patients: a randomised controlled pilot and feasibility study. Pilot Feasibility Stud. 2016;2:70. https://doi.org/10.1186/s40814-016-0111-x.
29. Archie P, Bruera E, Cohen L. Music-based interventions in palliative cancer care: a review of quantitative studies and neurobiological literature. Support Care Cancer. 2013;21:2609–24. https://doi.org/10.1007/s00520-013-1841-4.

Chapter 14
Barriers to Advance Care Planning (ACP) in the Hospital: A Review and Case Study

Christian Goodwin and Kevin Conrad

What Is Advance Care Planning?

Advance care planning (ACP), in its simplest form, is a conversation between patients, their loved ones, and their providers about goals, values, and preferences for care [1]. ACP is defined as "a process that supports adults at any age or stage of health in understanding and sharing their personal values, life goals, and preferences regarding future medical care" [2].

Many individuals associate ACP with advance directives (ADs) or other legal documents that capture patients' treatment wishes. ACP is distinct from an AD. Unlike ADs, which are forms that document patient wishes, ACP is a process and series of conversations that helps patients identify and understand their values and preferences. ACP is a continual and longitudinal process involving ongoing conversations and revisions as an individual's health status changes.

Benefits and Purpose of ACP

ACP serves multiple purposes in clinical practice. ACP helps ensure that patients' wishes are respected once they can no longer make decisions for themselves and aids surrogate decision-makers in making decisions on their loved one's behalf [3, 4]. ACP promotes patient autonomy and facilitates care that aligns with the patient's goals and preferences. ACP also provides an opportunity for individuals to reflect

---

C. Goodwin
University of North Carolina Medical School at Chapel Hill, Chapel Hill, NC, USA

K. Conrad (✉)
Ochsner Health, New Orleans, LA, USA
e-mail: kconrad@ochsner.org

© The Author(s), under exclusive license to Springer Nature Switzerland AG 2022
K. Conrad (ed.), *Clinical Approaches to Hospital Medicine*,
https://doi.org/10.1007/978-3-030-95164-1_14

on their own values and goals. When begun early, ACP allows individuals to reflect on these values and goals without the duress of life-threatening conditions. While conversations are the core of ACP, documenting the outcomes of ACP in an accessible way that follows individuals through the health system is a goal of ACP [5].

The benefits of ACP are numerous. ACP has been associated with improved provider-patient communication, fewer hospitalizations at the end of life, less unwanted medical care, improved quality of life, and increased patient autonomy [6–8]. The benefits extend to family, providers, and health systems too. ACP can increase cost-effective care by decreasing aggressive and unwanted interventions near the end of life [9]. Family members may experience less intense grieving and have a lower likelihood of developing certain psychiatric conditions after their loved one's death [10, 11]. Providers experienced decreased levels of moral distress when discussing or removing life-sustaining treatments when their patient had participated in ACP [12].

A Snapshot of ACP in America

ACP is a complex process that can look different for every individual. Given the heterogeneity of ACP, measuring how and where ACP occurs is difficult. Tracking AD completion is often used as a proxy for ACP.

The majority of people in America have not completed an AD. A 2017 study found that only 37% of US adults had completed an AD [13]. Older Americans are more likely to complete an AD. Studies estimate that roughly 50% of older adults have completed an AD [13, 14]. AD completion is not a perfect measure of ACP, since patients can participate in ACP without documenting the conversations in and AD. Thus, rates of ACP may be higher. Two studies estimated that 70% of older adults in the USA have participated in ACP [15, 16].

Most ACP happens in outpatient settings. Studies of billable claims for ACP encounters found 70–90% of claims come from the outpatient setting [17, 18]. Skolarus et al. found that internal medicine and family medicine providers were the most likely to participate in ACP in the outpatient setting [18].

Multiple demographic factors are associated with increased rates of AD completion. UpToDate identifies older age, white race, history of chronic disease, high disease burden, high socioeconomic status, prior knowledge about AD, higher education level, and higher levels of functional impairment as being associated with increased likelihood of AD completion [19–25]. Conversely, certain populations are less likely to have participated in ACP. Racial and ethnic minorities, incarcerated populations, the homeless, and LGBTQ+ individuals are all less likely to have participated in ACP [26–31].

Hospital Medicine and ACP

Hospitalists play a critical role in ACP. Given the low rates of ACP, many hospitalized individuals will not have participated in ACP when they are admitted. With the shortage of palliative care providers and because of hospitalists' role in inpatient care, the Society of Hospital Medicine (SHM) has identified ACP as a core competency for hospitalists. SHM has developed numerous resources to help hospitalists conduct ACP [32–34]. As experts and stewards of inpatient care, hospitalists have a unique opportunity to introduce and facilitate ACP for hospitalized patients. I an addition ACP is often a critical component of the care plan.

Barriers to Conducting ACP in Practice

While the importance of ACP and the role that hospitalists play is clear, there are numerous barriers that prevent better, earlier, and more frequent ACP.

ACP Is Uncomfortable Many physicians find ACP and goals of care conversations uncomfortable. Some physicians feel that broaching the ACP conversation constitutes giving up hope for the patient [35]. This is often reinforced by family members. Hospitalists have noted that the lack of long-standing relationship with hospitalized patients makes ACP conversations difficult to broach [36]. The demands of hospital throughput often make establishing a mutually respectful relationship challenging. Families and patients who are not ready to talk about death and end-of-life care can make ACP feel even more uncomfortable and difficult [37].

Lack of Time ACP can be a time-intensive process, and physicians note a lack of time for having ACP conversations with patients and families [35–37]. While most recognize ACP is important, some physicians don't feel fully supported by their institutions to invest the necessary time and resources into ACP [35].

Lack of Training and Experience Medical school curricula have not traditionally emphasized end-of-life care, ACP, and the communication skills necessary for ACP [37, 38]. Residents and medical students have reported a lack of confidence and preparation for navigating these conversations [39]. Some providers are unclear when to initiate conversations with patients and families about the dying process and end-of-life care [35, 40]. Other studies found that providers and trainees may lack of knowledge and clarity about the role of ADs and other ACP documents [36].

Cultural Competency Death and dying is often intimately tied to faith, spirituality, and cultural traditions. Many doctors report not knowing what end-of-life care practices are culturally appropriate for their patients [35]. A 2015 study found that 86% of doctors perceived ACP conversations with patients from different ethnicities as "quite a bit" or "a great deal" challenging [41].

This list is by no means is exhaustive but presents some of the common barriers to ACP for hospitalists.

Overcoming the Barriers to ACP

There are numerous programs, interventions, and frameworks designed to improve ACP [42–46]. These solutions target a variety of stakeholders and stages in the ACP process. However, there is no silver bullet solution for improving ACP. It will continue to require extensive effort, innovation, and honest evaluation of those efforts. Every clinic or hospital has a unique environment that creates context-specific barriers. Understanding the barriers at your institution is the first step in overcoming those barriers and improving ACP.

Ochsner Health Case Study: Understanding Barriers Across the Practice Spectrum

Ochsner Health has long recognized the value of ACP but also appreciated the significant barriers to improving the quality and frequency of ACP across the system. In this case study, we present the process our team went through to better understand the context-specific barriers to ACP and to identify strategies for improving ACP. We include the resources we developed to understand our ACP landscape and highlight key messages and themes that could help other institutions complete similar quality improvement projects.

The Institution

Ochsner Health is a nonprofit, multisite hospital system that spans multiple states across the gulf south. The system, whose flagship 767-bed hospital is located just outside of New Orleans, had more than 876,000 patient encounters in 2019 [47]. There are six other facilities within the Ochsner System. Ochsner maintains partnership with numerous other health systems across the region.

Project Setup and Methods

Ochsner tapped a public health researcher (CG) with health systems quality improvement experience to lead the project. CG created the project plan, devised the interview guide, conducted the interviews, and led the analysis. Next, the team identified a clinical champion, a hospitalist with over 30 years of experience in the system, to serve in a dyad relationship with CG. The champion was selected for his clinical experience and his deep relationships with providers and departments across the system. The champion provided clinical expertise and oversight, as well as connections to providers.

We began the project by identifying a clear research question and goal. After multiple meetings with representatives from population health, hospital medicine, and palliative medicine, we decided on two primary questions: first, what barriers do clinicians and APPs encounter when discussing end-of-life plans with patients? Second, how can we increase and better document the number of patients having conversations about end-of-life care?

We then drafted an interview plan. First, we identified the departments we wanted to interview stakeholders from:

- Hospital medicine
- Hematology and oncology
- Primary care
- Emergency medicine
- Palliative medicine
- Information technology

We aimed to speak with attending physicians, house staff, residents, nurses, (APPs), nurse aides, and case managers from each of these departments.

With our key stakeholders identified, we developed and piloted an interview guide. The guide went through numerous iterations, and the final version of the guide is included in Appendix 1. This guide can serve as a template for other institutions hoping to conduct similar work.

Working with the champion and the Ochsner team, we designed our interview approach. The champion identified key stakeholders to speak with. We reached out to each potential interviewee via email. If an individual agreed to speak with us, we set up a 30–45-minute interview. CG conducted all the interviews by phone or zoom. CG also took notes and analyzed each interview, identifying key themes and highlighting barriers and solutions for improving ACP that each interviewee identified. At the end of each interview, we asked interviewees to connect us with any colleagues that might have valuable insights to share. The barriers to ACP and solutions to improve ACP that the interviewees identified are discussed below.

Identified Barriers

Interviewees identified the following common barriers to more and better ACP within their organization.

Lack of Training and Education Many noted that medical school curricula and postgraduate training do not often emphasize ACP and related communication skills. Providers had to hone these skills on their own as they went through training. Interviewees felt there was a lack of training and knowledge around hospital policy and legal statutes. Some were unclear about billing practices (e.g., how often can I bill for ACP for a given patient?) or had questions about local and state-level statutes surrounding ACP and end-of-life care (e.g., what is the order of surrogate decision-makers in my state?) Some interviewees were not aware of features within the electronic health record (EHR), like smart phrases and special tabs for ACP.

Provider Discomfort with ACP Many said that they and their colleagues experienced discomfort having ACP conversations. Some felt fellow clinicians began avoiding ACP conversations after having unpleasant experiences with them early in their training. Some thought that limited opportunities to practice ACP conversations also contributed to provider discomfort.

Low Perceived Value While all providers thought ACP was valuable for acutely ill and dying patients, some did not feel ACP was appropriate or valuable for other, less ill individuals. Some felt that the emphasis on widespread ACP was not medically appropriate or a good use of clinicians time.

Lack of Perceived Value of Palliative Care Some felt that engaging palliative care for ACP conversations was not valuable. One interviewee felt that consulting palliative care "just slowed the process [of patient care] down." Some hospitalists felt that they could provide sufficient palliative care without consulting the palliative care team. "Why would I call them in to do something I can do? The defined role of palliative care was different to different providers.

Patients Are Not Ready for ACP Many patients who need ACP are not "ready" to have these conversations when clinicians broach the topic. Interviewees noted that contacting the necessary family members and surrogate decision-makers can be difficult, especially if those individuals are not present during rounds. Even when the family is present, the family may have unrealistic expectations for goals of care or may not be ready to have these conversations.

Lack of Incentives ACP conversations can be time-consuming and may not be billable or generate many RVUs. Providers lamented not being able to bill for shorter ACP conversations. While most interviewees felt ACP was important, they often felt it was not well incentivized or that there were higher-priority competing demands during patient encounters. As one doctor said, "I know it's important, but

I only get to it when I can get to it." Many felt that department quality metrics did not create sufficient incentives either. Departments and teams often tracked ACP conversations at the department level, instead of the individual level.

Lack of Guidelines for ACP Suitability Interviewees disagreed on who should receive ACP, and many felt a lack of clear guidelines led to less ACP by leaving the decision to clinical judgment. Some felt the lack of guidelines allowed providers to avoid ACP more easily and kept it from becoming routine for providers. "The things we don't do often enough, we tend to never do."

Identified Solutions

Interviewees identified the following improvements or changes that could help facilitate ACP within their system.

Guidelines for Who Should Receive ACP Creating clear guidelines for who should receive ACP would reduce ambiguity and cognitive load for physicians. Many interviewees suggested creating an algorithm in the EHR based on risk scores, diagnoses, age, or other criteria that would automatically identify patients who should receive EHR. It was expressed that this initiative would be challenged by an already overburdened EHR.

Increase Partnership with Outpatient Clinics While hospitalists play a critical role in ACP, interviewees noted that primary care and outpatient settings often provide better environments for ACP. Strengthening ACP programs in the community and ambulatory settings would alleviate the burden for hospitalists.

Better Provider Education and Training Increasing the amount of training for medical students and residents and providing more opportunities to practice these skills was a common suggestion. For current providers, many thought more targeted educational programs and more opportunities to practice and role-play ACP conversations would help address physicians' discomfort with ACP.

Standardized Rounding Times More formal rounding schedules would help families know when the doctor would be present and could facilitate ACP conversations by allowing family and surrogate decision-makers to be present at a specific time. COVID-19 has aggravated this situation.

Dedicated Clinical Extender for ACP To alleviate the burden of ACP on the attending clinicians, some interviewees wanted to create a new role on the inpatient team to manage ACP. This designated clinical extender for ACP who would review each patient's chart to identify individuals who need ACP and facilitate the ACP conversations. This would alleviate the ACP burden for physicians and help ensure all patients who needed ACP received it.

Better Incentives for ACP Since many providers' ACP conversations are too short to bill insurance for, many wanted a better incentive scheme for ACP. Providing RVUs or incentive metrics for these shorter conversations was a common suggestion. Others suggested financially compensating hospitalists for each ACP conversation they completed.

Standardize Tools and Language for ACP The language, tools, and approaches that providers use for ACP conversations vary greatly. Standardizing the way providers conduct ACP could help ensure quality control across the system and provide consistency for patients and families.

Lessons Learned

In addition to the solutions above, these conversations highlighted four key takeaways for organizations and health systems looking to improve ACP. First, many providers perceived ACP as important but rarely had ACP conversations with their patients. It was not a lack of interest or perceived importance but rather a lack of training, time, and comfort that kept providers from conducting ACP. Additionally, ACP is often not as pressing as other concerns during a patient encounter. Unlike specific clinical conditions, a lack of ACP does not require immediate intervention. The hospitalists' world is increasingly being filled with urgent fires to be put out. This can lead clinicians to skip a potentially uncomfortable ACP conversation when time gets tight. It was clearly communicated by all that ACP is valuable. The message has gotten through. Taken together, these interviews showed our organization that we need to focus on eliminating the time, comfort, and training barriers instead of communicating the value of ACP.

Second, ACP conversations are not routine practice for many providers. ACP was not emphasized in medical school or residency for many interviewees. Unlike history-taking or the physical exam, ACP is not a part of routine patient interaction. It does not become habit for providers like other skills that has been engrained for our early years of training. We need to work upstream to make these conversations more comfortable and more routine for providers.

Third, community education could help facilitate ACP. Many providers expressed concerns that patients and families would not be ready to talk about death and dying. These fears are often justified; talking about death provokes anxiety in many people [48]. If we want to improve ACP, we need to help patients and families get more comfortable talking about death and dying and help everyone feel better prepared to have these conversations.

Fourth, creating a systematic way to identify patients who should receive ACP is incredibly important. Death is emotional. Especially for providers who have strong relationships with their patients, admitting to themselves and to their patients that they are dying is incredibly difficult. Creating a systematic way for identifying patients that need ACP can limit the impact of that emotion and make the right decision an easier decision. Simple systems-level interventions, like the "surprise question," can be easily implemented and can help identify patients who need ACP [49].

Appendix 1 Barriers to Advance Care Planning Interview

Introduction

1. Can you briefly walk me through your role at (*institution name*)?
2. What roles and responsibilities does your job involve on a daily basis?
    Now I'd like to talk about your experience with advance care planning (ACP). For this project, we're defining ACP as documented conversations with patients about their wishes for end-of-life care and management. ACP can be documented through different means including advance directives, POLST, 5 Wishes, or others. Do you have any questions about how we've defined ACP?
3. On a scale of 1–10 with 1 being not important at all and 10 being very important, how important is ACP for hospitalized patients? Please explain your choice.

    (a) How important is ACP for ambulatory patients? Please explain your choice.

4. Have you participated in advance care planning conversations? (If no, skip to question 8).
5. Can you tell me about your experience with advance care planning?
    (a) What was your role(s)?
    (b) How frequently did you participate?
    (c) Who participated in the ACP conversation? What about the broader ACP process?
    (d) What ACP conversation training have you received?

    Now I'd like to ask a few questions about the process of ACP.
6. To start, can you walk me through a typical ACP interaction? What does that process look like from start to finish?
    (a) In your current role, what might prompt you to start an ACP conversation with a patient?
    (b) How do you or your team identify patients for ACP?
    (c) How do you or your team approach patients about ACP?
    (d) How do you or your team document the ACP conversation?
    (e) How can you access a patient's ACP once it's in the system?
    (f) How easy/difficult?
    (g) How can you see if a patient has had ACP in another clinical setting? A previous encounter?

7. In your opinion, how do these conversations affect patient care, if at all?

    (a) How does ACP affect the discharge process, if at all?

8. Are you compensated for having these conversations?
9. How do you engage with the palliative care service for ACP conversations, if at all?
10. Tell me about an ACP conversation you participated in that went well. What contributed to the conversation going well?

    (a) What factors help make an ACP conversation go well/easy?

11. Can you think of an ACP conversation that didn't go well? What contributed to the conversation going poorly?

    (a) What factors make an ACP conversation difficult?

    Now I'd like to ask you for your opinion about ways to improve ACP here at your organization.

12. What are the biggest barriers to ACP in your current role?

    (a) Initiating?
    (b) Conducting?
    (c) Recording and documenting?

13. What barriers have you seen across your spectrum of practice?
14. What changes would make it easier to initiate ACP?
15. What changes would make it easier to conduct and record ACP?
16. What changes would make it easier to access ACP information?
17. What other changes could help make ACP better for patients?
18. Do you have any other comments or questions?
19. Who else should I speak to about the topics?

References

1. Advance Care Planning: Health Care Directives | National Institute on Aging [Internet]. [cited 2021 Jul 12]. Available from: https://www.nia.nih.gov/health/advance-care-planning-health-care-directives.
2. Sudore RL, Lum HD, You JJ, Hanson LC, Meier DE, Pantilat SZ, et al. Defining advance care planning for adults: a consensus definition from a multidisciplinary delphi panel. J Pain Symptom Manag. 2017;53(5):821–832.e1.
3. Myers J, Cosby R, Gzik D, Harle I, Harrold D, Incardona N, et al. Provider tools for advance care planning and goals of care discussions: a systematic review. Am J Hosp Palliat Care. 2018;35(8):1123–32.
4. Fried TR, Zenoni M, Iannone L, O'Leary J, Fenton BT. Engagement in advance care planning and surrogates' knowledge of patients' treatment goals. J Am Geriatr Soc. 2017;65(8):1712–8.
5. Hickman SE, Hammes BJ, Moss AH, Tolle SW. Hope for the future: achieving the original intent of advance directives. Hast Cent Rep. 2005:Spec No:S26–30.

6. Brinkman-Stoppelenburg A, Rietjens JAC, van der Heide A. The effects of advance care planning on end-of-life care: a systematic review. Palliat Med. 2014;28(8):1000–25.
7. Houben CHM, Spruit MA, Groenen MTJ, Wouters EFM, Janssen DJA. Efficacy of advance care planning: a systematic review and meta-analysis. J Am Med Dir Assoc. 2014;15(7):477–89.
8. Martin RS, Hayes B, Gregorevic K, Lim WK. The effects of advance care planning interventions on nursing home residents: a systematic review. J Am Med Dir Assoc. 2016;17(4):284–93.
9. Klingler C, in der Schmitten J, Marckmann G. Does facilitated advance care planning reduce the costs of care near the end of life? Systematic review and ethical considerations. Palliat Med. 2016 May;30(5):423–33.
10. Lum HD, Sudore RL, Bekelman DB. Advance care planning in the elderly. Med Clin North Am. 2015 Mar;99(2):391–403.
11. Jimenez G, Tan WS, Virk AK, Low CK, Car J, Ho AHY. Overview of systematic reviews of advance care planning: summary of evidence and global lessons. J Pain Symptom Manag. 2018;56(3):436–459.e25.
12. Elpern EH, Covert B, Kleinpell R. Moral distress of staff nurses in a medical intensive care unit. Am J Crit Care. 2005 Nov;14(6):523–30.
13. Yadav KN, Gabler NB, Cooney E, Kent S, Kim J, Herbst N, et al. Approximately one in three US adults completes any type of advance directive for end-of-life care. Health Aff (Millwood). 2017;36(7):1244–51.
14. McMahan RD, Tellez I, Sudore RL. Deconstructing the complexities of advance care planning outcomes: what do we know and where do we go? A scoping review. J Am Geriatr Soc. 2021;69(1):234–44.
15. Silveira MJ, Wiitala W, Piette J. Advance directive completion by elderly Americans: a decade of change. J Am Geriatr Soc. 2014;62(4):706–10.
16. Silveira MJ, Kim SYH, Langa KM. Advance directives and outcomes of surrogate decision making before death. N Engl J Med. 2010;362(13):1211–8.
17. Ashana DC, Chen X, Agiro A, Sridhar G, Nguyen A, Barron J, et al. Advance care planning claims and health care utilization among seriously ill patients near the end of life. JAMA Netw Open. 2019;2(11):e1914471.
18. Skolarus LE, Lin CC, Kerber KA, Burke JF. Regional variation in billed advance care planning visits. J Am Geriatr Soc. 2020;68(11):2620–8.
19. Detering KM, Buck K, Ruseckaite R, Kelly H, Sellars M, Sinclair C, et al. Prevalence and correlates of advance care directives among older Australians accessing health and residential aged care services: multicentre audit study. BMJ Open. 2019;9(1):e025255.
20. Evans N, Bausewein C, Meñaca A, Andrew EVW, Higginson IJ, Harding R, et al. A critical review of advance directives in Germany: attitudes, use and healthcare professionals' compliance. Patient Educ Couns. 2012;87(3):277–88.
21. Aw D, Hayhoe B, Smajdor A, Bowker LK, Conroy SP, Myint PK. Advance care planning and the older patient. QJM. 2012;105(3):225–30.
22. Bullock K. The influence of culture on end-of-life decision making. J Soc Work End Life Palliat Care. 2011;7(1):83–98.
23. Kwak J, Haley WE. Current research findings on end-of-life decision making among racially or ethnically diverse groups. Gerontologist. 2005;45(5):634–41.
24. Teno JM, Gruneir A, Schwartz Z, Nanda A, Wetle T. Association between advance directives and quality of end-of-life care: a national study. J Am Geriatr Soc. 2007;55(2):189–94.
25. UpToDate [Internet]. [cited 2021 Jul 12]. Available from: https://www.uptodate.com/contents/advance-care-planning-and-advance-directives#H2094860.
26. Hughes M, Cartwright C. Lesbian, gay, bisexual and transgender people's attitudes to end-of-life decision-making and advance care planning. Australas J Ageing. 2015;34(Suppl 2):39–43.
27. Kaplan LM, Sudore RL, Arellano Cuervo I, Bainto D, Olsen P, Kushel M. Barriers and solutions to advance care planning among homeless-experienced older adults. J Palliat Med. 2020;23(10):1300–6.

28. Choi S, McDonough IM, Kim M, Kim G. The association between the number of chronic health conditions and advance care planning varies by race/ethnicity. Aging Ment Health. 2020;24(3):453–63.
29. Sudore RL, Landefeld CS, Barnes DE, Lindquist K, Williams BA, Brody R, et al. An advance directive redesigned to meet the literacy level of most adults: a randomized trial. Patient Educ Couns. 2007;69(1–3):165–95.
30. Europe PMC. Europe PMC.
31. Ekaireb R, Ahalt C, Sudore R, Metzger L, Williams B. "We take care of patients, but we don't advocate for them": advance care planning in prison or jail. J Am Geriatr Soc. 2018;66(12):2382–8.
32. Everything We Say and Do: Discussing advance care planning | The Hospitalist [Internet]. [cited 2021 Jul 16]. Available from: https://www.the-hospitalist.org/hospitalist/article/134791/transitions-care/everything-we-say-and-do-discussing-advance-care.
33. Palliative Care | Clinical Topics | Society of Hospital Medicine [Internet]. [cited 2021 Jul 16]. Available from: https://www.hospitalmedicine.org/clinical-topics/palliative-care/.
34. Hospitalists Play Key Role in Advance Care Planning [Internet]. [cited 2021 Jul 14]. Available from: https://www.medscape.com/viewarticle/951987.
35. Fulmer T, Escobedo M, Berman A, Koren MJ, Hernández S, Hult A. Physicians' views on advance care planning and end-of-life care conversations. J Am Geriatr Soc. 2018;66(6):1201–5.
36. Vanderhaeghen B, Van Beek K, De Pril M, Bossuyt I, Menten J, Rober P. What do hospitalists experience as barriers and helpful factors for having ACP conversations? A systematic qualitative evidence synthesis. Perspect Public Health. 2019;139(2):97–105.
37. Travers A, Taylor V. What are the barriers to initiating end-of-life conversations with patients in the last year of life? Int J Palliat Nurs. 2016;22(9):454–62.
38. Sutherland R. Dying well-informed: the need for better clinical education surrounding facilitating end-of-life conversations. Yale J Biol Med. 2019;92(4):757–64.
39. Sullivan AM, Lakoma MD, Block SD. The status of medical education in end-of-life care: a national report. J Gen Intern Med. 2003;18(9):685–95.
40. Smeenk FWJM, Schrijver LA, van Bavel HCJ, van de Laar EFJ. Talking about end-of-life care in a timely manner. Breathe (Sheff). 2017;13(4):e95–102.
41. Periyakoil VS, Neri E, Kraemer H. No easy talk: a mixed methods study of doctor reported barriers to conducting effective end-of-life conversations with diverse patients. PLoS One. 2015;10(4):e0122321.
42. Leah Rogne PD, editor. Advance care planning: communicating about matters of life and death. Springer Publishing Company; 2013.
43. Bernacki R, Hutchings M, Vick J, Smith G, Paladino J, Lipsitz S, et al. Development of the serious illness care program: a randomised controlled trial of a palliative care communication intervention. BMJ Open. 2015;5(10):e009032.
44. Schickedanz AD, Schillinger D, Landefeld CS, Knight SJ, Williams BA, Sudore RL. A clinical framework for improving the advance care planning process: start with patients' self-identified barriers. J Am Geriatr Soc. 2009;57(1):31–9.
45. Fortin G, Dumont S. Goals of care conversations at the end-of-life: perceived impact of an Interprofessional training session on professional practices. J Soc Work End Life Palliat Care. 2021;15:1–21.
46. Ho AHY, Lall P, Tan WS, Patinadan PV, Wong LH, Dutta O, et al. Sustainable implementation of advance care planning in Asia: an interpretive-systemic framework for national development. Palliat Support Care. 2021;19(1):82–92.
47. Online Newsroom [Internet]. [cited 2021 Jul 23]. Available from: https://news.ochsner.org/facts-statistics.
48. Is the Fear of Death Controlling Your Anxiety? [Internet]. [cited 2021 Aug 23]. Available from: https://www.healthline.com/health/death-anxiety-talk-about-grieving.
49. Moss AH, Lunney JR, Culp S, Auber M, Kurian S, Rogers J, et al. Prognostic significance of the "surprise" question in cancer patients. J Palliat Med. 2010;13(7):837–40.

Chapter 15
Value-Based Care in the Hospital

Jason B. Hill, Santoshi M. Kandalam, and Sneha Panganamamula

What Is Value?

In traditional economics, value is defined as a measure of the benefit provided by a specific good or service. Value is inherently subjective and can be ascertained by asking how much money a person is willing to pay for a certain commodity. For example, a long distance runner might find a $200 pair of sneakers to be worth the price, whereas the average person may not be willing to spend this sum for his or her pedestrian purposes.

What Is Value-Based Care?

Value-based care is defined as "health outcomes achieved per dollar spent" [1]. It is critical to note that value is referring to benefits measured on a population level rather than an individual level. Most people do not have a maximum amount of money they would spend in order to save their own or a loved one's life. Demand for healthcare services is generally thought to be price inelastic, meaning that demand will exist independent of cost; therefore it is extremely difficult to ascertain

---

J. B. Hill (✉)
Ochsner Medical Center - North Shore, Ochsner, New Orleans, LA, USA
e-mail: jahill@ochsner.org

S. M. Kandalam
University of Queensland, Faculty of Medicine, QLD, Australia

S. Panganamamula
New York University, New York, NY, USA

© The Author(s), under exclusive license to Springer Nature Switzerland AG 2022
K. Conrad (ed.), *Clinical Approaches to Hospital Medicine*,
https://doi.org/10.1007/978-3-030-95164-1_15

a specific value per individual. However, when looking at our healthcare system as a whole, the amount of dollars we spend compared to the population-wide quality of care delivered can serve as a measure of the overall value of our system.

How Do We Measure Value?

The accepted definition for value among the medical community is health outcomes achieved per dollar spent. Determining how to measure health outcomes is a multi-part process: choosing which health outcomes to measure, determining a uniform method of measuring the outcomes, comparing outcomes to a defined baseline, and repeating the process for negative outcomes.

Per the Agency for Healthcare Research and Quality, healthcare quality can be measured by the parameters of structure, process, and outcome [2]. A structural measure of quality would quantify organizational capacity to deliver healthcare services. For example, the ratio a healthcare system has of providers to patients is one indicator of structural quality. Procedural measures of quality would be used to evaluate what an organization does to provide care. For instance, the percentage of women eligible for mammograms that actually receive them is a measure of procedural quality. Lastly, an outcome measure of quality would assess what impact organizational interventions have had on the health status of patients [3]. The mortality rate of patients within 30 days of leaving the hospital is one example of an outcome measure [2].

Outcome measures are the ideal type of parameter to evaluate whether the care a system delivers is value-based. However, there are several challenges present in measuring healthcare outcomes. Most notably, healthcare outcomes are widely understood to largely be a consequence of socioeconomic factors, such as race, income, education, immigration status, food insecurity, housing status, etc. [4]. Thus health systems that serve communities of lower socioeconomic status might have poorer health outcomes despite delivering quality healthcare. Other challenges include the fact that patients may see several different providers within a fragmented healthcare system, such that measuring the value of a single provider may be challenging. Patient self-reported satisfaction with a provider may not directly correlate with health benefits, and there is a lack of standardization in the existing ways that hospitals are rated on quality [5].

With regard to our healthcare system as a national aggregate, the World Health Organization has a comprehensive list of health status indicators used to compare health outcomes between nations [6]. Some of the most frequently referenced indicators include life expectancy from birth, infant mortality rate, and maternal mortality rate. Assessing the amount of money spent as a nation on the healthcare sector in relation to these indicators is a commonly used way to determine the overall value of our healthcare system [7].

Current Value of Healthcare in the United States

The Organization for Economic Co-operation and Development (OECD) is an organization consisting of 37 nations, including the United States, with the aim of collecting and publishing healthcare data. Compared to other OECD countries, the United States spends the most money per capita on healthcare at $10,966 per person as of 2019 [8]. The second highest nation was Switzerland at $7732–which is 42% less than the United States spends. On average, OECD nations spend $5697 per capita on healthcare which is approximately half of what the United States spends [9].

Of course, the high cost of healthcare would be justified if the outcomes achieved were markedly better as well. However, this is decidedly not the case. The United States had an average life expectancy of 78.5 years in 2019–lower than the OECD average and about 5 years lower than Switzerland [8]. The United States also has a higher burden of chronic disease and obesity, higher maternal and infant mortality, and a higher rate of mortality from preventable causes compared to similar nations.

If value-based care is health outcomes achieved per dollars spent, then the fact that the United States spends the most money among developed nations for relatively poor outcomes signals that our system is less valuable to patients than other developed nations.

How Did We Get Here?

In order to understand why we currently do not have great value in our healthcare, it is essential to look back at the historical foundations leading to the current system we have today. Healthcare was largely an unorganized endeavor practiced by physicians without standardized licenses from the pre-colonial era until the Great Depression. The advent of health insurance was the first major milestone paving the road to the current system we have today.

Early Models of Health Insurance

The first time insurance was applied to the healthcare sector was in 1929 when a group of teachers in Dallas, Texas, contracted with Baylor University Hospital to pay 6 dollars a year in exchange for 21 days of inpatient care [10]. This was considered an affordable way to guarantee hospital-based care if needed during the Depression era. This model of insurance is known as capitation–when patients pay a certain amount of money to receive certain defined health benefits within a specified period of time.

This idea was expanded upon by Henry J. Kaiser who hired tens of thousands of workers for steel and construction projects in the 1930s [11]. At this time, many hospitals were at risk of closing due to revenue loss during the Great Depression. An agreement was reached between Mr. Kaiser and a physician named Dr. Sidney Garfield to the terms that Mr. Kaiser would pay 7 cents per worker per day to Dr. Garfield, and in return Dr. Garfield would provide necessary health services to workers. This model was expanded to numerous construction project sites in the state of California as well as to include workers' families, and the Kaiser-Permanente Medical Group was born from this form of capitated payments.

At the same time during the Depression era, hospitals began to form "Blue Cross" programs in which patients could pay a monthly premium in the event that they may require medical care. These premiums kept hospitals open with steady income while unpredictable fee-for-service revenue declined during the economic downturn. Physicians, most of whom were primary care providers, soon began forming "Blue Shield" plans in which patients paid premiums to access these outpatient medical services. This format of patients paying premiums in exchange for access to healthcare when needed is the cornerstone of the system we have today.

Employer-Based Commercial Health Insurance

During World War II, the United States began mobilizing and redirecting all resources toward a total war effort. Food and other goods were rationed, employment rates soared, and the Stabilization Act of 1942 allowed all wages and salaries to be frozen in order to avoid postwar inflation [12]. In order to attract potential employees to jobs during the labor shortage while also not being able to offer increased salaries, employers turned to offering fringe benefits such as health insurance. This quickly grew as a popular option because employers were able to offer benefits that were tax-deductible and employees received benefits that were exempt from taxes.

In the pre-war era, less than 10% of people had some form of health insurance, but by 1946 almost a third of the nation had coverage [12, 13]. Employer-sponsored insurance, a vestigial byproduct of World War II wage loopholes, remains the most common form of health coverage today with about 50% of Americans obtaining their policy through an employer in 2019 [14].

Medicare and Medicaid

In the 1950s, the cost of medical care began to rise sharply. Healthcare spending was about 4% of the GDP from the Great Depression to the postwar era but was rising to above 5% by the 1960s [15]. This was partly due to incredible advances in medical technology–such as the first cardiac pacemakers and kidney transplants–but also due to a lack of centralized government regulation of prices. Healthcare was becoming unaffordable to many, and efforts to initiate a single payer healthcare system by the federal government were unsuccessful. President Truman proposed a plan for universal coverage, but the American Medical Association and several members of Congress decried this as an attempt of having socialized medicine in the midst of the Cold War [16].

Health-associated costs continued to rise without restraint, and in 1965 President Johnson signed into law the amendments into the Social Security Act that would render Medicare and Medicaid into existence. The intent was to provide coverage for people deemed most vulnerable to the effects of rising costs of healthcare–namely, the elderly, poor, and disabled.

The positive health impacts of Medicare have been substantial. After implementation, the financial burden of healthcare on elderly people was significantly reduced, and life expectancy for adults older than 65 went up after 1965 at a faster rate than the rest of the population as a whole [17]. At the same time, costs accrued by the government to maintain Medicare have also risen exorbitantly. In fact, costs for Medicare have risen faster than virtually any other major federal program [18].

Medicaid, the safety net insurance program, originally covered low-income families with children, pregnant women, disabled people, and low-income elderly people. The impact of Medicaid on health has been more difficult to study as people who are eligible for Medicaid tend to be poorer and sicker at baseline compared to the general population. In the landmark Oregon Health Insurance Experiment, Medicaid enrollees who were randomly selected off a waiting list were compared to subjects who were not selected over time. The study showed improved access to primary and preventative care, better mental health, and reduced risk of medical debt but no improvements in major health conditions such as hypertension or diabetes [19]. Similar to Medicare, costs of maintaining Medicaid have risen since the advent of the program in 1965. Medicaid spent 4 dollars per US resident in 1966, 750 dollars in 2000, and 1869 dollars in 2019 [20].

The Rise and Fall of Managed Care

By the 1970s, healthcare spending was consuming almost 9% of the nation's GDP, leading the federal government to pass the Health Maintenance Organization (HMO) Act of 1973 [21]. This act provided federal funding to expand HMOs–the prototype of what came to be known as managed care–and also required employers of over 25 people to offer an HMO plan as an option. Under an HMO plan, patients could pay lower premiums and have lower cost-sharing but were subjected to regulations that were intended to cut the cost of healthcare overall. Patients could only see doctors that were contracted with the health plan, they could only see specialists with a referral from their primary care doctor, and most medications, imaging, or procedures were subject to utilization review by the plan.

Between the late 1980s and 1990s, managed care became the dominant form of health insurance, and this had a clear impact on the overall cost of healthcare which, for the first time in decades, remained a steady portion of the GDP from 1993 to 2000 [22]. Despite finally achieving lowered costs in the national healthcare system, there was a large backlash against the managed care revolution by the late 1990s. Patients were not appreciative of the red tape and denied care by insurance plans and physicians perceived far too much interference into medical care. In addition, many HMOs paid providers in their networks through capitation which shifted risk onto doctors rather than on the plans–a feature doctors were not fond of. Throughout the early 2000s, there was a massive shift away from managed care and toward plans like Preferred Provider Organizations (PPOs) which did not have the same burdens of utilization review and limitations of in-network providers as HMOs did. Between 2000 and 2010, the proportion of people insured through their employer with PPO plans rose from 39% to 58% [23].

As a result, throughout the 2000s, healthcare costs began to rise at an exorbitant rate as they had before. The cost of premiums on individuals and families soared higher and higher every year, and several tactics by for-profit health insurance companies made it more difficult to obtain coverage. For example, health plans would charge higher premiums for individuals with preexisting conditions or only provide coverage for a limited set of medical benefits. This ultimately led to one in every six Americans being uninsured in the early 2000s with several more being underinsured as well [24]. The end result was that a significant proportion of the population lacked access to needed care and faced unaffordable medical bills when they did seek care. These unpayable costs subsequently would get shifted onto the premiums of the insured and the vicious cycle of rising costs continued.

The Affordable Care Act

In 2010, President Barack Obama signed the Patient Protection and Affordable Care Act (ACA) into law–a gargantuan attempt to rectify some of these major deficits in the several moving, disjointed parts that comprised the national healthcare system. The three large goals of this legislation were to increase access to care, decrease the cost of care, and increase the quality of care.

In terms of access, a key feature of the ACA was the individual mandate requiring everyone to carry health insurance or pay a tax penalty. In order to make this a reasonable mandate, the ACA also expanded employer requirements for providing insurance, created a federal exchange where people could purchase individual insurance with income-based subsidies, expanded Medicaid to cover people living with an income of up to 138% of the federal poverty level, and made it so that health insurance companies had to cover certain benefits deemed essential and could not charge higher premiums for preexisting conditions [25]. The effect of these reforms on insurance levels was indeed substantial; the number of Americans without insurance dropped from 49 million in 2010 to an all-time low of 27 million in 2016.

The impact of the ACA on the overall cost of healthcare has been difficult to fully determine. The main ways this legislation attempted to reduce costs were through reducing Medicare Advantage payments, incentivizing comprehensive and cost-saving primary care through Accountable Care Organizations (ACOs), and tying payments from Medicare to quality measures rather than traditional fee-for-service [25, 26]. Costs of healthcare have risen every year since the passage of the ACA. However, there have been significant reductions in the rate of increase [27]. This has been attributed in part to the aftermath of the 2008 economic recession rather than specific provisions in the law itself. The rest of the impacts of the ACA on cost has been a mixed bag of positive and negative changes. For instance, although costs of healthcare premiums and out-of-pocket spending for the average family have gone up, out-of-pocket spending as a percentage of total healthcare spending has not risen since 2010.

Several new programs were encoded into the ACA with the intent to improve the overall quality of our healthcare system. One notable example is the Hospital Readmissions Reduction Program (HRRP) which reduced Medicaid and Medicare payments to hospitals for patients with certain conditions that were readmitted within 30 days of discharge. Though on the surface intended to incentivize hospitals to provide better-quality care and avoid readmission, safety net hospitals serving patient populations with lower socioeconomic status and a higher burden of disease were disproportionately penalized without any overall improvement in quality of health [28]. Another example is the Hospital Value-Based Purchasing Program (HVBP) which provided incentives to hospitals for meeting certain structural-, process-, and outcome-based quality measures. To date, there have been no significant improvements in quality for hospitals that have been subject to HVBP.

Although access to the healthcare system has markedly improved due to the Affordable Care Act, the impact of this legislation on cost and quality is still to be determined. It is important to note that there have been a few major changes since the original bill was signed into law. In the landmark 2012 case *National Federation of Independent Business v. Sebelius*, the Supreme Court ruled that expansion of Medicaid to all people eligible under federal law was excessively coercive of states [29]. Thus, states had the choice to opt into Medicaid expansion, and 36 states have chosen to do so as of 2021.

Transition to Value-Based Care

As the ACA grew, the government started experiencing the impact of rising healthcare costs, and there was increased motivation to create programs that cut costs. Simultaneously, the medical community arrived at their own conclusions, understanding that creating a healthcare system that operates like a regular corporation or industry was not in the best interest of the population that it served. Creating health systems using the basic economic principle of supply and demand not only ran counter to medical ethics but, as people discovered, was not necessary to turn a profit. Initially, organizations such as the Institute for Health Improvement and the Agency for Healthcare Research and Quality created initiatives that tackled public health policies and focused on population health. It was not until 2010 that the realization that profits in healthcare relied upon people becoming ill took hold, and systems started to recognize that they should have a vested interest in the health of the communities they were serving. The Institute for Health Improvement created the Triple Aim, "a framework focused on the health of the population, the experience of care for individuals within that population, and the per capita cost of providing that care." The ACA was one of the first steps of pursuing the Triple Aim [30].

Since that time, there have been many more initiatives created with the intent to transition healthcare toward value-based care. For example, Institute for Health Improvement's current initiative pushes the emphasis on population care to include equity. The vision for their "Pursuing Equity" initiative is motivated by the urgency of eliminating inequities that were brought to the front due the pandemic. As with all their initiatives, the organization will focus on raising awareness, educating, and creating networks to accomplish their goals. More recently the IHI changed the Triple Aim to the quadruple aim, including improving clinician experience as one of the core objectives in creating a better, more valuable, healthcare system [31].

Agency for Healthcare Research and Quality

Funded by the US Department of Health and Human Services, the Agency for Healthcare Research and Quality (AHRQ) is a federal agency that focuses on improving the healthcare system in the United States by collecting evidence and providing research data to practitioners across the United States. As stated on their home page, the organization develops the knowledge, tools, and data needed to improve the healthcare system and help patients, healthcare professionals, and policymakers make informed health decisions. It was developed in response to the issues laid out in the landmark paper "To Err is Human," published in November 1999. The paper extensively discussed the then current state of medical errors and outlined the importance of awareness and education [32]. This report significantly changed the culture of medicine, encouraging providers to be accountable for the "ugly" side of medicine nobody wanted to acknowledge.

Starting in 2010, the AHRQ monitored the incidence of different hospital-acquired conditions (HACs) that led to deaths, such as adverse drug events, catheter-associated urinary tract infections, central line-associated bloodstream infections, falls, obstetric adverse events, pressure ulcers, surgical site infectious, ventilator-associated pneumonias, and post-op venous thromboembolism. Through the implementation of both awareness and educational programs, the rate of HACs dropped dramatically over a period of 4 years. Cumulative deaths avoided due to HACs were nearly 87,000 by 2014 [33]. This data was proof that improvements can be made to decrease preventable deaths within the healthcare system. This highlighted the need for quality improvement (QI) projects and for changes that incorporate an "improvement culture" within medical education. Medical education is also evolving to increase awareness and understanding of the importance of quality care [34].

Patient-Centered Medical Homes

The role of primary care has evolved significantly over the last two decades. Understanding that primary care providers play one of the most important roles in a patient's health and satisfaction, there has been a push toward creating a model where the primary care doctor also had the responsibility of coordinating patient care. The Patient-Centered Medical Home (PCMH) model of healthcare was created with the intent of establishing a set of guidelines for communication between primary care and other providers involved in caring for a mutual patient. Before the guidelines were set, a few primary care providers had already started to develop structures with results that looked promising for better health outcomes and lower overall healthcare costs. Studies during that time reached a consensus that improving coordination decreases costs and hospital admissions, improves patient experiences and staff satisfaction rates, and distributes healthcare costs more evenly [35].

PCMHs are regulated by the National Committee for Quality Assurance (NCQA) and are required to focus on six main areas as listed on their website: team-based care and practice organization, care management and support, evidence-based clinical decisions, care coordination and care transitions, patient-centered access and continuity, and performance measurement and quality improvement [36]. Studies have repeatedly shown the benefit in cost reduction as well as outcomes for a patient within a PCMH system as compared to traditional primary care practices. This has not only allowed innovators to see the value in improving the healthcare system but has also shed insight into the effectiveness of having structured guidelines and incentives.

The focus on primary care also meant increasing primary interventions such as screening and regular follow-up with a physician. The PCMHs have been able to execute this successfully; one commonly used example is the improvement of diabetes control within their patient population. However, they had difficulties translating that to improving the health of the community. This was largely due to lack of access to medical care. The biggest landmark policy created to combat that issue is the ACA. While this act has covered many more Americans than previously, there were and still are barriers to access that disproportionately affect poorer, less healthy people in need of regular medical care [37].

Now responsible for a larger portion of national medical costs, Medicare and Medicaid policymakers were motivated to create solutions that would make medical services more economical. Many attempts to solve the crisis of high healthcare costs built upon the idea of increasing coordination through primary care, placing uniform guidelines and benchmarks for providers, and increasing financial risk for healthcare professionals to incentivize them to cut costs and improve quality.

Accountable Care Organizations

The ACA formally introduced Accountable Care Organizations (ACOs) to the healthcare landscape in another attempt to decrease healthcare costs and further the value-based care movement. ACOs are groups of primary care doctors, specialists, and healthcare systems that voluntarily operate as one unit to increase coordination, decrease medical errors, and improve value. ACOs are centered around a primary care physician who is responsible for coordinating care and gathering and sharing information within the ACO. It's important to note that patients in an ACO must be informed and have the option to decline sharing their data. Other requirements for ACOs include having at least 5000 Medicare fee-for-service beneficiaries under their care each year to qualify for shared savings. As long as the ACO fulfills these requirements and maintains quality of care as dictated by CMS, the entity will receive back its savings, thus incentivizing physicians to think about both costs and quality [38].

The difference between ACOs and previous initiatives is the addition of financial risk taken by healthcare systems, meaning that not only are payments tied to quality but also that healthcare systems are penalized for excess spending. ACOs have been evolving for the past decade, starting as Medicare Shared Savings Programs (MSSP) with low financial risk and transitioning to the Next-Generation ACO (NGACO) model. This model has the largest financial risk for healthcare providers.

In 2014, 3 years after the implementation of shared savings ACOs, Centers for Medicaid and Medicare Services (CMS) reported that the shared savings program had 338 ACOs with 4.9 million beneficiaries. The total shared savings was $341 million, and the average overall quality score was 83%. In 2018, 561 ACOs with 10.5 million beneficiaries were part of the program, with a shared savings of $938 million and a 93% average overall quality score. As of January 2021, there are around 10.7 million assigned beneficiaries [39]. Although there is a general consensus that ACOs decrease healthcare spending, the effect on Medicare spending is highly debated. According to the CMS benchmark calculation, in the first few years of implementing MSSP ACOs, the overall Medicare spending increased by $344.2 million; however, other studies report a decrease in spending of around $541.7 million [40]. One argument for why shared savings don't automatically translate to decreased spending for Medicare is the accountability placed on organizations; little to no organizations increased the amount of risk they were taking by joining. The main takeaway is that by correctly motivating healthcare providers and systems, it is possible to both decrease spending and increase quality [41].

The newer ACO model, the NGACO, built upon the initial MSSP and pioneer models by increasing the downside risk for organizations. In the initial years of implementation, NGACOs achieved a $349 million reduction, a change of −0.9%, before accounting for shared savings and payouts to providers. However, according to CMS data, there was a nonsignificant increase in net spending of 0.3% accounting for both shared savings and payments [42]. Despite observing direct cost reductions for Medicare, some providers advocate for the continuation of this program.

They believe that more recent data and a deeper analysis will provide more favorable financial results, also noting that patients in NGACO systems have dramatically better care experiences.

The ACO Investment Model (AIM) was a slightly different initiative that provided payments upfront for certain ACOs to get staffing and resources. This model was also targeted toward rural areas and smaller systems. Unlike some of the other models, CMS data showed that the AIM ACO was successful in reducing Medicare costs, with no change in quality [43].

Although ACOs have not been shown definitively to decrease costs for Medicare, there is a consensus that ACO models have been successful at reducing the overall cost of healthcare [44]. While ACOs may not be able to single-handedly decrease costs and increase quality, many providers are encouraged at the current results. Most also agree that other initiatives, possibly paired with ACOs, are required to address the rising costs of healthcare.

Medicaid Bundled Payments

In 2013, bundled payment systems were created by CMS in an attempt to decrease spending and increase coordination of care among the multitude of providers that a patient sees during an "episode" of care. CMS believed that the previous status quo, a fee-per-service-provided model, did not give providers enough incentive to be resourceful and efficient when deciding how to treat and who to involve in the patient's care. The Bundled Payments for Care Improvement (BCPI) initiative gave providers and hospitals incentives to decrease their expenditure and increase coordination between different providers. This transition shifted the responsibility of choosing efficient, quality, care from patients, and the government to hospitals and providers. Although the evaluation did not show a significant cost reduction for Medicare or Medicaid services nor a significant change in patient outcomes, there was evidence of hospitals reducing their overall costs and improving the quality of care. However, it is important to note that the cost reductions and quality improvements were not isolated to hospitals that participated in BCPI programs. A possible explanation for this is that the trend of healthcare delivery even outside of these programs was toward more sustainable and value-based spending at the time the initiative was implemented [45].

While developing this initiative, CMS wanted to ensure that cost cutting did not decrease the quality of healthcare delivered. Many studies assessed the impact of decreasing Medicare and Medicaid spending on private payments. The literature at the time showed that hospitals did not compensate the decrease in public payments by increasing private income, in fact they have been shown to decrease costs across the board [46].

The first bundled payment model targeted acute care hospitals and defined an episode of care as a single inpatient stay. Hospitals that opted to participate would be paid a target price per episode of care, determined by the Inpatient Prospective

Payment System. This payment was based on diagnosis, regardless of the number of services actually utilized. If the hospital was able to effectively treat a patient with less than the provided amount, they were allowed to keep the revenue; if they spent more, the costs would not be reimbursed. In order to ensure that reduced costs did not adversely affect patient outcomes, CMS conducted a thorough analysis of quality metrics such as 30-day all-cause mortality, 30-day all-cause readmissions, 30-day post episode, and patient discharge destination. The annual report done by Econometrica, Inc. concluded that "no consistent negative or positive impacts on claims-based health outcomes were observed" with the implementation of Model 1 [45]. Models 2–4 differed in the definition of episode as well as the incentives for providers.

The primary goals of the program as listed in the proposal are to increase the following: promotion of care coordination and data sharing, efficient and appropriate staffing models, patient risk stratification, patient and family engagement throughout care, data-driven program management, and continuous quality improvement. Bundling payments for episodes created a financial incentive for providers to strive toward achieving these goals. Prior to the push toward value-based care, large hospital systems did not have specific metrics or incentives in place to motivate their providers to think about the amount of resources they were utilizing and the overall cost of care for the patient and government.

Although we learned a lot from this initiative, the results did not show a significant reduction in cost for Medicare. There are multiple hypotheses as to why this was the case. A significant portion of research shows that bundled payments should in theory lower costs, leading to the consensus that the result of this initiative had more to do with implementation.

A 2020 study suggested that CMS would have had a higher chance of saving costs and seeing improvement if the BPCI was mandatory rather than voluntary. They found that the hospitals that chose to participate in the program had higher targeted prices assigned by CMS; on average, they received approximately $1000 more than non-BPCI hospitals [47]. The majority of hospitals who opted to be a part of the initiative were hospitals that had enough resources to cut costs, therefore benefiting from the bundled payment. The study further noted the importance hospitals place on making the decision to join certain payment plans, only joining if they are fairly confident about increasing their revenue.

Hospital Value-Based Purchasing Programs

The Hospital Value-Based Purchasing (VBP) program was developed under the hypothesis that tying payments to outcomes by providing both rewards and penalties would increase value. The budget for this initiative is designed to be neutral; Medicare redistributes payments to hospitals based on their ability to meet benchmarks. This initiative is both nonvoluntary and national in scope, making it very different from previous initiatives. If hospitals meet or exceed benchmarks, created via comparisons to other hospitals, they are rewarded; however, if hospitals have increased rates of HACs or lack of consistent discharge instructions, they are penalized. As an example, in 2015, if a hospital was found by the HAC Reduction Program to be in the lowest quartile as compared to other hospitals, that hospital could face a reduction in their CMS payments of 1%, or approximately $330 million [48]. The challenge with tying payments to performance is the difficulty in creating benchmarks and tools to assess the way providers deliver care. The scoring methodology for all the initiatives within Hospital VBP programs are constantly updated, improved, and made public so hospitals can set their own goals.

Another criticism of the program is the lack of evidence showing decreased mortality or improved quality as a direct result of either the benefits or penalties. A study comparing hospitals both within and without the VBP program resulted in similar, even slightly decreased improvement in mortality in hospitals that are paid through the VBP program [49].

The last CMS-developed quality initiative, the Hospital Readmissions Reductions Program (HRRP), relies entirely on penalties to encourage hospitals to decrease readmission rates after receiving treatment for six common conditions in the hospital. Although determining hospital performance is complicated, the concept of this initiative is simple. The goal is to have fewer readmissions compared to hospitals not participating in the HRRP. The biggest assumption in this theory is that hospitals are able to control the majority of factors that cause a patient to get readmitted.

CMS not only publishes the results of evaluating their own quality-based programs, but they also have initiatives that aim to publish the quality of healthcare provided by different institutions [50]. These programs are primarily targeted toward improving patient experience by allowing them to make more informed decisions about the care they are receiving.

Education

Apart from designing healthcare models with the aim of making significant structural changes, organizations like the AHRQ, IHI, and CMS also promote education to inspire healthcare professionals at an individual level to understand the importance of quality, innovation, and public health.

The AHRQ used to host an Innovations Exchange website that allowed medical professionals to share the development, implementation, outcomes, impact, and generalizability of innovative initiatives. The aim was to drive the creation and distribution of evidence-based projects that may eventually be adopted by numerous institutions in the United States. Though the initiative was discontinued due to lack of funding, the AHRQ website contains a downloadable, open-source, spreadsheet contains initiatives started at various different hospital systems [51]. The IHI has also created an open school for students, allowing them to familiarize themselves with the Triple Aim, improving quality, and patient safety [52].

The organization acknowledges the challenges of integrating innovation and dynamic changes into a curriculum that is known to be slow adopting new principles; however, the organizations strongly believe that the benefits are vital to the sustainability of healthcare. As previously described, there is a common understanding that the costs of our current system are continuing to increase. Some initiatives have shown the capability of decreasing the rate at which costs increase, showing hope for a more sustainable system.

Conclusion

Innovation is at the root of American culture and may be the only answer to combating the challenges the United States' unique healthcare system faces. Other countries in the OECD spend less on healthcare and are able to have better life expectancy for their citizens. These countries have increased access to healthcare and spend more money managing common diseases rather than focusing on specialized care. Hospitalists in the United States spend significant amounts of time working on secondary and tertiary prevention methods, shifting the focus away from primary prevention. Many studies have shown that the impact of healthcare is much less significant than factors such as genetic disposition, social circumstances, and behavioral patterns. In fact, a CDC study showed that healthcare has an impact of 10% on premature mortality; allowing us to understand why more advanced, specialized care at the expense of primary prevention reduces both our quality and quantity of life [53].

The IHI makes it clear that understanding and intentionally addressing patients' social determinants of health is a key factor in adding value to healthcare. Hospitalists, though generally not thought to have a huge role in primary prevention, do have a large impact on value. Approximately one-third of the money spent on healthcare goes toward inpatient services. Government programs Medicare and Medicaid pay for 66.3% of hospital costs. Since value, as defined earlier in the chapter, increases as costs decrease, we can see why hospitalists have a large role in determining the value of healthcare [53]. Therefore, focusing on quality within hospital systems is key to increasing value.

QI projects that aim to increase value are currently being run by most major hospital systems in the United States. Although it is difficult to determine the exact amount spent on QI projects, a recently conducted systematic review shows that QI projects that achieve their quality goal generally do tend to decrease costs, despite the added cost of implementation [54]. Government-led projects have the potential to decrease costs at a much larger scale than individualized hospitals; however, large-scale operations are significantly harder to implement, as witnessed by the initial bundled payment plans. Despite the challenges, some studies have found that participation in voluntary value-based reforms and meaningful use of electronic health records in addition to HRRP did have greater reductions in cost than participating in HRRP alone [55]. This strengthens the argument that the initiatives run by CMS could have greater impacts in combination with each other.

The main question of whether the projects developed to drive value-based care have directly improved patient outcomes both in quality and quantity of life still remains to be determined. However, the problems that value-based care attempts to solve are undeniable and universally accepted as important issues to resolve.

References

1. Porter ME. What is value in health care? N Engl J Med. 2010;363(26):2477–81. https://doi.org/10.1056/NEJMp1011024.
2. Pittet D. Infection control and quality health care in the new millennium. Am J Infect Control. 2005;33(5):258–67. https://doi.org/10.1016/j.ajic.2004.11.004.
3. Dallolio L, Raggi A, Sanna T, Mazzetti M, Orsi A, Zanni A, Farruggia P, Leoni E. Surveillance of environmental and procedural measures of infection control in the operating theatre setting. Int J Environ Res Public Health. 2018;15(1):46. https://doi.org/10.3390/ijerph15010046.
4. Braveman P, Gottlieb L. The social determinants of health: it's time to consider the causes of the causes. Public Health Rep (Washington, DC : 1974). 2014;129(Suppl 2):19–31. https://doi.org/10.1177/00333549141291s206.
5. Suchy K. A lack of standardization: the basis for the ethical issues surrounding quality and performance reports. J Healthc Manag. 2010;55(4):241–51.
6. Carey G, Crammond B. Action on the social determinants of health: views from inside the policy process. Soc Sci Med. 2015;128:134–41. https://doi.org/10.1016/j.socscimed.2015.01.024.
7. Pham H. Modeling US mortality and risk-cost optimization on life expectancy. IEEE Trans Reliab. 2011;60(1):125–33. https://doi.org/10.1109/tr.2010.2103990.
8. World Health O. World health statistics 2020: monitoring health for the SDGs, sustainable development goals. Geneva: World Health Organization; 2020.
9. Anderson GF, Hussey P, Petrosyan V. It's still the prices, stupid: why the US spends so much on health care, and a tribute to Uwe Reinhardt. Health Aff. 2019;38(1):87–95. https://doi.org/10.1377/hlthaff.2018.05144.
10. Moseley GB The u.s. Health care non-system, 1908–2008. (1937–7010 (Print)).
11. Zinner MJ, Loughlin KR. The evolution of health care in America. Urol Clin North Am. 2009;36(1):1–10. https://doi.org/10.1016/j.ucl.2008.08.005.
12. Hoffman B. Health care reform and social movements in the United States. Am J Public Health. 2003;93(1):75–85. https://doi.org/10.2105/ajph.93.1.75.
13. Hirshfield DS. The Lost Reform â Daniel S. Hirshfield | Harvard University Press. Harvard University Press; 1970. https://www.hup.harvard.edu/catalog.php?isbn=9780674498082. Accessed February 2021.
14. Duggan M, Goda GS, Jackson E. The effects of the affordable care act on health insurance coverage and labor market outcomes. Natl Tax J. 2019;72(2):261–322. https://doi.org/10.17310/ntj.2019.2.01.
15. Getzen TE. The growth of health spending in the United States from 1776 to 2026. Oxford University Press; 2019. https://doi.org/10.1093/acrefore/9780190625979.013.488.
16. Markel H. 69 years ago, a president pitches his idea for national health care. Health; 2014.
17. Moon M Medicare. (0028–4793 (Print)).
18. Manton KG, Gu X, Lamb VL. Long-term trends in life expectancy and active life expectancy in the United States. Popul Dev Rev. 2006;32(1):81–105. https://doi.org/10.1111/j.1728-4457.2006.00106.x.

19. Allen H, Baicker K, Taubman S, Wright B, Finkelstein A. The Oregon health insurance experiment: when limited policy resources provide research opportunities. J Health Polit Policy Law. 2013;38(6):1183–92. https://doi.org/10.1215/03616878-2373244.
20. Klemm JD. Medicaid Spending: A Brief History. vol 22; 2000.
21. Fox P. A history of managed health care and health insurance in the United States. In: Kongstvedt P, editor. The essentials of managed health care. 6th ed. Burlington, MA: Jones and Bartlett Learning; 2021.
22. Pinkovskiy ML. The impact of the managed care backlash on health care spending. Rand J Econ. 2020;51(1):59–108. https://doi.org/10.1111/1756-2171.12306.
23. Kaiser HSoE-SHB. Distribution of Health Plan Enrollment for Covered Workers, by Plan Type, 1988–2012. The Henry Kaiser Family Foundation; 2013.
24. Tolbert J. Key facts about the uninsured population. 2020.
25. Adler H. A short primer on the affordable care act. Technol Innov. 2013;15(3):265–7. https://doi.org/10.3727/194982413x13790020922022.
26. Weiner J, Marks C Fau, Pauly M, Pauly M. Effects of the ACA on Health Care Cost Containment. (1553–0671 (Electronic)).
27. Manchikanti L Fau, Helm Ii S, Helm Ii S Fau, Benyamin RM, Benyamin RM Fau, Hirsch JA, Hirsch JA. A critical analysis of obamacare: affordable care or insurance for many and coverage for few? (2150–1149 (Electronic)).
28. Blumenthal D, Abrams M. The affordable care act at 10 years - payment and delivery system reforms. N Engl J Med. 2020;382(11):1057–63. https://doi.org/10.1056/NEJMhpr1916092.
29. Frohnen BP. Waivers, federalism, and the rule of law. Perspect Polit Sci. 2016;45(1):59–67. https://doi.org/10.1080/10457097.2015.1050306.
30. Whittington JW, Nolan K, Lewis N, Torres T. Pursuing the triple aim: the first 7 years. Milbank Q. 2015;93(2):263–300. https://doi.org/10.1111/1468-0009.12122.
31. Arnetz BB, Goetz CM, Arnetz JE, Sudan S, VanSchagen J, Piersma K, Reyelts F. Enhancing healthcare efficiency to achieve the quadruple aim: an exploratory study. BMC Res Notes. 2020;13(1):362. https://doi.org/10.1186/s13104-020-05199-8.
32. Institute of Medicine Committee on Quality of Health Care in A. In: Kohn LT, Corrigan JM, Donaldson MS, editors. To err is human: building a safer health system. Washington: National Academies Press (US); 2000. Copyright 2000 by the National Academy of Sciences. All rights reserved. Washington (DC). 10.17226/9728.
33. Saving Lives and Saving Money: Hospital-acquired conditions update. 2021.
34. Akdemir N, Peterson LN, Campbell CM, Scheele F. Evaluation of continuous quality improvement in accreditation for medical education. BMC Med Educ. 2020;20:308. https://doi.org/10.1186/s12909-020-02124-2.
35. Epperly T. The patient-centred medical home in the USA. J Eval Clin Pract. 2011;17(2):373–5. https://doi.org/10.1111/j.1365-2753.2010.01607.x.
36. Massa I, Miller BF, Kessler R. Collaboration between NCQA patient-centered medical homes and specialty behavioral health and medical services. Transl Behav Med. 2012;2(3):332–6. https://doi.org/10.1007/s13142-012-0153-4.
37. Hefner JL, Wexler R, McAlearney AS. Primary care access barriers as reported by nonurgent emergency department users: implications for the US primary care infrastructure. Am J Med Qual. 2015;30(2):135–40. https://doi.org/10.1177/1062860614521278.
38. Harolds JA. Will accountable care organizations deliver greater quality and lower cost health care? Clin Nucl Med. 2010;35(12):935–6. https://doi.org/10.1097/RLU.0b013e3181fb5194.
39. Shared Savings Program Fast Facts. Centers for Medicare and Medicaid Services. 2021.
40. Schulz J, DeCamp M, Berkowitz SA. Spending patterns among medicare ACOs that have reduced costs. J Healthc Manag. 2018;63(6):374–81. https://doi.org/10.1097/jhm-d-17-00178.
41. Ouayogode MH, Colla CH, Lewis VA. Determinants of success in shared savings programs: an analysis of ACO and market characteristics. Healthcare J Deliv Sci Innov. 2017;5(1–2):53–61. https://doi.org/10.1016/j.hjdsi.2016.08.002.

42. Next Generation Accountable Care Organization: Evaluation of the first three years. Centers for Medicare and Medicaid Services, Baltimore, MD; 2019.
43. Trombley M, Fout B, Zhou C, Brodsky S, Morefield B, McWilliams M, Nyweide D. Factors associated with reduced medicare spending in the accountable care organization (ACO) investment model. Health Serv Res. 2020;55:123–4.
44. Wilson M, Guta A, Waddell K, Lavis J, Reid R, Evans C. The impacts of accountable care organizations on patient experience, health outcomes and costs: a rapid review. J Health Serv Res Policy. 2020;25(2):130–8. https://doi.org/10.1177/1355819620913141.
45. McClellan SR, Trombley MJ, Marshall J, Kahvecioglu D, Kummet CM, LaRocca C, Dummit L, Hassol A. Bundled payment episodes initiated by physician group practices: Medicare beneficiary perceptions of care quality. J Gen Intern Med. https://doi.org/10.1007/s11606-021-06848-9.
46. Frakt AB. The end of hospital cost shifting and the quest for hospital productivity. Health Serv Res. 2014;49(1):1–10.
47. Berlin NL, Gulseren B, Nuliyalu U, Ryan AM. Target prices influence hospital participation and shared savings in Medicare bundled payment program. Health Aff. 2020;39(9):1479–85. https://doi.org/10.1377/hlthaff.2020.00104.
48. Soltoff S, Koenig L, Demehin AA, Foster NE, Vaz C. Identifying poor-performing hospitals in the medicare hospital-acquired condition reduction program: an assessment of reliability. J Healthc Qual. 2018;40(6):377–83. https://doi.org/10.1097/jhq.0000000000000128.
49. Figueroa JF, Tsugawa Y, Zheng J, Orav EJ, Jha AK. Association between the value-based purchasing pay for performance program and patient mortality in US hospitals: observational study. BMJ. 2016;353:i2214. https://doi.org/10.1136/bmj.i2214.
50. Jung JK, Wu BX, Kim H, Polsky D. The effect of publicized quality information on home health agency choice. Med Care Res Rev. 2016;73(6):703–23. https://doi.org/10.1177/1077558715623718.
51. Health Care Innovations Exchange. 2021.
52. Tartaglia KM, Walker C. Effectiveness of a quality improvement curriculum for medical students. Med Educ Online. 2015;20(1):27133. https://doi.org/10.3402/meo.v20.27133.
53. Kaplan RM, Milstein A. Contributions of health care to longevity: a review of 4 estimation methods. Ann Fam Med. 2019;17(3):267–72. https://doi.org/10.1370/afm.2362.
54. de la Perrelle L, Radisic G, Cations M, Kaambwa B, Barbery G, Laver K. Costs and economic evaluations of quality improvement collaboratives in healthcare: a systematic review. BMC Health Serv Res. 2020;20(1):1–10. https://doi.org/10.1186/s12913-020-4981-5.
55. Ryan AM, Krinsky S, Adler-Milstein J, Damberg CL, Maurer KA, Hollingsworth JM. Association between hospitals' engagement in value-based reforms and readmission reduction in the hospital readmission reduction program. JAMA Intern Med. 2017;177(6):862–8. https://doi.org/10.1001/jamainternmed.2017.0518.

Chapter 16
Wellness in Physicians in the Era of the COVID-19 Pandemic

Kevin Conrad and Rula Saeed

Introduction

At the time of this publication, the area of the Southern United States where I and the co-author of this chapter practice hospital medicine is in the midst of the fourth surge of COVID-19 infections. Despite aggressive ongoing efforts, vaccination rates remain among the lowest in the country, and the end of the pandemic is very uncertain. Each wave brings similar but new challenges. With each surge, an increasing sense of futility begins to creep in and the wellness of both hospitalists other providers is challenged.

As in previous surges, the emergency room is at capacity, the hospital is running low on beds, staff is stretched to its limits, and fatigue is setting in. At this time, it is impossible to fully measure both the short-term and long-term effect of the pandemic on our mental well-being. Equally difficult is to assess the effectiveness of measures taken to improve providers' well-being during the pandemic. However, the pandemic has lasted too long to not take some measure of its impact on the mental health and what measures have been undertaken both initially and on an ongoing basis to promote wellness during this crisis. This surge will end as the others have, but as we transition from survival mode, how will the healthcare community emotionally process the pandemic and what impact will it have on the future delivery of healthcare?

As the pandemic approaches its second year, wellness of healthcare workers has become increasingly important as we acknowledge the chronicity of the current

---

K. Conrad (✉)
Ochsner Health, New Orleans, LA, USA
e-mail: kconrad@ochsner.org

R. Saeed
University of Queensland School of Medicine, Ochsner Clinical School, New Orleans, LA, USA

situation. Indeed it has become essential as staff shortages fostered by burnout play a key role in dealing with the overwhelmed healthcare system. It is increasingly recognized that the finite collective mental health reserves of our providers is as important as the physical challenges such as hospital beds and ventilators in dealing with the pandemic. Resources, human capital being the most important, are limited, and wellness is an essential factor in maintaining a viable workforce.

At the time of this publication, the COVID-19 virus has infected 212 million people worldwide and shows little indication of slowing down [1]. One of its most vulnerable targets has been healthcare workers—ED physicians, hospitalists, respiratory therapists, nurses, and many others, who risk their lives daily to care for those infected. Healthcare workers have been uniquely impacted by COVID-19 infections, with those living in the United States facing an increased chance of infection and death compared with other countries [2]. The risk is amplified in those of color and advanced age.

Equally important is the mental stress placed on healthcare providers. As the pandemic advanced, significant dilemma was encountered among physicians. Physicians with preexisting burnout were suddenly exposed to a sudden surge of rapidly deteriorating patients compounded by a lack of capacity and supplies.

Early on, several specific COVID-19 stressors were discovered. In the United States, investigators at Stanford Medicine and Mount Sinai Health System initially found that frontline workers had eight major COVID-19-related anxieties: (1) competence in providing appropriate care, (2) ability to keep up with up-to-date information, (3) ability to not get infected and keep families not infected, (4) timely access to PPE, (5) access to rapid testing, (6) assistance with personal tasks, (7) access to family care, and (8) healthcare for their families.

For physicians already struggling to find a balance between work and mental health at baseline, the added fear of treating a novel pandemic impaired usual coping mechanisms. Those with extended direct contact with COVID-19 patients, such as hospitalists, critical physicians and nursing staff, and support staff have had the added emotional weight of repeatedly witnessing family members unable to say their final goodbyes. Many providers report that they don't have time to process the emotional impact of what they have been through and are concerned about what the future mental accounting of this time may bring.

These factors have left many asking—at what point does the psychological burden of endless workload, fear, anxiety, and lack of physical support overwhelm the mental health of those at the front lines and of the healthcare system as a whole?

Wellness Among Healthcare Workers During the First Year of the Pandemic

Early in the pandemic, significant psychological repercussions were found in many healthcare workers in some of the initial hotspots. This was reported in the countries of China and Italy. As expected, much of the initial excitement of the call to action and duty was replaced by fear and uncertainty. It was reported that there was a

50.4% incidence of depression, a 44.6% incidence of anxiety, and a 34% incidence of insomnia among Chinese healthcare workers [3]. For 39.1% of healthcare workers living in areas impacted heavily by the pandemic, experiencing feelings of isolation and concern for family members contributed to their distress.

A commonly used scale to assess the mental health of healthcare workers during the pandemic was the Depression, Anxiety, and Stress-21 (DAS-21). In 1 study, it was determined that of 286 participants in 1 initial location, 64.7% had symptoms of depression, 51.6% had symptoms of anxiety, and 41.2% had stress [4]. Many of these symptoms were extensive and were ranked as moderate to severe. It was also found that increased weekly working hours, increased number of COVID-19 patients cared for, lower level of support from peers and supervisors, lower logistic support, and lower feelings of competence during COVID-19-related tasks were correlated with a higher score on the scale [4]. The greater an individual area was affected, the greater the degree of burnout was noted among providers.

A decrease in quality of sleep, decreased self-efficacy, and depression was also noted in physicians who lacked a reliable support system compared to non-healthcare workers. For many the isolation of the practice of medicine was compounded by the nature of treating an infectious pandemic [5]. For many, these support systems served as a refuge from the physical and mental constraints of their job. Isolation, due to fear of spreading the virus to loved ones, led many into feelings of isolation and to a loss of time to decompress with their support systems, perpetuating an already strained coping mechanism.

Factors Contributing to Burnout in Providers Caring for COVID-19 Patients in Early Outbreaks

In studies from the areas first affected by a COVID-19-related virus, 2003 Severe Acute Respiratory Syndrome (SARS 2003) shed some light on the most critical factors which played into mental health deterioration. Fear of transmission to loved ones and colleagues was easily the most important stressor. SARS 2003, while limited in its scope, provided some insight into some of the mental challenges that would occur with the COVID-19 pandemic.

Similarly, during the COVID-19 pandemic, physicians exposed to the COVID-19 virus had distress over their health and over the possibility of transmitting the virus to family living in the same household. Subsequently, 88.3% of physicians reported significant emotional fluctuations and stress during their required isolation time [5].

Initially physicians were suddenly faced with a virus that did not have a standardized treatment regimen. Guidance at the national level and local was limited and in a constant state of flux. Treatment was often determined by the supplies on hand and at the local area. This included standards in which to initiate palliative care, which varied for one institution to another. Although not specifically measured, this uncertainty among all aspects of care was repeatedly reported as a major factor in burnout [5].

Healthcare workers had to rapidly acquire new skills to treat a novel respiratory infection and had to adjust to the transience and futility of these skills on the outcome of their patients. This led to feelings of helplessness and failure. Skill and the confidence to implement these skills, which had once been a protective factor for physicians, had abruptly disintegrated, leading to a tremendous amount of uncertainty over the future. Stigmatization of healthcare workers for either not doing enough or for seemingly spreading the virus led to feelings of fear and a desire to leave the healthcare profession [4].

False theories and conspiracies applied through social media infiltrated many communities and impeded healthcare workers' efforts to promote scientific facts. The general public's backlash to masks caused many physicians to feel that their efforts to contain the spread were futile and underappreciated. The lack of personal protective equipment (PPE) also played an enormous role in physician fear and made many feel abandoned and neglected. Not having adequate protection to do one's job played a large part in distrust in the community and the government, leading to a psychological shift in mentality. Immense and widespread media coverage made it difficult for any attempt at providing a consistent message to patients. Likewise, the media's lack of transparency about vaccinations, finances, businesses, and a plan for returning to the norm made it impossible to systematically provide public health guidance.

It is reasonable to conclude that healthcare workers and medical staff were ill-equipped and untrained when it came to suddenly having to provide mental healthcare for families, patients, and themselves. The mass casualty of the pandemic, feelings of guilt, and ineffectiveness for not being able to do more to help their patients contributed to this.

Unexpected social media condemnation of healthcare workers and feelings of a general loss of control took a mental and physical toll on many physicians, causing several to take their own lives [6]. Although support was offered by most of the public, a unique aspect of this pandemic has been the skepticism of healthcare by a sector of society. Obviously this has been tied into partisan politics of the current era.

The high rate of suicide among physicians predated the COVID-19 pandemic, being approximately 50% higher than in the general public [6]. The addition of a sudden and unexpected health crisis amplified such instances. In late April, Dr. Lorna Breen, a 49-year-old emergency room physician in New York City, died by suicide after experiencing weeks of grueling work hours and fatigue during the pandemic [7]. Due to the immense number of cases flooding the East Coast, she had endured the sight of her colleagues sleeping in hallways and working extended shifts up to 18 hours. After contracting the virus, Dr. Breen felt guilty for taking the necessary time to rest and quarantine. Her story and others like her worldwide prove the vulnerability of healthcare workers and the traumatic physical and mental repercussions that come with a system that commands maximum productivity with finite support.

Historical Perspective of Burnout Among Healthcare Workers

To understand the swift and intense mental stress with which the COVID-19 pandemic afflicted healthcare workers across the world, one must first take into consideration the baseline levels of exhaustion that existed among physicians long before the pandemic. Burnout has been defined as a long-term response to stress, marked by emotional and physical exhaustion, depersonalization, and a lack of sense of personal accomplishment [8].

The concept of healthcare worker burnout is not new and not limited to healthcare providers of this era. As far back as 1922, the director of the Bureau of Public Health Education for New York City published in the American Journal of Public Health that the "occupational strain is greater in medicine than in any of the other professions" and noted that physicians were more than twice as likely to commit suicide than any other profession [9]. In the Journal of Social Issues in 1975, the cycle of burnout was depicted as feeling cornered and targeted from all sides, recounting, "we work too much, too long and too intensely. We feel pressure from within to work and help, and we feel pressure from the outside to give. When the staff member then feels an additional pressure from the administrator to give, even more, he is under a three-pronged attack" [10]. It was found that a degree in medicine, whether MD or DO, increased the prospect of burnout in the United States, with those in emergency medicine, general internal medicine, and family medicine being most at risk [11].

The way in which healthcare workers rapidly found themselves exhausted during the COVID-19 pandemic came as no surprise, given the alarming level of physician burnout in the United states predating the pandemic; after all, it has been said—"to burn out, one has to be burning" [10].

Prior to the pandemic, surveys found that rates of physical and mental exhaustion among healthcare workers were between 40% and 60% [12]. Burnout has been associated with poor outcomes, long posthospital recovery, poor medication adherence, and poor blood pressure control [12]. The risk of substance use disorders and the suicide rate was found to be 25× higher than that in the general population, with an estimate of 200–400 physicians dying by suicide in the United States annually [12]. Modern medicine has been stressed by several factors. In particular, the increasing complexity of patient billing and finances has required that physicians spend more time on clerical duties, which have been shown to increase the rate of burnout [12].

Even prior to establishing independent practices, medical students are introduced to the culture of fast-paced productivity with little time for themselves and are at times applauded for how quickly and successfully they can assimilate to such a culture. It was shown that in comparison with US college graduates ages 22–32, medical students had a higher prevalence of high emotional exhaustion, high depersonalization, and burnout with a worse physical and emotional quality of life [13]. Although some progress has been made, medical training continues to be a high stress environment as compared to other professions.

Although it is expected that some amount of stress is necessary in such a demanding profession with the lives of so many at stake, research has shown that the relationship between stress and performance is an inverted U-shaped curve [14]. Stress initially begins as an energizing and motivating process. Much of this sentiment was appreciated in the early days of the pandemic. Unfortunately the excitement of anew medical challenge was replaced by the realities of system ill prepared for this pandemics scale. Stress can eventually evolve over time over time and become paralyzing for those who do not possess sufficient coping mechanisms. Ultimately stress can cause the downward spiral of cognitive impairment, mental illness, and overall physiologic deterioration.

The term burnout had not been used as effectively as it has in the past several years. The concept of healthcare workers struggling mentally and physically due to the taxing trials and tribulations of their occupation was often overlooked as hospitals overflowed. The COVID-19 pandemic brought to light the seriousness of well-being and the cycle which had perpetuated physicians' mental and physical deterioration for decades.

Coping Mechanisms at the Individual Level

Physicians have long learned to utilize coping mechanisms to deal with the fast-paced and demanding environment they work in. Coping mechanisms are regarded as either problem-focused, which aims to change the climate causing stress, or emotion-focused, which aim to manage the emotional response one has to the stressor. Wellness among physicians has been studied to be maintained by a certain element of psychological resilience, a "process of positive adaptation in the face of adversity that can emerge at different life stages depending on the situation" [15]. A study by O'Dowd et al. showed that for some, the positives of their work-life, such as the patient-doctor relationship, is enough to provide them with the resilience to productively function. Job satisfaction is considered to be a major protective factor for those experiencing burnout and provided immense gratification as it often represented medical efficacy at the hands of the physician. The study also detailed other "resilience strategies" or protective practices that physicians often utilize to protect their mental health such as engaging in leisurely activities, leaving work at work in order to have protected home time, and knowing when to ask for and receive help. A key component of psychological resilience (PR) found in the study was maintaining boundaries with patients and developing interests outside of medicine.

Coping mechanisms are not always healthy and sometimes destructive. It has been reported that 45% of physicians cope with burnout by isolating themselves from others, 33% turn to junk food, 25% turn to alcohol, and 20% turn to binge eating, while 6% of others turn to tobacco, prescription drugs, or marijuana [16]. Having unhealthy coping mechanisms perpetuates the cycle of burnout and undoubtedly sets up healthcare workers into seeking more readily available methods of relaxation. Additionally, because one of the issues at hand is the limited leisure time physicians have, they are more likely to seek out quick outlets to decompress rather than implore the more time-consuming methods of building psychological resilience.

In response to these factors, healthcare workers must be educated on the consequences of utilizing quick-fix unhealthy coping mechanisms and how to incorporate simple changes into their daily lives in order to reduce mental baggage. Making changes at an individual level solves only one side of the problem, but it is essential as it provides a self-owned level of protection for inevitable times of struggle as well as during unexpected worldwide health crises such as the COVID-19 pandemic.

System-Level Promotion of Physician Wellness During the COVID-19 Pandemic

In order to truly address the issue of physician burnout and foster an environment of wellness, change must not only occur at an individual level but at a systemic level as well. Healthcare systems must start taking ownership of the health of their employees and prioritizing a safe mental working environment. It has been reported by many public health experts that supporting the mental well-being and resilience of frontline healthcare workers is not just a good business practice; it is imperative to ensure global recovery from the COVID-19 pandemic [17].

In the recent pandemic, several system-wide development of protocols were found to be essential. This includes adequate storage and display of PPE. There should be crisis training for explaining accurate current information of the disease. Risk of contagion and ways of protections should be clearly demonstrated. An effort should be made to establish systemic diagnostic and treatment protocols and updated in a timely manner. This includes appropriately evolving guidelines for palliative care [4].

Encouraging conversation with colleagues and sharing stories about emotional and physical burdens faced by physicians could be helpful in reducing feelings of isolation and loneliness. Physicians may be initially resistant to this concept, and many early efforts were met with little participation. Attitudes can change with system support.

These efforts should be supported by administrations utilizing federal funding to provide support groups and therapy, either using social media or telemedicine. This will ensure that it is easily accessible [18]. Consequently, normalizing conversations around emotions like grief and guilt, especially during public health emergencies, is imperative to providing support. Not only does emotional support need to be accessible, but it should be provided without consequences. Sufficient protected time off should be given so that healthcare workers are not left struggling to choose between their mental health and work. Encouraging things such as individualized emotional support plans has been suggested as mental health needs differ from person to person [17].

The Agency for Healthcare Research and Quality (AHRQ) Guidelines for Emergency Providers of Healthcare

Other than reducing stress, it is important to understand that the entire system must be reworked in order to address the factors which led to burnout initially. The Agency for Healthcare Research and Quality, a division of the United Sates Department of Health and Human Services, determined some clinician-chosen interventions which would help make the workplace more satisfactory and reduce burnout in times of normal and emergent situations. These interventions included scheduling monthly provider meetings which focused on work issues or clinical topics and enhancing team functioning through depression screening quality improvement projects. This would engage office staff, enhance teamwork, and reduce the pressure on physicians to be responsible for all aspects of care. It was also suggested that medical assistants enter patient data into electronic health records, track forms, and send faxes to give doctors more face-to-face time with patients [8].

Other suggested interventions include hiring floating clinicians which could assist in covering unexpected time off for those who need it, ensuring enough time during the day for physicians and residents to address required documentation, and entering data into the electronic health record [8]. Offering flexible or part-time work schedules to those who requested it is also thought to be beneficial [8].

Although somewhat more difficult to implement in times of emergency, when community needs overwhelm hospital capacity, the AHRQ also suggested developing a backup force of healthcare workers that would be readily available to take on the pressures that hospital workers cannot handle. This could include retired physicians, nurses, and students close to graduation. The point of such backup workers would be to prepare for catastrophic events which bring on masses of patients, similar to what happened in the early days of the COVID-19 pandemic. Many such plans were enacted at healthcare facilities and may serve as a template for future relief efforts.

During emergency times, use of military resources should be considered including workers, hospitals, and potentially even ships that be incorporated as needed. This may include military-style triage that could also help streamline patient care [17].

At the minimum, during this pandemic healthcare workers need clear instructions, up-to-date information, adequate PPE, screening tests, logistical support, transport, accommodation, education, and dissemination of reliable advice on stress management from their respective institutions [6].

Formal training is needed in meeting the emotional needs of not only patients but families as well. This includes both their emotions and physical needs, which is critical for ensuring both the caregivers and the patients are equally attended to. If possible, shorter shifts allow for physicians to have adequate rest and have been shown to reduce attentional failures by 18% [17]. It has been found that interventions, whether through mindfulness training or through workplace reprogramming, reduced overall burnout from 54% to 44%, emotional exhaustion from 38% to 24%, and depersonalization from 38% to 34% .[19].

Importantly, it has never been a better time for healthcare professionals to develop team building skills. Unit cohesion has been found to promote social support, facilitate help-seeking, and reduce the stigma of stress which in turn improves coping adaptation and fosters resilience [20].

System Solutions: Establishing a Chief Wellness Officer

The National Academy of Medicine and other professional societies have called for system-level interventions to promote clinician well-being. In response to this, many healthcare organizations (HCOs) have introduced a new senior leadership position seen in other industries—the healthcare chief wellness officer (CWO). During the pandemic this has proven to be a highly influential position. By incorporating CWOs into the emergency command structure, these HCOs have been able to rapidly identify and address healthcare worker needs throughout the pandemic. The CWO enables efforts to proceed in focused and efficient manner. Unproven mental health interventions can often be time-consuming with little return. A centralized office allows for the constant review and modification of initiatives.

The CWOs at a number of institutions played an important role in understanding and addressing the real time concerns of the healthcare workforce. This has occurred by on site interviews and rapidly deployed surveys. For many HCOs the CWOs is not seen as a luxury but a necessity in retaining and efficiently utilizing a limited workforce. It is vital to have a single point person accountable for implementing the various interventions mentioned in this chapter. Academic institutions have utilized them as well to meet the unique needs of medical students and residents in training.

It has been suggested that the first goal of the chief wellness officer position is shifting the organizational framework from promoting the triple aim of healthcare of improving patient experience, reducing cost, and improving population health to embracing the quadruple aim which prioritizes organizational efforts to improve the well-being of the healthcare team. The pandemic will certainly define and advance this objective. This is reflected by the increasing numbers of academic articles being produced by CWOs and hopefully will continue to grow in the future.

Conclusion

Burnout among physicians is not a new issue. Prior to the pandemic, it affected one in every two US physicians [11]. It must not only be addressed during pandemics but daily due to its effect on millions worldwide and its inevitable path to serious consequences, including suicide. The more healthcare workers are ignored and dismissed, the harder it will be for this group to provide adequate care for patients. This inevitably will lead to a tragic cycle where neither the patient nor the caregiver can form sustainable relationship. To ensure there is adequate healthcare in a post-pandemic world, the system must change by proactively addressing healthcare workers' mental health needs. A new paradigm must be developed that does not accept that providers are immune to stress and mental health is consider as essential in maintaining sustainability among all working in patient care.

Key Points
- The COVID-19 pandemic has drastically affected the mental health of healthcare workers in all specialties, increasing the incidence of depression, anxiety, and insomnia due to lack of PPE, fear of spread, helplessness of treatment, and the emotional weight of mass casualty.
- Burnout is a long-term stress reaction characterized by emotional decline, depersonalization, and loss of confidence that had been afflicting healthcare workers long before the COVID-19 pandemic and played a large role in amplifying their mental and physical distress.
- Change must occur on an individual and systemic level, including hospital administration and government funding to ensure physicians, residents, and nurses have appropriate shift hours, rest time, access to therapy, and adequate backup staff and crisis plans to take over when hospitals become overwhelmed.
- Many healthcare organizations have introduced a new senior leadership position seen in other industries—the healthcare chief wellness officer. This single point person can coordinate and maximize wellness efforts in real time.

References

1. CSSE J. Coronavirus Resource Center; 2021.
2. Gold J. We need to talk about the Covid-19 deaths of healthcare workers. Forbes. https://www.forbes.com/sites/jessicagold/2020/12/22/we-need-to-talk-about-the-covid-19-deaths-of-healthcare-workers/?sh=28e2a5d3707b.
3. Lai J, Ma S, Wang Y, Cai Z, Hu J, Wei N, Wu J, Du H, Chen T, Li R, Tan H, Kang L, Yao L, Huang M, Wang H, Wang G, Liu Z, Hu S. Factors associated with mental health outcomes among health care workers exposed to coronavirus disease 2019. JAMA Netw Open. 2020;3(3):e203976. https://doi.org/10.1001/jamanetworkopen.2020.3976.
4. Elbay RY, Kurtulmus A, Arpacioglu S, Karadere E. Depression, anxiety, stress levels of physicians and associated factors in Covid-19 pandemics. Psychiatry Res. 2020;290:113130. https://doi.org/10.1016/j.psychres.2020.113130.
5. Shreffler J, Petrey J, Huecker M. The impact of COVID-19 on healthcare worker wellness: a scoping review. West J Emerg Med. 2020;21(5):1059–66. https://doi.org/10.5811/westjem.2020.7.48684.
6. El-Hage W, Hingray C, Lemogne C, Yrondi A, Brunault P, Bienvenu T, et al. Health professionals facing the coronavirus disease 2019 (COVID-19) Pandemic: What are the mental health risks? L'Encephale. 2020.
7. Romine T. 2020. https://www.cnn.com/2020/04/28/us/er-doctor-coronavirus-help-death-by-suicide-trnd/index.html. CNN.
8. AHRQ. Physician burnout. Agency for Healthcare Research and Quality; 2017.

9. Marchalik D. Physician burnout in the modern era. Lancet. 2019;393(10174):868–9. https://doi.org/10.1016/S0140-6736(19)30399-X.
10. Freudenberger HJ. Staff burn-out. J Soc Issues. 1974;30(1):159–65. https://doi.org/10.1111/j.1540-4560.1974.tb00706.x.
11. Shanafelt TD, Boone S, Tan L, Dyrbye LN, Sotile W, Satele D, West CP, Sloan J, Oreskovich MR. Burnout and satisfaction with work-life balance among US physicians relative to the general US population. Arch Intern Med. 2012;172(18):1377–85. https://doi.org/10.1001/archinternmed.2012.3199.
12. Stewart MT, Serwint JR. Burning without burning out: a call to protect the calling of medicine. Curr Probl Pediatr Adolesc Health Care. 2019;49(11):100655. https://doi.org/10.1016/j.cppeds.2019.100655.
13. Dyrbye LN, West CP, Satele D, Boone S, Tan L, Sloan J, Shanafelt TD. Burnout among U.S. medical students, residents, and early career physicians relative to the general U.S. population. Acad Med. 2014;89(3):443–51. https://doi.org/10.1097/acm.0000000000000134.
14. Lebares CC, Guvva EV, Ascher NL, O'Sullivan PS, Harris HW, Epel ES. Burnout and stress among US surgery residents: psychological distress and resilience. J Am Coll Surg. 2018;226(1):80–90. https://doi.org/10.1016/j.jamcollsurg.2017.10.010.
15. O'Dowd E, O'Connor P, Lydon S, Mongan O, Connolly F, Diskin C, McLoughlin A, Rabbitt L, McVicker L, Reid-McDermott B, Byrne D. Stress, coping, and psychological resilience among physicians. BMC Health Serv Res. 2018;18(1):730. https://doi.org/10.1186/s12913-018-3541-8.
16. Kane L. Medscape national physician burnout & suicide report 2020: the generational divide; 2020.
17. Santarone K, McKenney M, Elkbuli A. Preserving mental health and resilience in frontline healthcare workers during COVID-19. Am J Emerg Med. 2020;38(7):1530–1. https://doi.org/10.1016/j.ajem.2020.04.030.
18. Shechter A, Diaz F, Moise N, Anstey DE, Ye S, Agarwal S, Birk JL, Brodie D, Cannone DE, Chang B, Claassen J, Cornelius T, Derby L, Dong M, Givens RC, Hochman B, Homma S, Kronish IM, Lee SAJ, Manzano W, Mayer LES, McMurry CL, Moitra V, Pham P, Rabbani L, Rivera RR, Schwartz A, Schwartz JE, Shapiro PA, Shaw K, Sullivan AM, Vose C, Wasson L, Edmondson D, Abdalla M. Psychological distress, coping behaviors, and preferences for support among New York healthcare workers during the COVID-19 pandemic. Gen Hosp Psychiatry. 2020;66:1–8. https://doi.org/10.1016/j.genhosppsych.2020.06.007.
19. Epstein RM, Privitera MR. Doing something about physician burnout. Lancet. 2016;388(10057):2216–7. https://doi.org/10.1016/s0140-6736(16)31332-0.
20. Jun J, Tucker S, Melnyk BM. Clinician mental health and Well-being during global healthcare crises: evidence learned from prior epidemics for COVID-19 pandemic. Worldviews Evid Based Nurs. 2020;17(3):182–4. https://doi.org/10.1111/wvn.12439.

Chapter 17
LGBTQ Healthcare Issues

Leise Knoepp and Olivia Mirabella

Members of the LGBTQ+ community are diverse and definitions are evolving. Some may fall in multiple of these categories, as noted in Table 17.1, while others do not strictly fit in any. Each patient should be treated as an individual with their own unique needs, history, and identity, while keeping in mind the overall healthcare challenges that face the LGBTQ+ community.

Epidemiology of LGBTQ+ and Healthcare

Recent polling estimates that 5.6% of the American population identifies as LGBTQ+, which is more than 1% higher than previous estimates from 2017. More specifically, these percentages are higher among younger people, and the data for Generation Z (people aged 18–23 in 2020) shows that one in six people identify as LGBTQ+ [2]. As this percentage increases, a growing number of physicians and healthcare workers are going to be involved in the care of patients identifying as a part of this group. Therefore, it is important to understand this population's unique medical needs and relationship with the healthcare system.

Individuals identifying as LGBTQ+ are more likely to experience discrimination in healthcare settings as compared to their cisgender and heterosexual counterparts, and as many as 70% of transgender people and 56% of lesbian, gay, or bisexual people report experiencing discrimination when pursuing healthcare [3]. Not only

L. Knoepp (✉)
Ochsner Health, New Orleans, LA, USA
e-mail: lknoepp@ochsner.org

O. Mirabella
University of Queensland School of Medicine, Ochsner Clinical School, New Orleans, LA, USA

© The Author(s), under exclusive license to Springer Nature Switzerland AG 2022
K. Conrad (ed.), *Clinical Approaches to Hospital Medicine*,
https://doi.org/10.1007/978-3-030-95164-1_17

Table 17.1 Definitions

LGBTQ+	An abbreviation for lesbian, gay, bisexual, transgender, and queer. The addition of the "+" allows for the inclusion of other identities along the gender and sexual spectrums
Gender	A social construct used to classify a person as a man, woman, or some other identity. Fundamentally different from the sex one is assigned at birth, gender encompasses a set of social, psychological, and emotional traits, often influenced by societal expectations
Queer	This term can include, but is not limited to, gay, lesbian, bisexual, transgender, intersex, and asexual people and has different meanings to different people. Some still find it offensive, while others reclaim it to encompass the broader sense of history of the gay rights movement. "Queer" can also be used as an umbrella term like LGBT, as in "the queer community"
Sex	Defines a categorization based on the appearance of the genitalia at birth
Sexual orientation	Defines an enduring emotional, romantic, or sexual attraction. Sexual orientation is fluid
Transgender	This is used most often as an umbrella term, but some commonly held definitions include (1) someone whose gender identity or expression does not fit (dominant-group social constructs of) assigned birth sex and gender. (2) A gender outside of the man/woman binary. (3) Having no gender or multiple genders
Transfeminine	This is a term used to describe an individual assigned male sex at birth (AMAB) but who identifies with a more feminine gender
Transmasculine	This is a term used to describe an individual assigned female sex at birth (AFAB) but who identifies with a more masculine gender

Source: [1]

Disclaimer: *members of the LGBTQ+ community are diverse. Some may fall in multiple of these categories, while others do not strictly fit in any. Each patient should be treated as an individual with their own unique needs, history, and identity, while keeping in mind the overall healthcare challenges that face the LGBTQ+ community*

does this negatively impact the LGBTQ+ faction, but witnessing these negative outcomes can promulgate similar fears within the greater community. In fact, distrust of biased medical professionals can propagate avoidance of healthcare, with a 2018 study noting that 23% of LGBTQ+ people eschewed healthcare all together due to the fear of being mistreated [4].

Paucity of health insurance also plays a role limiting healthcare access for LGBTQ+ people, and the transgender faction is most impacted, as they are less likely to have insurance than their cisgender counterparts, even after controlling for sociodemographic factors [5]. Those who are insured still often face additional barriers, including adequate cost coverage of hormone therapy and gender-affirming surgeries.

Although many social determinants of health are not unique to the LGBTQ+ population, some are seen at disproportionate rates. These include prevalence of mental health disorders, sexual assault and domestic violence, homelessness, and certain health conditions. In fact, LGBTQ+ people are two times more likely to be diagnosed with a mental health disorder, the most common of which are depression, anxiety, and substance misuse. Overall, suicidal ideation rates are higher in the

LGBTQ+ population as compared to their non-LGBTQ+ counterparts, with the highest rates in transgender and adolescent contingent [6]. While mental health disorders may reported at a higher frequency in this population, it is important to understand that identifying as LGBTQ+ is not a mental health disorder, and not all within this group will have mental health diagnoses.

Members of the LGBTQ+ community are at 120% higher risk of facing homelessness during their lifetime compared to heterosexual and cisgender individuals [7], and there is a higher rate among younger members. This higher prevalence of homelessness may be impacted by the often deficient social support commonly faced by the LGBTQ+ population.

Sexual assault and intimate partner violence are reported at higher rates among certain members of the LGBTQ+ community, with transgender and bisexual constituents affected most commonly. Lamentably, nearly half of transgender people will experience assault in their life [8].

Many members of the LGBTQ+ community also identify with a minority group, which may compound existing healthcare disparities and barriers to care. Considering this, as well as the other aforementioned inequalities, it is crucial that healthcare professionals understand the unique needs and challenges of the LGBTQ+ community to improve quality of care and the relationship between providers and members.

Creating a Safe Space for LGBTQ+ Patients

Making patients feel safe, heard, and comfortable is an important part of all aspects of healthcare and patient interactions. With patients who have historically experienced discrimination, such as LGBTQ+ individuals, this becomes even more important, beginning from the first moment of care.

Environment

Whether a patient is scheduling an outpatient appointment or arriving for inpatient hospital admission, initial interactions are vital to ensuring patient trust and comfort. Accordingly, members of the LGBTQ+ community have reported that their impression of the quality of healthcare they receive is influenced by the environment in which it takes place [9].

In the clinic setting, visual cues, including reading materials and informational pamphlets on LGBTQ+ topics, can help make patients feel more comfortable and welcome. Many places may choose to have nondiscrimination statements posted or pride symbols displayed, and in both clinic and hospital settings, designating restrooms as gender-neutral is important. Training all staff to use correct names and pronouns when communicating with patients and ensure patient confidentiality can also help create a more trusting atmosphere, allowing medical care to regain primary focus of the visit.

Not only do patients risk facing discrimination from healthcare providers, but they may experience discrimination from other patients, as well. Thus, care and consideration should be taken if placing patients in shared rooms, especially those with shared bathrooms. For example, a transmasculine individual who requires cervical cancer screening may feel uncomfortable in the waiting area of a gynecologist's office. Appropriate measures to alleviate this unease, such as performing testing a more gender-neutral environment (a primary care physician who performs screening) or scheduling the patient as the first or last appointment of the day to avoid peak traffic hours, should be made to help encourage compliance with preventive health measures.

Forms and Documentation

Similarly, using nondiscriminatory forms and documentation is important. Patients who do not perceive correct representation in this format may feel more uncomfortable and be deterred from seeking care. Inclusive documentation provides space for legal and preferred names, sex, and gender identity. Notation of preferred and legal information is necessary and respectful, as a patient may not have changed their preferred identifying information legally and it may not match their legal information. This distinction not only helps validate patient identity, but it also helps avoid any confusion among staff and providers.

Introductions, History Taking, and Vocabulary Use

Using a patient's correct preferred pronouns is one of the most effective ways to show a patient respect and help make them feel comfortable. Medical professionals who are not regularly working with LGBTQ+ patients may not be as aware of this practice, and there are some strategies to simplify and standardize this process. A simple introduction such as "Hello, my name is Dr X. My pronouns are she/her/hers. How do you prefer to be addressed?" can be extremely useful. It is demonstrative that the provider understands the importance of defining this nomenclature and further validates the patient. Visibly designating preferred provider pronouns on hospital badges or as wearable stickers/pins can also convey inclusivity [10].

Aside from pronouns, providers should also be mindful of general vocabulary used during conversation. One strategy to insure this is mirroring the language used by the patient. For example, if a patient uses the terms "partner" or "spouse," the provider knows the patient is comfortable with that specific terminology. During uncertain situations, like transmasculine patients who still require breast and cervical screening, using gender-neutral terms is usually acceptable. To increase patient comfort and compliance, one should also avoid gender-specific labeling of exam components, like "well-woman exam." Use of preferred terminology is also imperative when referring to body parts. For example, using a gender-neutral term like "chest" when discussing breast screening may be more agreeable for patients. However, when in doubt, asking the patient their preferred vocabulary, can easily clarify the situation in a respectful manner.

When obtaining a medical history from transgender patients, there are several things to keep in mind. Care should focus on attending to patient's physical, mental, and social health needs and well-being while respectfully affirming their gender identity. For example, older terms such as "sex reassignment" should be avoided. Asking open-ended questions can build rapport while gaining relevant medical information. For example, asking a patient to describe any gender-affirming care they have had allows them to better steer the conversation with their own words and language. Likewise, when more specific clarification is needed, it can be helpful to explain why that information is relevant. For example, in trying to decide if a pap smear needs to be considered during your exam, one might ask, "To help me know if we need to be screening you for certain types of cancer, would you mind telling me if you have a cervix?" Phrasing questions in such a way both demonstrates medical relevance and may feel less confrontational. Thorough documentation of all response details is important both for continuity and preventing the patient from having to answer potentially distressing questions multiple times. Thus, as with any patient, once initial gender-specific information is recorded, subsequent encounters usually only require review of previously recorded details, increasing overall patient comfort with the visit.

When treating the LGBTQ+ population, there are certain aspects of history that are especially important to obtain, and physicians should be aware of these. Due to the higher prevalence of depression, suicidal ideation, and domestic abuse among this group, a careful social history should be recorded, and specific screening should be implemented when appropriate. This can help identify any barriers to care and assess needed follow-up and referrals. To better facilitate these needs, LGBTQ+ care, as with many emerging healthcare models, is likely to be multidisciplinary, and a typical care team may include endocrinologists, surgeons, psychiatrists, counselors, social workers, primary care providers, and others.

Special Considerations for the LGBTQ+ Patient

Hormone and Other Gender-Affirming Therapies

Hormone therapy may be part of gender-affirming care, and adeptness in this management or referral to a managing specialist is imperative, as hormone therapy can help LGBTQ+ patients achieve gender-specific goals. The following sections will discuss different types of hormone therapy, potential side effects, and considerations of these treatments in the hospital setting. As with any therapy, it is important to review the benefits, risks, and alternatives of hormone therapy and to obtain informed consent before initiating treatment.

Estrogen

Estrogen may be requested and prescribed as part of feminizing hormone therapy. Estradiol (17-beta estradiol) is the most widely utilized form and can be administered in a variety of ways: transdermal patches/sprays/creams/gels, oral or sublingual tablets, or injections. Other estrogen formulations, such as ethinyl estradiol, carry increased risks of adverse events, like venous thromboembolism (VTE), and are not as commonly used. However, it is important to be aware that these forms do exist and of their potential risks [1, 4]. As any estrogen therapy may increase risk of thromboembolic events, behaviors that can potentiate these risks, like tobacco use, should be addressed, and lifestyle modifications, like smoking cessation, should be encouraged [1].

Additionally, the following are considerations for hospitalists treating transfeminine patients on estrogen therapy [1]:

- Active sex hormone-sensitive cancer is a contraindication to estrogen therapy.
- Side effects of estrogen include new or worsening migraines, exacerbation of already-present autoimmune conditions, hot flashes, mood changes, and weight gain.
- Transdermal estrogen has been shown to have lower risk of VTE compared to oral medication and should be used when possible in those with risk factors.
- Having a history of VTEs (personal or family) is not a frank contraindication to estrogen therapy in transfeminine patients, but risk of VTE may increase with estrogen use. Therefore, risks and benefits should be weighed, and modifiable risk factors should be adjusted when possible. Pathways for managing VTE in transfeminine patients estrogen therapy can be found through University of California, San Francisco's Transgender Care and Treatment Guidelines: https://transcare.ucsf.edu/guidelines/feminizing-hormone-therapy.
- Patients presenting with a VTE may have estrogen therapy held during the acute treatment, but it can be resumed after weighing risks and benefits with the patient.
- Patients in hypercoagulable states on estrogen therapy can choose to stay on estrogen therapy and can be managed with standard anticoagulation protocols either episodically or long term.

Anti-Androgens

Another treatment commonly used in the transfeminine patient population is the anti-androgen class of medications, which block or reduce the masculinizing effects of testosterone and may be used if patients want or need to avoid estrogen therapy.

Examples include the potassium-sparing diuretic spironolactone; 5-alpha reductase inhibitors, like finasteride and dutasteride; and gonadotropin-releasing hormone (GnRH) analogues. Any patient taking spironolactone may experience limited polydipsia, polyuria, and orthostasis because of the diuretic effects. Hyperkalemia, due to the potassium-sparing mechanism, can be a more significant issue with spironolactone treatment, but this outcome may be reduced by avoiding this treatment in those with renal insufficiency. Five-alpha reductase inhibitors are usually reserved as second-line agents, as they achieve less feminization due to mechanism of action but may be used due to patient preference or in those unable to tolerate spironolactone. GNRH analogues have some anti-androgen use but are mainly used for pubertal delay in transgender adolescents [1].

Testosterone

The use of testosterone is a common part of masculinizing hormone therapy, and preparations of testosterone approved in the United States are identical to human testosterone. Routes of administration of testosterone include subcutaneous and intramuscular injection and topical creams, patches, and gels.

Concerns have been raised about the impacts of testosterone on the cardiovascular system and lipid profiles, but the data from studies have shown mixed results. Alterations of lipid profiles (increased LDL and triglycerides and decreased HDL) have been observed, but these changes do not correlate with an overall increased risk of cardiovascular disease and mortality [11].

Important considerations for hospitalists with transmasculine patients on testosterone include [1]:

- Active sex hormone-sensitive cancer is a contraindication to testosterone therapy.
- Hemoglobin and hematocrit (H&H) should be considered in the context of the patient's testosterone level and menstrual status, rather than standard gender-specific ranges. The H&H for a transmasculine man with cessation of menstruation and a physiological testosterone level should be within the normal cis-male range.
- The cis-male upper limit of normal should be used for interpretation of creatinine and alkaline phosphate, with no defined lower limit of normal.
- Patients with underlying polycystic ovary syndrome may have increased symptoms and increased insulin resistance.
- Side effects of testosterone include new or worsening migraines, changes to autoimmune conditions, mood changes, and hair loss.
- Pregnancy is possible and cannot be missed in patients taking testosterone and/or with cessation of menstruation.

Lesbian, Gay, and Bisexual Care

There are certain conditions and risk factors that are seen at higher rates in the lesbian, gay, and bisexual (LGB) population specific to men who have sex with men (MSM) and women who have sex with women (WSW). Awareness of these is important in the care of these patients. Many of these risks may be related to societal minority status and increased by previous negative healthcare experiences.

Women who have sex with women [12, 13]:

- Lower rates of human papillomavirus (HPV) vaccination
- Lower rates of regular HPV/Papanicolaou testing
- Lower rates of breast cancer screening
- Increased rates of obesity
- Increased rates of mental health disorders (anxiety and depression)
- Increased rates of smoking, alcohol, and illicit drug use

The guidelines for breast and cervical cancer screening of WSW are the same as all other women. In theory, due to the higher prevalence of nulliparity, obesity, and smoking and the lower rates of hormone-based contraception, there may be a higher risk of ovarian cancer; however, at this time, there are no additional, recommended screenings for ovarian cancer in this population [14].

Men who have sex with men [12, 15]:

- Increased rates of sexually transmitted infections (human immunodeficiency virus, gonorrhea, chlamydia, herpes, syphilis)
- Increased risk of HPV
- Increased risk of hepatitis A and B
- Increased rates of mental health disorders (anxiety, depression, and eating disorders)

Due to these increased risks, it is recommended that MSM patients receive immunization for hepatitis A and B. These individuals are also eligible for the HPV vaccination [16].

Incorporating LGBTQ+ Education into Medical School, Residency, and Other Allied Health Professional Training

Formally educating healthcare providers about the needs and challenges faced by the LGBTQ+ community is a starting point for addressing healthcare disparities. After completion of education, healthcare professionals are responsible for implementing this into daily patient care. This comes with continued practice and review, which may be an area continuing education that needs improvement.

A 2018 study which surveyed 308 primary care physicians in the United States found that 85.7% of those surveyed were willing to provide care to transgender people; however, only 68.6% felt capable of providing care, and 47.9% reported feeling they lacked training in transgender health [17]. Similarly, a study of 658 medical students in New England found that 92.7% of students felt comfortable treating sexual minority patients, but only 76.7% felt competent [18]. Studies like these show the problem seems to stem more from a lack of knowledge than intentional discrimination. Therefore, increased education and training regarding the care of LGBTQ+ patients is needed to help those physicians who want to provide care prepare to do so.

While incorporating LGBTQ+ curriculum is important, it is also important to remember that LGBTQ+ individuals will exist in the healthcare system outside LGBTQ+ specific needs. For this reason, there have been recent recommendations by experts in the field to integrate LGBTQ+ patient care strategies throughout the whole of medical education [19].

With the recent increase in the number of LGBTQ+ identifying individuals, there has never been a better time to start focusing on improving the care of these patients. Healthcare providers need to take initiative in learning about this population and make strides in reducing the disparities and discriminations that have impacted them and, thus, their medical care.

Key Points
- Being aware of the social determinants and relationship with the healthcare system, the LGBTQ+ population can help physicians address barriers to care.
- Creating a welcoming, safe, and judgment-free environment is an important part of healthcare, especially for the LGBTQ+ population.
- Knowing the common risk factors, side effects, and changes (i.e., laboratory values) that may be associated with different hormone therapies can help providers optimize management of patients on these treatments. Likewise, it is important to weigh the risks and benefits of any therapy with a patient's input and understanding.
- LGBTQ+ patients face the same health problems as cisgender and heterosexual patients.

References

1. UCSF Transgender Care DoFaCM, University of California San Francisco. Guidelines for the primary and gender-affirming care of transgender and gender nonbinary people. 2nd edn; 2016. transcare.ucsf.edu/guidelines.
2. Jones J. LGBT identification rises to 5.6% in latest U.S. estimate; 2021.
3. Healthcare Equality Index 2019. In: Human Rights Campaign Foundation; 2019.
4. Rosendale N, Goldman S, Ortiz GM, Haber LA. Acute clinical care for transgender patients: a review. JAMA Intern Med. 2018;178(11):1535–43. https://doi.org/10.1001/jamainternmed.2018.4179.
5. Gonzales G, Henning-Smith C. Barriers to care among transgender and gender nonconforming adults. Milbank Q. 2017;95(4):726–48. https://doi.org/10.1111/1468-0009.12297.
6. Mental Health Disparities: LGBTQ. American Psychiatric Association; 2017. psychiatry.org.

7. Morton MH, Dworsky A, Samuels GM. Missed opportunities: youth homelessness in America. National estimates. 2017. voicesofyouthcount.org.
8. Brown TNT, Herman JL. Intimate partner violence and sexual abuse among LGBT people: a review of existing research. The Williams Institute, UCLA School of Law. 2015. https://williamsinstitute.law.ucla.edu/.
9. McClain Z, Hawkins LA, Yehia BR. Creating welcoming spaces for lesbian, gay, bisexual, and transgender (LGBT) patients: an evaluation of the health care environment. J Homosex. 2016;63(3):387–93. https://doi.org/10.1080/00918369.2016.1124694.
10. Brown C, Bsn RN, Frohard-Dourlent H, Wood B, Saewyc E, PhD RN, Fsahm F, Eisenberg M, ScD MPH, Porta C, PhD MPH, Rn F. "It makes such a difference": an examination of how LGBTQ youth talk about personal gender pronouns. J Am Assoc Nurse Pract. 2020;32(1):70–80. https://doi.org/10.1097/JXX.0000000000000217.
11. Seal LJ. Cardiovascular disease in transgendered people: a review of the literature and discussion of risk. JRSM Cardiovasc Dis. 2019;8:2048004019880745. https://doi.org/10.1177/2048004019880745.
12. Moll J, Krieger P. Lesbian, gay, or bisexual (LGB): caring with quality and compassion. In: Martin ML, Heron SL, Moreno-Walton L, Jones AW, editors. Diversity and inclusion in quality patient care. Cham: Springer International Publishing; 2016. p. 101–12. https://doi.org/10.1007/978-3-319-22840-2_9.
13. Knight DA, Jarrett D. Preventive health care for women who Have sex with women. Am Fam Physician. 2017;95(5):314–21.
14. Carroll N. Medical care of sexual minority women. In: Barbieri R, Elmore J, Eckler K (eds). UpToDate, Waltham, MA; 2020. Accessed on 26 Feb 2021.
15. Knight DA, Jarrett D. Preventive health care for men who have sex with men. Am Fam Physician. 2015;91(12):844–51.
16. Dhanireddy S. Primary care of gay men and men who have sex with men. In: Elmore J, Kunins L (eds). UpToDate. Waltham, MA; 2019. Accessed on 26 Feb 2021.
17. Shires DA, Stroumsa D, Jaffee KD, Woodford MR. Primary care clinicians' willingness to care for transgender patients. Ann Fam Med. 2018;16(6):555–8. https://doi.org/10.1370/afm.2298.
18. Zelin NS, Hastings C, Beaulieu-Jones BR, Scott C, Rodriguez-Villa A, Duarte C, Calahan C, Adami AJ. Sexual and gender minority health in medical curricula in new England: a pilot study of medical student comfort, competence and perception of curricula. Med Educ Online. 2018;23(1):1461513. https://doi.org/10.1080/10872981.2018.1461513.
19. Streed CG Jr., Siegel J, Davis JA. Keeping our promise to LGBTQ+ patients; 2019.

Chapter 18
Racial Disparities in Healthcare

Veronica Gillispie and Ryan Abrigo

Introduction

Racial disparities in medicine have been acknowledged for decades and continue to persist across healthcare systems. These disparities appear throughout every domain in medicine, from heart disease to maternal mortality. Multiple factors influence the rise of racial disparities in healthcare, including racism, discrimination, unequal healthcare access, income inequality, and social determinants of health. Efforts have been made to try to reduce the amount of racial disparity seen in hospitals, but the disparity still exists in many areas.

Reported Disparities

Minority groups face disparities in many domains, including morbidity, mortality, and prevalence of various diseases. The Center for Disease Control published a 2013 report detailing the health disparities of different groups. The report found that people of color are more likely to suffer from hypertension, diabetes, asthma, HIV/AIDs, and tuberculosis. Infant mortality rates are statistically higher in Black Americans, Hispanic Americans, and Native Americans than White Americans. In self-reported surveys, minority groups were more likely to self-report poorer health ratings and increased days of feeling physically unwell [1]. A literature review conducted by the Institute of Medicine [2] stated that minority patients are less likely to receive necessary medical services when compared to White patients. The National Healthcare Quality and Disparities Report by the US Department of Health and Human Services found that Black Americans, Native Americans, Alaska Natives, and Hispanic Americans all received worse quality of care than White Americans [3].

A literature review conducted by the Veteran's Health Administration reported that most studies comparing Black American and White American veterans found similar or worse mortality in Black American veterans [4]. The Veteran's Health Administration found that mortality disparities for Black American veterans existed in a number of areas, including chronic kidney disease, diabetes, HIV/AIDS, stroke, and colorectal cancer [4].

Cardiovascular Disease

Cardiovascular disease is currently the leading cause of death in the United States. Rates of cardiovascular disease are known to be higher in minority groups, especially Black Americans. The premature mortality rate, defined as a measure of unfulfilled life expectancy, of cardiovascular disease including heart attack and stroke was highest in Black Americans out of all races [3]. Black Americans also have the highest rates of hypertension of all ethnic groups [5]. Black Americans are twice as likely to have strokes as non-Hispanic White Americans [6]. Ethnic minorities overall have higher rates of coronary artery disease, myocardial infarction, and death from acute coronary syndrome [6]. Minority patients have also been shown to be less likely to be treated with potentially lifesaving treatments such as percutaneous coronary intervention and angiography [6]. Among Asian American patients, some subgroups including Asian, Indian, and Filipino men had higher mortality burdens of hypertension and strokes [7]. Native Americans and Alaska Natives are more likely to have coronary artery disease and hypertension than White Americans [8].

Diabetes

Compared to White Americans, the prevalence of diabetes mellitus is higher across minority groups including Black Americans, Hispanic Americans, Asian Americans, and Native Americans [9]. Individuals in minority groups with diabetes are more likely to develop complications and require lower limb amputations than nonminority groups [9]. These complications often lead to significant disability in these patients.

Breast Cancer

Breast cancer is the one of the most common and second most deadly cancer suffered by American women. Technological and medical advances in screening, detection, and treatment for breast cancer have helped reduce morbidity and mortality; there still appears to be disparities when comparing minority groups to nonminority groups. White American women are actually the most likely group to be diagnosed with breast cancer; however, Black American women have higher rates of death from breast cancer [10]. While many confounders may explain this disparity, one theory is that lack of access to mammography and breast cancer treatment may be leading factors [11]. Hispanic women appear to have a lower incidence of breast cancer than White women, but it has been shown that breast cancer is often diagnosed at an advanced stages compared to White women [10].

HIV/AIDS

Racial disparities are seen in HIV/AIDS diagnoses, with Hispanic American and Black American groups having the highest rates of HIV infection [12]. Some posit that these groups are more likely to engage in risky behaviors than other groups, but studies offer data to dispute this belief. In a study of young Black American and Hispanic American adults, behavioral patterns and risk engagement alone were not enough to predict HIV risk Williams et al. [12]. HIV-positive Black Americans are also less likely to be treated with antiretroviral therapy and prophylaxis for pneumocystis jiroveci (PCP) infection [13].

Analgesia

In regard to analgesia, minority patients' pain is often dismissed or undertreated when compared to White patients. This racial disparity has been noted in numerous studies and in both acute and chronic care settings. In one study, Black American patients with fractures were less likely to receive analgesics in the emergency department when compared to White American patients [5]. Another study looking at emergency department patients with kidney stones showed that Black American and Hispanic American patients were less likely to receive opioid analgesia than White American patients [14]. An Oregon study found that Hispanic American and Asian American patients who requested ambulances for trauma were less likely to have their pain assessed by providers, and all minority patients in this study were less likely to be given analgesics for trauma [15]. Regarding chronic noncancer pain, Black American patients in the Veteran's Affairs system were less likely to be treated with opioids than White Americans [16]. Regarding pregnancy and delivery, Black American and Hispanic American women were less likely to be given epidural analgesia [17]. The factors that contribute to these racial disparities in analgesic treatments are undoubtedly complex. The extensive literature on this topic proves that this is a problem that has always been present and continues to persist in our healthcare system. Provider attitudes, bias, and systemic policies must be researched and explored further in order to address this issue.

Provider Bias

Bias of healthcare professionals toward patients is a serious concern and known contributor to racial disparities. Although most providers believe bias is immoral and wrong, they may not always be able to recognize their own biases and prejudice. A provider's conscious and unconscious thoughts may ultimately affect their behaviors and judgment toward others, including their patients. For example, a provider may unconsciously believe a minority patient is less competent or more likely to abuse prescription drugs and thus will be less willing to prescribe a strong analgesic to minority patients.

A systemic review of healthcare literature found that implicit bias is prevalent in US healthcare providers, as providers tend to have positive attitudes toward White Americans and negative attitudes toward people of color [18]. Other studies found evidence that patient-physician communication differs between White and minority patients.

One study by Johnson et al. showed that physicians were more verbally dominant, less patient-centered, and less likely to ask for patient input regarding treatment plans when talking to Black American patients compared to White American patients. In addition, Black American patients and their physicians both displayed reduced levels of positive affect compared to the White American patients and their physicians [19].

Oliver et al. conducted another study exploring physician bias where researchers surveyed physicians who were given case scenarios involving patients with severe osteoarthritis. The patients in the scenarios were virtually identical aside from race, with some patients being White and others Black. The study found that physicians believed that the Black patients were less medically cooperative than the White patients. While this study did not show that biases predicted different treatment recommendations, the authors suggest that implicit bias may still affect treatment decisions in the real world [20]. An additional study published in *Academic Emergency Medicine* found that physicians, especially White physicians, tended to have an implicit racial bias in favor of White patients and were more likely to treat White patients for a myocardial infarction than Black patients with thrombolysis [21]. In contrast to the last study, this study found a tangible difference in treatment plans based on the patient's race.

These studies show that the field of medicine is not immune to bias and that this bias can be quantified and visualized at least somewhat. More efforts should be made to help healthcare professionals acknowledge and challenge their biases, as these biases may be directly harmful to patient care.

Access to Health Insurance

One example of socioeconomic disparity can be seen in health insurance coverage. Black American and Hispanic Americans have been shown to have lower insurance coverage rates compared to non-Hispanic White Americans [22]. Minority groups are also more likely to work in lesser paying jobs where they are often offered substandard health insurance benefits [23]. With less access to comprehensive health insurance, minority individuals may be more hesitant to seek medical care for both preventative health and acute conditions requiring hospitalization. Over time, this lack of insurance can cascade to disability and death for thousands of minority Americans.

Children of minority groups also have higher rates of being uninsured. Hispanic American children and Black American children are twice as likely to be uninsured when compared to non-Hispanic White children [24].

Poverty

Poverty is another factor that must be acknowledged when addressing racial disparities. It is known that minority groups suffer from poverty at significantly higher rates than nonminority groups. The US Census Bureau reported that 18.8% of Black Americans, 15.7% of Hispanic Americans, and 23% of Native Americans had incomes below the poverty line in 2019 [25]. In contrast, the census bureau reported that only 7.3% of White Americans fell below the poverty line. Poverty hinders one's access to health education, healthy food, transportation to medical appointments, health insurance, and safe housing. The effects of poverty often commence in childhood and may have lasting effects throughout life. Children living in poverty have worse medical outcomes and have higher rates of conditions such as obesity, asthma, and learning disability [26]. One recent study by Taylor et al. found that childhood poverty may even cause structural changes to the brain during development [27]. In that study, decreases in prefrontal and hippocampal volume were observed in children living in poverty, based on their neighborhood disadvantage including areas of greater unemployment, lower levels of education, percent living in poverty, and controlled for household income [27].

At least some degree of racial disparity in hospital medicine is directly or indirectly linked to the socioeconomic inequalities seen in minority groups. The Pew Research Center reports that in 2016, White households had four times as much wealth in comparison to Black American families and three times as much wealth as Hispanic American families [28].

Life Expectancy

There is an established relationship between income and life expectancy. One study by Taylor et al. found the gap of life expectancy between the richest 1% and poorest 1% of individuals was a difference of 10.1 years for women and 14.6 years for men [27]. This study found that life expectancy decreased linearly as individual's incomes fell and vice versa. As noted earlier, income and poverty disparity are exacerbated in minority groups, and thus income disparity may be a possible factor contributing to lower life expectancies in these groups [28]. Education is another factor, and minority status combined with low education has been related to significantly lower life expectancies [29].

Notable Examples of Racial Disparities in Recent Years

Black Maternal and Infant Health

In recent years, substantial racial disparities in maternal health and pregnancy have caused national attention. The CDC reports that pregnancy-related death rates for Black women are over three times that of White women in America [30]. In the CDC report, in women over 30, Black women had four to five times the rates of pregnancy-related deaths as White women. Hemorrhage and hypertensive disorders of pregnancy were more likely to cause maternal deaths in Black women than White women. For Black women with college degrees, the maternal death rate was 5.2 times that of White women with college degrees. These disparities appear to be persistent and unchanging since at least 2007 based on CDC data [30].

Racial Disparities in COVID-19

The COVID-19 pandemic has undoubtedly caused unprecedented stress and grief among the world. Many have been hospitalized or lost their lives due to COVID-19. In the United States, stark disparities have been identified in the way COVID-19 affected minority communities.

In one retrospective cohort study conducted in Louisiana [31], researchers in the Ochsner healthcare system found that 76.9% of patients hospitalized with COVID-19 and 70.6% of patients who died due to COVID-19 were Black American. 80% of patients who were given mechanical ventilation or critical care were Black American. Black Americans only comprise 31% of the patients in the Ochsner Health System, so these statistics may have appeared to show a sharp disparity in outcomes within this hospital system. However, when adjusting for differences in socioeconomic statuses and comorbid conditions, it was found that Black patients did not have a higher inpatient mortality compared to White patients. This study suggests that racial differences in COVID-19 outcomes may be due to multifactorial causes, including the types of jobs that minority groups work in possibly being more associated with increased person-to-person contact, socioeconomic statuses, and comorbid conditions that may affect minority groups disproportionately.

Another study found that 52% of COVID-19 diagnoses and 52% of COVID-19 deaths were in counties with disproportionately Black American populations despite the fact that these counties make up around 20% of all US counties [32].

The racial disparities do not only affect Black American populations. In a New York study, it was found that Hispanic patients had two times the age-adjusted death rate from COVID-19 [33]. In the state of Arizona, Native Americans were found to make up 3% of COVID-19 cases and 18% of COVID-19 associated deaths, despite making up only about 5% of the population. In Hawaii, native Hawaiians and Pacific Islanders are also disproportionately being affected by COVID-19 [34]. Asian Americans have faced prejudice and overt racism due to the so-called China flu, and some Asian subgroups are more susceptible to COVID-19 hospitalization and death compared to White American counterparts [35].

Socioeconomic disparity, structural racism, social conditions, and many other factors may explain why the COVID-19 pandemic is ravaging minority populations.

What Can Be Done to Reduce Racial Disparities in Hospital Care?

To reduce racial disparities in medicine, changes must be made on both an individual personal level and systemic level. On an individual level, we must first acknowledge the disparities and educate ourselves and fellow providers on them. Providers must be aware of their own internal biases and be encouraged to catch themselves and reflect on their thoughts when they realize their thinking may be biased. Providers should be encouraged to broaden their exposure to different cultures by meeting people of different backgrounds. Even simply delving into media from other cultures can help broaden cultural exposure. Staff must be encouraged to step up and speak out when they feel a patient is being unfairly treated. On a systemic level, online and in-person diversity training can help providers learn about biases and stereotypes. Policies should be made to help address health inequities by providing more health education and resources to minority groups in need.

Key Points
- Minority groups face racial disparities in a multitude of healthcare domains, including higher morbidity and mortality of certain diseases.
- Provider bias can contribute to racial disparities and should be addressed on both a personal and systemic levels.
- Socioeconomic disparities are one of the many factors contributing to racial disparities in healthcare.
- Significant disparities in Black maternal and infant health have been known for decades and continue to persist.
- Racial disparities have contributed to disproportionate COVID-19 hospitalizations and deaths in minority groups.

References

1. Centers for Disease C, Prevention. CDC health disparities and inequalities report; 2013. p. 1–187.
2. Institute of M. Unequal treatment: confronting racial and ethnic disparities in health care. Washington (DC): National Academies Press (US); 2003.

3. Agency for Healthcare R, Quality. 2019 National Healthcare Quality and Disparities Report; 2019.
4. Peterson K, Anderson J, Boundy E, Ferguson L, McCleery E, Waldrip K. Mortality disparities in racial/ethnic minority groups in the veterans health administration: an evidence review and map. Am J Public Health. 2018;108(3):e1–e11. https://doi.org/10.2105/AJPH.2017.304246.
5. Musemwa N, Gadegbeku CA. Hypertension in African Americans. Curr Cardiol Rep. 2017;19(12):129. https://doi.org/10.1007/s11886-017-0933-z.
6. Graham G. Disparities in cardiovascular disease risk in the United States. Curr Cardiol Rev. 2015;11(3):238–45.
7. Jose Powell O, Frank Ariel TH, Kapphahn Kristopher I, Goldstein Benjamin A, Eggleston K, Hastings Katherine G, et al. Cardiovascular disease mortality in Asian Americans. J Am Coll Cardiol. 2014;64(23):2486–94. https://doi.org/10.1016/j.jacc.2014.08.048.
8. Dept of H, Human Services - Office of Minority H. Heart disease and American Indians/Alaska natives; 2021.
9. Spanakis EK, Golden SH. Race/ethnic difference in diabetes and diabetic complications. Curr Diab Rep. 2013;13(6):814–23. https://doi.org/10.1007/s11892-013-0421-9.
10. Yedjou CG, Sims JN, Miele L, Noubissi F, Lowe L, Fonseca DD, et al. Health and racial disparity in breast cancer. Adv Exp Med Biol. 2019;1152:31–49. https://doi.org/10.1007/978-3-030-20301-6_3.
11. Hirschman J, Whitman S, Ansell D. The black: white disparity in breast cancer mortality: the example of Chicago. Cancer Causes Control. 2007;18(3):323–33. https://doi.org/10.1007/s10552-006-0102-y.
12. Williams C, Eisenberg M, Becher J, Davis-Vogel A, Fiore D, Metzge D. Racial disparities in HIV prevalence and risk behaviors among injection drug users and members of their risk networks. J Acquir Immune Defic Syndr. 2013;63(Suppl 1):S90–S4. https://doi.org/10.1097/QAI.0b013e3182921506.
13. Moore RD, Stanton D, Gopalan R, Chaisson RE. Racial differences in the use of drug therapy for HIV disease in an urban community. 2010. https://doi.org/10.1056/NEJM199403173301107.
14. Berger AJ, Wang Y, Rowe C, Chung B, Chang S, Haleblian G. Racial disparities in analgesic use amongst patients presenting to the emergency department for kidney stones in the United States. Am J Emerg Med. 2021;39:71–4. https://doi.org/10.1016/j.ajem.2020.01.017.
15. Kennel J, Withers E, Parsons N, Woo H. Racial/ethnic disparities in pain treatment: evidence from Oregon emergency medical services agencies. Med Care. 2019;57(12):924–9. https://doi.org/10.1097/MLR.0000000000001208.
16. Burgess DJ, Nelson DB, Gravely AA, Bair MJ, Kerns RD, Higgins DM, et al. Racial differences in prescription of opioid analgesics for chronic noncancer pain in a national sample of veterans. J Pain. 2014;15(4):447–55. https://doi.org/10.1016/j.jpain.2013.12.010.
17. Glance Laurent G, Wissler R, Glantz C, Osler Turner M, Mukamel Dana B, Dick AW. Racial differences in the use of epidural analgesia for labor. Anesthesiology. 2007;106(1):19–25. https://doi.org/10.1097/00000542-200701000-00008.
18. Hall WJ, Chapman MV, Lee KM, Merino YM, Thomas TW, Payne BK, et al. Implicit racial/ethnic bias among health care professionals and its influence on health care outcomes: a systematic review. Am J Public Health. 2015;105(12):e60–76. https://doi.org/10.2105/AJPH.2015.302903.
19. Johnson RL, Roter D, Powe NR, Cooper LA. Patient race/ethnicity and quality of patient–physician communication during medical visits. Am J Public Health. 2004;94(12):2084–90.
20. Oliver MN, Wells KM, Joy-Gaba JA, Hawkins CB, Nosek BA. Do physicians' implicit views of African Americans affect clinical decision making? J Am Board Fam Med. 2014;27(2):177–88. https://doi.org/10.3122/jabfm.2014.02.120314.
21. Dehon E, Weiss N, Jones J, Faulconer W, Hinton E, Sterling S. A systematic review of the impact of physician implicit racial bias on clinical decision making. Acad Emerg Med. 2017;24(8):895–904. https://doi.org/10.1111/acem.13214.

22. Sohn H. Racial and ethnic disparities in health insurance coverage: dynamics of gaining and losing coverage over the life-course. Popul Res Policy Rev. 2017;36(2):181–201. https://doi.org/10.1007/s11113-016-9416-y.
23. Williams DR, Rucker TD. Understanding and addressing racial disparities in health care. Health Care Financ Rev. 2000;21(4):75–90.
24. Pfizer. A profile of uninsured persons in the United States; 2008.
25. Semega J, Kollar M, Shrider EA, Creamer JF. Income and poverty in the United States. 2019. 2019:88.
26. Chaudry A, Wimer C. Poverty is not just an indicator: the relationship between income, poverty, and child well-being. Acad Pediatr. 2016;16(3):S23–S9. https://doi.org/10.1016/j.acap.2015.12.010.
27. Taylor RL, Cooper SR, Jackson JJ, Barch DM. Assessment of neighborhood poverty, cognitive function, and prefrontal and hippocampal volumes in children. JAMA Netw Open. 2020;3(11):e2023774. https://doi.org/10.1001/jamanetworkopen.2020.23774.
28. Rakesh K, Anthony C. How U.S. wealth inequality has changed since Great Recession. Pew Research Center; 2017.
29. Olshansky SJ, Antonucci T, Berkman L, Binstock RH, Boersch-Supan A, Cacioppo JT, et al. Differences in life expectancy due to race and educational differences are widening, and many may not catch up. Health Aff. 2012;31(8):1803–13. https://doi.org/10.1377/hlthaff.2011.0746.
30. Centers for Disease C. Racial and ethnic disparities continue in pregnancy-related deaths; 2019.
31. Price-Haywood EG, Burton J, Fort D, Seoane L. Hospitalization and mortality among black patients and white patients with Covid-19. N Engl J Med. 2020;382(26):2534–43. https://doi.org/10.1056/NEJMsa2011686.
32. Millett GA, Jones AT, Benkeser D, Baral S, Mercer L, Beyrer C, et al. Assessing differential impacts of COVID-19 on black communities. Ann Epidemiol. 2020;47:37–44. https://doi.org/10.1016/j.annepidem.2020.05.003.
33. Macias Gil R, Marcelin JR, Zuniga-Blanco B, Marquez C, Mathew T, Piggott DA. COVID-19 pandemic: disparate health impact on the Hispanic/Latinx population in the United States. J Infect Dis. 2020;222(10):1592–5. https://doi.org/10.1093/infdis/jiaa474.
34. Kaholokula JK, Samoa RA, Miyamoto RES, Palafox N, Daniels S-A. COVID-19 special column: COVID-19 hits native Hawaiian and Pacific islander communities the hardest. Hawaii J Health Soc Welf. 2020;79(5):144–6.
35. Wang D, Gee GC, Bahiru E, Yang EH, Hsu JJ. Asian-Americans and Pacific islanders in COVID-19: emerging disparities amid discrimination. J Gen Intern Med. 2020;35(12):3685–8. https://doi.org/10.1007/s11606-020-06264-5.

Chapter 19
Gender and Racial Disparities in Career Advancement in the United States

Anna Garbuzov, Jessica Koller-Gorham, and Tamika Webb-Detiege

Introduction

Medical education strives to create doctors who are compassionate, knowledgeable, and capable of delivering the best care to their patients. Employing the most qualified people to become doctors is crucial to ensure excellent patient outcomes, yet women and minorities have been historically underrepresented as healthcare providers. Women now comprise 51.6% of medical school matriculants, but as the career ladder continues, women progressively compose a smaller percentage of leadership positions, comprising 46% of residents to only 18% of deans and 25% of full professors (Fig. 19.1) [1]. This discrepancy may be due in part to a lag as women catch up to men in leadership positions. In 2017, women surpassed men in medical school matriculants for the first time in history [2]. There are other factors at play though, and if no actions are taken now, this cycle can be perpetuated and allowed to continue for generations.

In addition to gender imbalance, physicians have faced prejudice based on race and ethnicity. In particular, Black physicians have faced discrimination in the workplace throughout our history. They were prohibited from attending many White medical schools, had limited access to specialized training, and were often denied privileges at hospitals [3]. There continue to be racial and ethnic differences in the United States between the general population and the physicians who care for them.

A. Garbuzov, B.A.
University of Queensland-Ochsner Clinical School, New Orleans, LA, USA

J. Koller-Gorham, M.D.
Department of Surgery, Ochsner Health, New Orleans, LA, USA
e-mail: jessica.kollergorham@ochsner.org

T. Webb-Detiege, M.D. (✉)
Department of Rheumatology, Ochsner Health, New Orleans, LA, USA
e-mail: twebbdetiege@ochsner.org

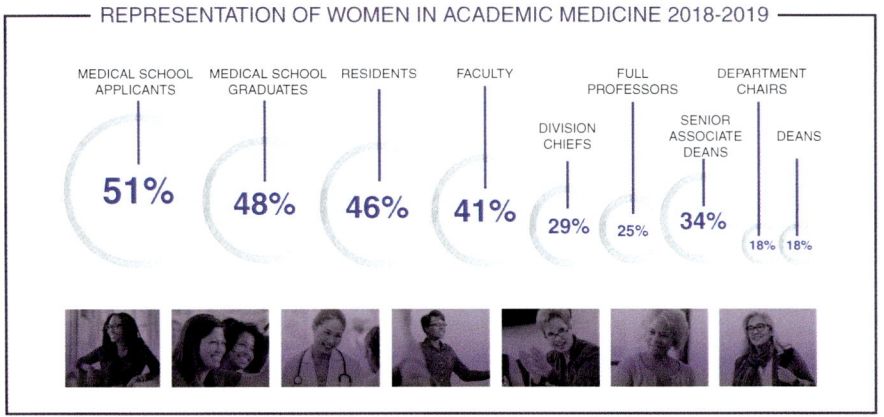

Fig. 19.1 Representation of women in academic medicine [1]

Black, Hispanic, and Native American people constitute 30% of the general population but only 10% of practicing physicians [4]. Conversely, 61% of the general population in the United States is White, and 79% of all full professors of surgery identify as White [5]. This gap exists across many medical fields; in 2018, only 3.6% of full-time medical academic faculty in the United States were Black [6]. In 2006, just 2.2% of physicians and medical students were Black, which is a smaller percentage than in 1910, when the Flexner Report was published (2.5%) [7]. This difference is particularly significant in certain fields, such as radiation oncology, where only 1.7% of full-time faculty were Black in 2018 [6].

Physicians from ethnic and racial minorities provide an important role in healthcare. They are more likely than their White counterparts to work in underserved communities and have minority patients seek out their care [5]. While Black newborns are twice as likely to die in their first year of life as White newborns, having a Black physician deliver a Black baby was found to decrease this difference by half [8]. Women physicians have also been shown to achieve excellent outcomes for their patients. Patient 30-day mortality and 30-day readmission rates were lower for patients seen by women hospitalists as compared to those seen by men [9]. These differences may exist because women physicians are more likely to follow clinical guidelines, encourage preventative care, communicate better with patients, and provide more counseling to patients than their male peers [9].

Although gender and racial disparity has been a part of American history, the times are evolving in a positive trajectory. In acknowledging our past, we can fully understand the context in which individuals now work and live. The goal is not to perpetuate the past but to break the cycle by recognizing injustice and disparities, along with the benefits that everyone receives when we live in a truly equitable society. In medicine, we recognize that a patient's past health practices such as poor diet or smoking will impact their future. Physicians are similarly affected by the past of our society. By discussing the history of injustices, we allow for reflection and healing. We create space to mourn past and present injustices, with the hope that by acknowledging and facing these issues, we can avoid perpetuating them. As stated by Dr. Robert Baker et al.:

> "As leaders of the medical profession come together and move into the future, they should do so with a clear recognition of the effects of the past but also *an awareness that the story of African Americans and organized medicine is still being written.*" [7]

Discussions around diversity, equity, and inclusion in medicine can be uncomfortable. Some readers may believe that discussing these issues perpetuates inequality by dwelling on the past. Others may feel defensive and believe that these conversations are meant to negate their hard work. Our hope is that the readers who feel this way can put aside these concerns temporarily to appreciate a different viewpoint. We hope to inspire more thoughtful conversations that are cognizant and appreciative of a more diverse perspective, even beyond race and gender.

A Brief History of Black Physicians in the United States

Black physicians have faced tremendous adversity over the years in achieving parity with their White colleagues. The first Black American to obtain a medical degree was Dr. James McCune Smith (Fig. 19.2) in 1837; in fact, he had to receive his degree from the University of Glasgow because he was denied entry to US medical schools due to his race [10, 11]. In 1847, Dr. David Jones Peck was the first Black man to receive a medical degree from a US medical school [7]. That same year, the American Medical Association (AMA) was founded as an overarching conglomeration of medical societies to create a framework for the medical field and support physicians [7]. In 1854, Dr. John Van Surly DeGrasse was accepted into the Massachusetts Medical Society, making him the first Black physician to be accepted into a medical society in the United States [7].

In 1870, three Black physicians attempted to start their path to AMA membership [7]. They were members of the National Medical Society, which was a newer, racially integrated society [7]. All members of the National Medical Society were excluded from AMA membership when the all-White Medical Society of the District of Columbia disputed their admission, claiming that the National Medical Society tried to undermine them by addressing racial discrimination within their Society [7]. It is worth noting that this issue was brought to a vote, which excluded members of the National Medical Society and passed by a vote of 114 to 82 [7]. Meanwhile, the first Black woman physician in the United States to earn a medical degree was Dr. Rebecca Crumper Lee in 1873 [11].

In response to another integrated society attempting to join the AMA in 1872, new legislation in 1874 shifted the responsibility for society admission to state societies; however, many of the societies in the South, where most Black people lived, openly excluded Black physicians from joining, effectively absolving the AMA of

Fig. 19.2 Dr. James McCune Smith was the first Black American physician to have a medical degree and the first Black physician published in US medical journals [10]

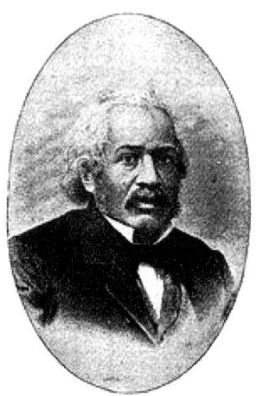

their responsibility to address discrimination while maintaining the status quo [7]. This policy was upheld again in 1939 [7]. This history of exclusion led to Black physicians forming their own societies, and in 1895 the National Medical Association (NMA) was founded [7]. While both societies formally denied race being a limiting factor, at the turn of the century, the AMA and the NMA were mostly composed of White physicians and Black physicians, respectively [7].

The 1910 *Flexner Report* highlighted the state of medical education. Commissioned by the AMA, it recommended men and women to attend medical school together while acquiescing to racial segregation, claiming that Black physicians required different training to serve "their" people [7]. The *Flexner Report* suggested that five Black medical colleges close, even though it recognized that the remaining two schools would be unable to train enough Black physicians to serve the 9.8 million Black patients in the United States [7, 12]. Further examples of racism that Black physicians faced included the need to build Black hospitals for Black patients turned away from other hospitals, as well as the separation of Black physicians in the AMA's *Directory* under the "colored" section, which made it more difficult for these physicians to receive bank loans and liability insurance (this section remained from 1906 to 1939, despite frequent protests from the NMA) [7].

Following World War II, many Americans saw parallels between Hitler's racist ideologies and White supremacism in the United States, prompting changes in social ideologies, which led some of the AMA's societies to allow entry to Black physicians for the first time in the late 1940s and 1950s [7]. Throughout the Civil Rights Movement, the NMA and AMA often took opposing stances, with the NMA pushing for civil reform and the AMA standing against federally organized health insurance, such as Medicare [7]. After the Civil Rights Act (1964) and Medicare and Medicaid Act (1965) passed, the AMA finally allowed a council to exclude societies based on their segregation policies in 1968 – a right which the council never exerted [7].

In 2008, the AMA formally apologized to Black physicians for the exclusionary practices of the organization [13]. The AMA eventually released a statement on racism in medicine in 2020 after the protests of the killing of George Floyd and other Black Americans. For the first time in history, the AMA recognized that racism is a public health threat and committed to working to take down racist practices and policies [14]. The policy also addressed the need to mitigate the effects of racism on providers [14]. Systemic racism has always affected public health. The history of the AMA demonstrates how deeply entrenched racism has been in the medical field and highlights the importance of promoting diversity with cultural humility.

A Brief Timeline of Women Physicians in the United States

Women have also faced adversity in joining the medical field. Dr. Elizabeth Blackwell was the first woman to be accepted and complete her medical degree at a US medical school [15]. She was rejected by all the medical schools she initially applied to in 1847, and she was even advised by one professor to disguise herself as a man and study abroad [15]. She was eventually accepted to Geneva Medical College later that year, but she continued to face discrimination after graduation [15]. In 1857, she founded the New York Infirmary for Women and Children in response to being denied work at hospitals because she was a woman, and in 1868, she opened the Women's Medical College of the New York Infirmary for Women and Children with her sister, Dr. Emily Blackwell [15].

Despite Dr. Elizabeth Blackwell's success in attaining a medical education, women that came after her continued to face formidable challenges. Soon after Dr. Blackwell received her degree, Geneva Medical College stopped allowing women to attend [16]. Women continued to apply and were granted admission to certain schools, making up around 5% of physicians by the end of the nineteenth century [16]. This number remained stable until the 1960s as women had to fight against Victorian ideals of purity and modesty, as well as the notion that a woman belonged in the home instead of the professional sphere [16].

Black women faced additional challenges in seeking a medical education, showing that individuals with multiple marginalized identities face further discrimination. While Black medical colleges were formed after the Civil War, paralleling the rise of a Black middle class, Black women were not welcomed [17]. At end of the nineteenth century, most Black women physicians attended and graduated from the Women's Medical College of Pennsylvania, which was a predominantly White institution [17]. Around this time, medical education was not standardized, and there were concerns regarding the quality of training. This changed in response to the 1910 *Flexner Report*, which created a framework to improve and standardize physician education [18]. The report addressed the education of Black men, but it only addressed Black women in the context of becoming nurses [18].

The road to equality has been slow, and there remains work to be done today. In 2003, women surpassed men in medical school applicants for the first time [17]. In 2020, fields like neurosurgery and orthopedics were projected to take another 47 and 138 years, respectively, for women representation to reflect the general population if the current trajectory continued [19]. This history provides a somber reminder of the challenges women, especially women of color, have faced in becoming physicians.

Important Terminology

At the end of 2020, the AMA adopted policies to recognize that race is a social construct and is a separate entity from biology, ethnicity, or genetics [20]. This system allows clinical practice and research to more accurately understand risk factors related to biology, genetics, the experience of racism, and social determinants of health [20]. The Association of American Medical Colleges (AAMC) collects data regarding the race and ethnicity of medical school applicants, students, and physicians [21]. In an effort to allow readers and authors to be on the same page, the terminology will be defined here.

To ensure consistency with the AAMC's reports, we will be including the same categories, such that race and ethnicity will be captured within the following categories:

- American Indian or Alaska native
- Black or African American
- Multiple race or ethnicity
- Unknown
- Asian
- Hispanic, Latino (Latinx), or Spanish origin
- Native Hawaiian or other Pacific Islander
- White [21]

We understand that this system does not fully capture the range of diversity present among the US population. For example, the category "Asian" includes a diverse group with people from many different cultural backgrounds and countries. Hopefully there will be a better and more accurate system in the future, but for now we will maintain uniformity with the AAMC in the interest of consistency.

Some important terms for discussing diversity are *implicit bias*, *white fragility*, and *structural racism*. *Implicit bias* refers to the subconscious biases that permeate thoughts and actions as a result of one's upbringing and social interactions [22]. These thoughts are often challenging to address as they can be contradictory to conscious beliefs [22]. Implicit biases are especially problematic because they have been shown to affect behavior [23]. These biases affect hiring patterns and can further disparities by perpetuating stereotypes [23]. By accepting that we all enter a space with biases, we create room to question these thoughts and improve our interactions with others.

In the book *White Fragility: Why It's So Hard for White People to Talk About Racism*, Dr. Robin DiAngelo coins the term w*hite fragility* to address some of the challenges in discussing race. White fragility describes the low threshold that certain individuals have for discussing racism, which can lead to defensiveness, feelings of guilt and anger, or avoidance of further conversations [24]. While conversations around race may be uncomfortable and laden with emotions, they are crucial for healing and leading to meaningful change. Addressing racism and bias is not meant to diminish the personal struggles that all individuals face in their daily life. Rather, it enhances our understanding of those around us and allows for a more caring society.

Education and the exploration of bias are important steps in addressing discrimination, but they do not fix everything. Dr. Deborah Plummer argues that as White people gain an increased understanding of racial dynamics, they can become complacent or self-congratulatory [25]. White fragility can also lead to a White savior complex, where people of color are assumed to be helpless and in need of rescuing, in the process undermining the success and resilience of these groups [25]. Dr. Plummer states that in order to truly make a difference, it is necessary to take concrete actions to support changes to policies that lead to structural racism, like promoting qualified minority applicants or advocating for changes to the criminal justice system [25].

Structural racism refers to how racism is more than just the prejudices an individual may have, as these beliefs play out in laws and policies, and they can become embedded in societal norms [26]. One famous example of structural racism is redlining. The Home Owners' Loan Corporation (HOLC) was established by the federal government in 1933 in response to the Great Depression to promote homeownership [26]. The HOLC drew red lines around areas with large Black populations to signal them as areas where people would not receive these government loans, resulting in less Black homeowners and capital [26]. As a result of these racist policies, real estate in Black neighborhoods lost value, and there was less investment in social programs to support good roads, transportation, schools, garbage collection, and employment [26]. Although redlining officially ended in 1968, the aftermath of these policies can still be seen today as directly affecting the health of residents in once redlined areas through higher rates of preterm birth, cancer, maternal depression, and other health issues [26]. In order to avoid perpetuating discriminatory policies, like redlining, everyone must address the biases they possess as a result of living within a biased culture. Equity can be promoted through education that is followed by behavioral and systemic changes.

Unique Challenges for Underrepresented Racial and Ethnic Minorities Today

In healthcare, those from underrepresented racial and ethnic groups face several obstacles to career advancement, including lack of opportunities for mentorship, implicit bias, and discrimination from colleagues [27]. These challenges lead to individuals underrepresented in medicine being less likely to be promoted and more likely to be part-time faculty [27]. A cross-sectional survey of trainees in MD/DO, MD/PhD, and DO/PhD programs in the United States found that trainees who identified as Black reported the lowest interest in academic medicine (40.8%) when compared to other racial and ethnic groups, with those who identify as White reporting 46.4% and Hispanic as 49.4% [27]. While loans were the primary source of funding for medical school for all medical students, trainees who identified as Black or Hispanic were less likely than their counterparts to be able to rely on family or partner support, with only 2.5% and 5.8%, respectively, to the 13.5% of White trainees and 24.3% of Asian trainees able to do so [27].

This difference leads to an increased financial burden among Black and Hispanic trainees, and it persists into their post-training careers [27]. The financial burdens faced by these groups may also prevent them from seeking more specialized training, which would further delay years of earning potential. Additional challenges occur due to the fact that Black trainees face 1.9 to 3.4 times higher rates of discrimination when compared to their counterparts [27]. This may account for the lower 10 year promotion rates seen for Black assistant professors [5].

Underrepresented minorities are also more likely to face *microaggressions*, with specific examples noted in Table 19.1. They are defined as the everyday, subtle interactions, which may be intentional or unintentional, that express derogatory or negative attitudes toward marginalized groups [28]. The person disseminating a microaggression is often unaware of the harm they are causing and may even mean to share a compliment. However, the underlying message is embedded with racism and stereotypes that can further alienate the individual [28]. Although these actions may be subtle, frequent microaggressions negatively affect the productivity and well-being of the individual [28].

Table 19.1 Examples of microaggressions faced by minority physicians in clinical medicine. Microaggressions in medicine can lead to qualified physicians feeling a decrease in confidence and exclusion from the field.

Patients or staff call a physician by first name instead of title
Asking "When will I see the doctor?" and assuming that the physician is the nurse or cleaning staff
Addressesing other team members, even if the minority physician is the senior on the team
Being told "you are so articulate," as if it is unusual for someone who looks like you to be intelligent [28]
"Where are you really from?," implying you are not American
Mispronouncing or not making an effort to learn your non-Anglican name

Another challenge racial and ethnic minorities often face in academic medicine is the *minority tax*, also frequently referred to as *cultural tax*, *Black tax*, or *Brown tax*, which is defined as the additional responsibilities that minorities are given in order to improve diversity, equity, and inclusion (DEI) in an institution [29, 30]. These tasks are often not compensated financially, are emotionally tiring, and serve to further drain the individuals most affected by bias [30]. These individuals are frequently part of a minority group at their institutions to begin with, further leading to a disproportionate workload compared to their peers [30]. Examples of responsibilities include serving on committees to promote DEI, being mentors to junior colleagues, or participating in panels on DEI [30]. One of the issues with the minority tax is that this work may not be recognized as valuable by the institution and siphons time away from the primary role assigned [30]. Furthermore, changes at an institutional level are often slow, leading to frustration and burn out [30]. People want to do the work because they know it as crucial, but they must be recognized, compensated, and allowed to set boundaries [30].

This tax can be further compounded for individuals who have multiple minority identities, including race, gender, disability, sexual orientation, or religion. When there are more mentees with a minority identity than mentors, mentors can be worn thin. Dr. Sophie Balzora, a Black woman gastroenterologist, succinctly shares, "We are tasked with creating, promoting, and leading diversity committees and recruiting efforts while we ourselves might be drowning in the same system we are burdened to improve" [31].

Gender in Medicine

Differences in Promotion Rates

A landmark study by Dr. Lynn Nonnemaker in 2000 showed that while the number of women at all levels of academic medicine was increasing, there were still few women being promoted [32]. Another study in 2014 showed that these differences in promotion remained even when accounting for differences in age, specialty, experience, and research [33]. In 2020, a study looked at 35 years of graduating cohorts of medical students to assess differences in promotion rates [34]. Women were still less likely to be promoted, even when adjusting for year of graduation, department, and race and ethnicity [34]. Even after becoming associate or full professors, women were half as likely as men of equal rank to be promoted to department chair [34]. A study looking at women surgeons among medical school faculty found that women progressively make up a smaller percentage as the career ladder progresses [22].

There are many possible explanations for these differences. While some may perceive that gender is not an issue in promotion, some women have stated that the higher up the ladder they went, the more of an "old boys club" they found it to be [35]. For others, success and inclusion can even vary within a single institution, based on department leadership or expectations [35]. Another challenge is addressing the pay gap. The lack of transparent salaries at many institutions both fosters an environment where women may be paid less, but also where women may believe they are paid less and sow distrust in the institution despite equitable pay [35].

There are many factors that may further play into promotion discrepancies for women. Women surgical residents have been found to be significantly less likely to receive awards than their male counterparts, particularly for teaching and clinical excellence, even when accounting for the smaller number of women residents [36]. Bias and perception of women's competence may play a role in why women were less likely to be evaluated well in teaching, but the difference disappeared in a more objective field like research [36]. Another reason for promotion discrepancy is the challenge women face due to family dynamics. Women may be more likely to desire to work part time to maintain traditional family responsibilities [35].

Confidence is another issue that can affect who gets promoted. A review conducted by Hewlett-Packard (HP) showed that women only applied for promotions when they thought they met 100% of the qualifications listed for a job, whereas men would apply if they met only 60% [37]. This confidence gap has also been identified in medicine. While men and women have similar performances on exams in medical school, female residents report less confidence overall and in procedures, although men and women report similar confidence in the patient-physician relationship [38]. This difference in confidence has also been noted among graduating surgical residents, where men had significantly higher levels of confidence than women [39]. It is important to note that confidence does not necessarily reflect competence, and understanding limitations is crucial to avoid performing procedures outside of one's scope [40]. If institutions recognize this confidence gap, they can increase women in leadership positions by encouraging women to apply and stating more concrete credentials for the job.

Letters of recommendation are also a key consideration during the hiring process, and in medicine, evaluations are important contributors. One study examining evaluations of surgical residents found that men were significantly more likely to be described with standout words, such as "exceptional" or "leader," than their women counterparts [41]. While evaluations are meant to be standardized, women can be unfairly impacted due to implicit bias about women's roles. These differences also affect letters of recommendation. One study looked at letters of recommendation for successfully promoted faculty in 37 different specialties at a large medical institution in the 1990s [42]. They found that women were significantly more likely to receive a letter of minimal assurance, which tended to be a shorter letter lacking specific details regarding the applicant's qualifications [42]. Women were also more likely to have at least one doubt raiser, which is defined as negative language negating an applicant's ability to fulfill a role [42]. Examples of doubt raisers include phrases like, "while Sarah has not done a lot of bench research" or "now that she has chosen to leave the laboratory," which sow doubt in the applicant's qualifications [42].

Lastly, differences were found in how men and women were described. Letter writers were more likely to discuss women's training but men's research, highlighting men's accomplishments but addressing women in more traditional roles [42]. The most common possessive phrases for women were "her teaching" and "her training," whereas letters for men commonly addressed "his research" and "his skills and abilities" [42]. While the study did not look into the reasons for these differences, recognizing that there are discrepancies can help letter writers and readers become more aware of biases and the context of women's accomplishments.

When evaluating the best applicants for a job, it is crucial to realize that evaluations and awards may not be reflective of the applicant's qualifications. Understanding the limitations of these tools can help recruiters use a more holistic approach in hiring, promoting, and retaining qualified women. The confidence gap should also be considered, as a woman's confidence may not accurately reflect her competence in her field.

The Gender Pay Gap in Medicine

Discrimination does not end with the hiring process; rather, it follows a woman for her entire career. The gender pay gap exists across many careers, and the medical field has not been immune. A report by Doximity in 2018 showed that full-time women physicians were earning 73% of men's income [43]. A 2020 study showed that even at the highest level of clinical department chair, women were still making $0.88 for every dollar that a man earned [44]. For women who are also ethnic and racial minorities, this pay gap has not been well documented. While Black women physicians have also been shown to earn 27% less than their non-Hispanic White men counterparts [31], more research is required to investigate whether a pay gap exists across different ethnicities.

The Johns Hopkins University School of Medicine (JHUSOM) discovered that there was a significant discrepancy in the career promotion of women faculty members and, in response, created a committee to review and address these findings [45]. By standardizing the process to promotion, prioritizing recruitment and retention of women faculty, and creating pathways for women to become leaders in their fields, JHUSOM was able to decrease their gender pay gap to 1.9% [45]. Through this effort, JHUSOM was able to decrease the difference in accumulated wealth between men and women from $501,416 to $210,829 [45]. While this is a smaller pay gap than the national average, there is still room to achieve parity.

People may believe that the reasons for the pay gap are not related to inherent sexism. Some argue that women work fewer hours than men, see fewer patients, or pursue less lucrative fields, often in order to have more time with their families [43]. This notion has been rebuked when looking at salary differences of full-time employees only [45]. A pay gap was found among academic physicians even when accounting for specialty, academic productivity, position, and work hours [46]. There should be absolutely no pay gap for equal work. A pay gap suggests that work by women is inherently less valuable. Hospitals receive equal compensation for work done by men and women, and they should compensate their employees appropriately. A survey of surgical residents found that women had lower salary expectations and felt less prepared to negotiate than men despite having similar career goals [47]. These concerns reveal potential areas that can be addressed in order to encourage and support women in academic medicine.

What About Burnout?

Burnout is defined as the chronic stress an individual experiences that is difficult to manage due to a lack of social support and resources, which leads to depersonalization and emotional fatigue, especially with regard to emotionally exhausting work [48]. Medical students and physicians are often highly driven, competitive, and perfectionists; when coupled with rigorous workload, this places them at high risk for burnout [48]. Burnout may present as depression, anxiety, a decrease in efficiency, and a decreased desire to help others [48]. It can also affect patients as burnout may lead to physicians having worse patient outcomes and lower patient satisfaction scores [49].

In a survey of 162 medical students, Black students reported significantly higher personal burnout scores, specifically physical and psychological fatigue [48]. Women were also more likely to report burnout related to work and had higher personal burnout scores than men [48]. It is worth considering that minority physicians may operate with higher baseline levels of stress due to the culmination of minority tax, microaggressions, and bias and therefore be more susceptible to burnout.

Promotion of well-being is a significant concern as physicians have turned to suicide at higher rates than the general population. Healthcare professionals, including physicians and dentists, of Asian and Pacific Islander descent were found to be 2.80 times more likely to die from suicide than the general population [49]. This may be related to stigma around discussing mental health in these communities, leading to lower rates of diagnosis and treatment [49]. Other significant risk factors include job difficulties, increasing age, and mental and physical health problems [49]. One population in particular identified as higher risk for dying by suicide was older, married men [49]. This finding may be due to challenges in the transition to retirement or senior positions around purpose, routine, and changes in family dynamics [49]. Men may be more affected because of a reluctance to be vulnerable and express the need for mental health services due to societal expectations around masculine traits [49].

In discussions concerned with gender, there may be an assumption that the main goal is to help women at the expense of men. The elevated risk for suicide among older men shows that promoting physician well-being and career success encompasses many distinct groups. In order to make medicine a truly equitable and diverse field, we need to address the barriers for all physicians. The elevated suicide risk for older men and Asian and Pacific Islander physicians highlights the need to address physician well-being and mental health screening for all physicians. Championing equity can benefit everyone by increasing support and confronting the stigma around mental health.

If you or a loved one is at risk for suicide, please contact the National Suicide Prevention Lifeline at 1-800-273-8255. For physician-specific care, including medical students, visit https://www.physiciansupportline.com or call 888-409-0141 [50].

The Intersectionality of Minority Identities: Sexuality, Gender Identity, Disability, and Religion

In this chapter, we have addressed some of the challenges that minorities in medicine face. Physicians who have multiple identities that are underrepresented and traditionally undervalued in medicine also have difficulties in career development. The term *intersectionality* was first coined in 1989 by Kimberlé Crenshaw to highlight that Black women face discrimination due to their race and gender in a way that is interdependent and complex [51]. The intersection of multiple identities can predispose individuals to discrimination that can be more than the summation of its parts [51].

In medicine, there are physicians with many different minority identities, such as identifying as LGBTQIA+ (lesbian, gay, bisexual, transgender, queer or questioning, intersex, asexual or allied, and others), having a disability, or practicing an underrepresented religion. These individuals face additional challenges, as they may have trouble finding a mentor with the same identities and may also experience more microaggressions. Physicians may struggle with the decision to disclose certain aspects of their identity, such as their sexuality or gender, to colleagues or patients due to fear of judgment and exclusion. Just as recruitment for diversity in race and gender improves the workforce, supporting other identities allows physicians to provide better care for patients who identify with various minority groups [52].

Individuals with disabilities also face challenges. While 19% of the American population lives with a disability, only 2% of physicians do, and many of those physicians developed their condition after residency training [53]. The medical model of disability views a disability as something to fix, whereas a social model can see the value of this variation [53]. For example, physicians with hearing loss may be better at communicating with hearing-impaired patients because they can relate to their challenges [53]. Additionally, living with a disability can help physicians reframe what pathologies need to be cured and be mindful of the full spectrum of treatment options [53]. However, the current hospital model is not welcoming to those who require accommodations, and this can negatively affect the ability for medical students with disabilities to enter and remain in the medical field. When applying to residencies, these students can be at a disadvantage as programs are able to discriminate against these students without outright stating why the applicant was rejected [53].

Physicians may also face discrimination based on their religious affiliations. In particular, Muslim Americans have been targeted with hate crimes and prejudice in the aftermath of the World Trade Center attacks on September 11, 2001. One study found that Muslim physicians who viewed religion as "most important" were the most likely to face discrimination at work, with 24% of respondents reporting frequent discrimination in their work [54].

To address the intersectionality of gender and race in career advancement, one study evaluated the trends among academic surgery leadership [55]. Their study found that while women faculty were increasing in representation, the representation of Black women remained constant, and Hispanic women were decreasing [55]. More research is required to address the extent that multiple minority identities have on career development, but making medicine more welcoming and supportive in general can help improve the promotion and retention of these individuals.

COVID-19 and Disparities
With the COVID-19 pandemic, it is important to briefly consider how this worldwide stressor has had disproportionate impacts. Minority individuals in the United States, especially Black Americans, have died at higher rates from the pandemic than their White counterparts [56]. Minority doctors tend to have specialties where they interact with patients more, and they may have had to work without adequate personalized protective equipment [57]. Women have also been impacted more, as the loss of childcare options has largely fallen on their shoulders [57].

Recommendations for Increasing Diversity in the Workforce

While this chapter has discussed some of the more discouraging aspects of discrimination in medicine, many leaders have addressed solutions for these concerns. In order to actively encourage diversity, equity, and inclusion, the medical field must increase the accessibility of leadership positions, decrease bias in the interview process, and improve the retention of minority physicians.

There are many existing solutions to increase accessibility for career advancement. Mentorship is important for creating connections and support for minority physicians and medical students. Coaching and sponsorship are vital for helping these individuals gain exposure and be more prepared to face the challenges of leadership. To encourage physicians who are underrepresented to enter and stay in medicine, a committee can be made, similar to the "We are SAGES (Society of American Gastrointestinal and Endoscopic Surgeons)" task force created in 2017 [53]. This task force assessed the organizational culture and identified barriers through a survey and identified concerns around nepotism and lack of transparency around promotion [58]. In response to these findings, they are creating formal leadership training and mentorship programs [58]. An additional issue that was recognized was discrimination within the organization that was based on factors in addition to gender and race, such as age, surgical specialty, and academic versus private practice [58]. These are being addressed by increasing the diversity of SAGES in the media and in committees [58].

In addition to increasing recruitment of minority physicians, the interview process can be adapted to increase diversity in medicine. One solution is to follow the example of symphony orchestras, which hired more women musicians when auditions were held behind a screen and the judges could not see the applicants [23]. Similarly, applicant information can be blinded in order to decrease bias [59]. Institutions will help encourage hiring and promotion of underrepresented minorities by placing value on advocacy work [27]. Advocating for minorities and remaining vigilant when biases emerge during hiring and promotion discussions are additional solutions [30].

Once minority physicians have been promoted, it is important to improve the retention of these individuals. We must recognize that the minority tax exists and provide financial compensation to those who lead the way in promoting equity within our organizations [31]. When promoting physicians to diversity, equity, and inclusion committees, there should be opportunities to negotiate for time, financial compensation, an assistant, or office space [30]. Ensuring that promotion will yield tangible and timely results can help physicians remain on track with career goals [30]. Finally, retention can improve by respecting boundaries consistent with contracts and personal values, as working after hours or on holidays imposes further pressures for others in marginalized positions to keep up [30].

Retention of women in particular can be improved by addressing the gender pay gap. By reporting salaries and providing regular performance reviews, institutions provide objective information, which makes it easier to ensure accountability for equal pay and increases women's trust in the institution [59]. Institutions can also implement bias trainings, improve access to coaching and mentorship, and provide negotiation trainings to support women [45]. Ensuring equal leave policies, regardless of gender or marriage status, will also help alleviate the burden that women experience due to expectations around childcare.

In order to address these concerns, physicians must collectively acknowledge the value that diverse minds bring to the table, including contributions to improved patient care. Those in positions of power must address their own biases to ensure more fair discussions around promotion.

Key Points
- The medical field has a long history of discriminating against minority physicians, and minority physicians continue to be underrepresented today, particularly in leadership positions.
- Hiring practices can be improved by learning about the challenges faced by minority physicians in order to recognize the limitations of awards, letters of

recommendations, and perceived confidence to accurately capture an applicant's competence.
- While challenges remain to ensuring an equitable society, leaders in the medical field have already begun to find ways to promote and retain more minority physicians, such as increasing mentorship opportunities, providing leadership training, and valuing advocacy work.

References

1. Lautenberger DM, Dandar VM. The state of women in academic medicine 2018–2019: exploring pathways to equity; n.d.
2. Heiser S. The majority of U.S. medical students are women, new data show | AAMC. In: AAMC. 2019. https://www.aamc.org/news-insights/press-releases/majority-us-medical-students-are-women-new-data-show. Accessed 24 Jun 2021.
3. Jordan K. The struggle and triumph of America's first black doctors. The Atlantic; 2016.
4. Flannagan M, Asfaw S, Ferrada P, Ford H. Race/ethnicity and surgery. In: Telem DA, Martin CA, editors. Diversity, equity, and inclusion. Springer; 2021. p. 89–95.
5. Abelson JS, Wong NZ, Symer M, et al. Racial and ethnic disparities in promotion and retention of academic surgeons. Am J Surg. 2018;216:678–82. https://doi.org/10.1016/j.amjsurg.2018.07.020.
6. Deville C. The suffocating state of physician workforce diversity. JAMA Intern Med. 2020;180:1418. https://doi.org/10.1001/jamainternmed.2020.3815.
7. Baker RB, Washington HA, Olakanmi O, et al. African American physicians and organized medicine, 1846–1968: origins of a racial divide. JAMA. 2008;300:306–13. https://doi.org/10.1001/jama.300.3.306.
8. Greenwood BN, Hardeman RR, Huang L, Sojourner A. Physician–patient racial concordance and disparities in birthing mortality for newborns. Proc National Acad Sci. 2020;117:21194–200. https://doi.org/10.1073/pnas.1913405117.
9. Tsugawa Y, Jena AB, Figueroa JF, et al. Comparison of hospital mortality and readmission rates for medicare patients treated by male vs female physicians. JAMA Intern Med. 2016;177:206. https://doi.org/10.1001/jamainternmed.2016.7875.
10. Haskins J. Celebrating 10 African-American medical pioneers. In: AAMC. 2019. https://www.aamc.org/news-insights/celebrating-10-african-american-medical-pioneers. Accessed 14 Feb 2021.
11. Morgan TM. The education and medical practice of Dr. James McCune smith (1813–1865), first black American to hold a medical degree. J Natl Med Assoc. 2003;95:603–14.
12. Savitt T. Abraham Flexner and the black medical schools. J Natl Med Assoc. 2006;98:1415–24.
13. CNN. AMA apologizes for racially biased policies. http://www.cnn.com/2008/HEALTH/07/10/ama.racism/index.html. 2008. Accessed 28 May 2021.
14. AMA. New AMA policy recognizes racism as a public health threat | American Medical Association. In: AMA. 2020. https://www.ama-assn.org/press-center/press-releases/new-ama-policy-recognizes-racism-public-health-threat. Accessed 15 Feb 2021.
15. Moore W. Elizabeth Blackwell: breaching the barriers for women in medicine. Lancet. 2021;397:662–3. https://doi.org/10.1016/s0140-6736(21)00260-9.
16. Morantz-Sanchez R. Sympathy and science: women physicians in American medicine. 2nd ed. The University of North Carolina Press; 1999.
17. Borst CG, Jones KW. As patients and healers: the history of women and medicine. OAH Mag Hist. 2005;19:23–6.

18. Bailey M. The Flexner report: standardizing medical students through region-, gender-, and race-based hierarchies. Am J Law Med. 2017;43:209–23. https://doi.org/10.1177/0098858817723660.
19. Bennett CL, Baker O, Rangel EL, Marsh RH. The gender gap in surgical residencies. JAMA Surg. 2020;155:893–4. https://doi.org/10.1001/jamasurg.2020.2171.
20. AMA. New AMA policies recognize race as a social, not biological, construct | American Medical Association. In: AMA. 2020. https://www.ama-assn.org/press-center/press-releases/new-ama-policies-recognize-race-social-not-biological-construct. Accessed 15 Feb 2021.
21. AAMC. Diversity in medicine: facts and figures 2019. In: AAMC. 2019. https://www.aamc.org/data-reports/workforce/report/diversity-medicine-facts-and-figures-2019. Accessed 15 Feb 2021.
22. Stephens EH, Heisler CA, Temkin SM, Miller P. The current status of women in surgery. JAMA Surg. 2020;155:876–85. https://doi.org/10.1001/jamasurg.2020.0312.
23. Bendick M, Nunes AP. Developing the research basis for controlling bias in hiring. J Soc Issues. 2012;68:238–62. https://doi.org/10.1111/j.1540-4560.2012.01747.x.
24. DiAngelo R. White fragility. Counterpoints. 2016;497:245–53.
25. Plummer DL. Why blacks are tired of hearing about white fragility…and why it matters. In: Medium. 2020. https://deborahlplummer.medium.com/why-blacks-are-tired-of-hearing-about-white-fragility-and-why-it-matters-62c16ef9df35. Accessed 28 May 2021.
26. Bailey ZD, Feldman JM, Bassett MT. How structural racism works — racist policies as a root cause of U.S. racial health inequities. New Engl J Med. 2020;384:768–73. https://doi.org/10.1056/nejmms2025396.
27. Siebert AL, Chou S, Toubat O, et al. Factors associated with underrepresented minority physician scientist trainee career choices. BMC Med Educ. 2020;20:422. https://doi.org/10.1186/s12909-020-02328-6.
28. Sue DW, Capodilupo CM, Torino GC, et al. Racial microaggressions in everyday life. Am Psychol. 2007;62:271–86. https://doi.org/10.1037/0003-066x.62.4.271.
29. Mensah MO. Majority taxes — toward antiracist allyship in medicine - ProQuest. NEJM. 2020;383:e23. https://doi.org/10.1056/nejmpv2022964.
30. Gewin V. The time tax put on scientists of colour. Nature. 2020;583:479–81. https://doi.org/10.1038/d41586-020-01920-6.
31. Balzora S. When the minority tax is doubled: being black and female in academic medicine. Nat Rev Gastroentero. 2021;18:1–1. https://doi.org/10.1038/s41575-020-00369-2.
32. Nonnemaker L. Women physicians in academic medicine — new insights from cohort studies. New Engl J Medicine. 2000;342:399–405. https://doi.org/10.1056/nejm200002103420606.
33. Jena AB, Khullar D, Ho O, et al. Sex differences in academic rank in US medical schools in 2014. JAMA. 2015;314:1149–58. https://doi.org/10.1001/jama.2015.10680.
34. Richter KP, Clark L, Wick JA, et al. Women physicians and promotion in academic medicine. New Engl J Med. 2020;383:2148–57. https://doi.org/10.1056/nejmsa1916935.
35. Carr PL, Gunn CM, Kaplan SA, et al. Inadequate progress for women in academic medicine: findings from the National Faculty Study. J Womens Health. 2015;24:190–9. https://doi.org/10.1089/jwh.2014.4848.
36. Kuo LE, Lyu HG, Jarman MP, et al. Gender disparity in awards in general surgery residency programs. JAMA Surg. 2021;156:60–6. https://doi.org/10.1001/jamasurg.2020.3518.
37. Kay K, Shipman C. The confidence gap. In: The Atlantic. 2014. https://www.theatlantic.com/magazine/archive/2014/05/the-confidence-gap/359815/. Accessed 28 Feb 2021.
38. Gavinski K, Cleveland E, Didwania AK, et al. Relationship between confidence, gender, and career choice in internal medicine. J Gen Intern Med. 2020:1–6. https://doi.org/10.1007/s11606-020-06221-2.
39. Fonseca AL, Reddy V, Longo WE, et al. Operative confidence of graduating surgery residents: a training challenge in a changing environment. Am J Surg. 2014;207:797–805. https://doi.org/10.1016/j.amjsurg.2013.09.033.
40. Babchenko O, Gast K. Should we train female and male residents slightly differently? JAMA Surg. 2020;155:373–4. https://doi.org/10.1001/jamasurg.2019.5887.

41. Gerull KM, Loe M, Seiler K, et al. Assessing gender bias in qualitative evaluations of surgical residents. Am J Surg. 2019;217:306–13. https://doi.org/10.1016/j.amjsurg.2018.09.029.
42. Trix F, Psenka C. Exploring the color of glass: letters of recommendation for female and male medical faculty. Discourse Soc. 2003;14:191–220. https://doi.org/10.1177/0957926503014002277.
43. Asgari MM, Carr PL, Bates CK. Closing the gender wage gap and achieving professional equity in medicine. JAMA. 2019;321:1665–6. https://doi.org/10.1001/jama.2019.4168.
44. Mensah M, Beeler W, Rotenstein L, et al. Sex differences in salaries of department chairs at public medical schools. JAMA Intern Med. 2020;180:789–92. https://doi.org/10.1001/jamainternmed.2019.7540.
45. Rao AD, Nicholas SE, Kachniarz B, et al. Association of a simulated institutional gender equity initiative with gender-based disparities in medical school faculty salaries and promotions. JAMA Netw Open. 2018;1:e186054. https://doi.org/10.1001/jamanetworkopen.2018.6054.
46. Jagsi R, Griffith KA, Stewart A, et al. Gender differences in the salaries of physician researchers. JAMA. 2012;307:2410–7. https://doi.org/10.1001/jama.2012.6183.
47. Gray K, Neville A, Kaji AH, et al. Career goals, salary expectations, and salary negotiation among male and female general surgery residents. JAMA Surg. 2019;154:1023–9. https://doi.org/10.1001/jamasurg.2019.2879.
48. Armstrong M, Reynolds K. Assessing burnout and associated risk factors in medical students. J Natl Med Assoc. 2020;112:597–601. https://doi.org/10.1016/j.jnma.2020.05.019.
49. Ji YD, Robertson FC, Patel NA, et al. Assessment of risk factors for suicide among US health care professionals. JAMA Surg. 2020;155:713–21. https://doi.org/10.1001/jamasurg.2020.1338.
50. Physician Support Line. n.d. https://www.physiciansupportline.com/. Accessed 2 May 2021.
51. Crenshaw K. Demarginalizing the intersection of race and sex: a black feminist critique of antidiscrimination doctrine, feminist theory and antiracist politics. University of Chicago Legal Forum 139–167; 1989.
52. Thadikonda KM, Gast KM, Chaiet SR. Sexual orientation and gender identity and surgery. In: Telem DA, Martin CA, editors. Diversity, equity, and inclusion. Cham: Springer; 2020. p. 97–104.
53. Keune JD. Disability and the surgical career. In: Telem DA, Martin CA, editors. Diversity, equity, and inclusion. Cham: Springer; 2020. p. 105–15.
54. Padela AI, Adam H, Ahmad M, et al. Religious identity and workplace discrimination: a national survey of American Muslim physicians. Ajob Empir Bioeth. 2015;7:1–11. https://doi.org/10.1080/23294515.2015.1111271.
55. Riner AN, Herremans KM, Neal DW, et al. Diversification of academic surgery, its leadership, and the importance of intersectionality. JAMA Surg. 2021;156. https://doi.org/10.1001/jamasurg.2021.1546.
56. Price-Haywood EG, Burton J, Fort D, Seoane L. Hospitalization and mortality among black patients and white patients with Covid-19. New Engl J Med. 2020;382:2534–43. https://doi.org/10.1056/nejmsa2011686.
57. Woodhams C, Dacre J, Parnerkar I, Sharma M. Pay gaps in medicine and the impact of COVID-19 on doctors' careers. Lancet. 2020;397:79–80. https://doi.org/10.1016/s0140-6736(20)32671-4.
58. Telem DA, Qureshi A, Edwards M, et al. SAGES climate survey: results and strategic planning for our future. Surg Endosc. 2018;32:4105–10. https://doi.org/10.1007/s00464-018-6149-5.
59. Krecko LK, Greenberg CC, Greenberg JA. Gender and surgery. In: Telem DA, Martin CA, editors. Diversity, equity, and inclusion. Cham: Springer; 2020. p. 79–87.

Chapter 20
Research in Medicine

Tonchanok Intaprasert, Audrey Lim, and Rob Eley

Hospital Medicine from the Research-Scientist Perspective

Ask the public how a research scientist contributes to hospital medicine and chances are they will describe someone sitting in a laboratory remote from the hospital developing a new drug. What they may not realize is that those of us who are hospital-based research scientists support the practice of hospital medicine by engaging with all three pillars of evidence-based medicine – current best clinical evidence, clinician experience and expertise, and patient preferences. Hospital medicine is thus supported from "bench to bedside."

The authors of this chapter provide examples of how research across this continuum has contributed to current clinical practice: from new diagnostic and predictive tools improving management of PE and stroke to advances in robotics providing opportunities for new surgical procedures. They also discuss how poor evidence removed droperidol from the clinician's toolbox for behavioral management, and how good evidence by hospital-based research scientists returned it. That return prompted a colleague to note that this was "the biggest game changer" in patient management and staff safety in his 35 years as an emergency physician.

T. Intaprasert · A. Lim
University of Queensland, Faculty of Medicine, Herston, QLD, Australia

R. Eley (✉)
Emergency Department, Princess Alexandra Hospital, and Southside Clinical Unit, Faculty of Medicine, University of Queensland, Brisbane, QLD, Australia
e-mail: r.eley@uq.edu.au

© The Author(s), under exclusive license to Springer Nature Switzerland AG 2022
K. Conrad (ed.), *Clinical Approaches to Hospital Medicine*,
https://doi.org/10.1007/978-3-030-95164-1_20

Introduction

The practice of modern medicine relies on a combination of compassionate care and expert knowledge developed through rigorous research principles and scientific discoveries [1]. This ongoing research forms the groundwork of modern clinical decision-making and distinguishes evidence-based medicine [2] from alternative medicine. This puts the impetus on physicians to guide their clinical practice based on clinical expertise, patient values, and the best research evidence available via critical appraisal of study methods for validity of results [2, 3].

Evidence-based medicine guides practice based on what has been shown to benefit patients and allows research to highlight objective measurements for quality-of-care outcomes. Examples of these outcome attributes can be measured through the Institute of Medicine's quality of care domains. These domains can be summarized and defined as follows [3]:

1. *Safe*: Care intended to help patients does not cause harm.
2. *Effective*: Scientific knowledge guides care for those who would most likely benefit to avoid underuse or misuse of services.
3. *Patient-centered*: Individual patient values guide clinical decisions.
4. *Timely*: Reduction of delays for care delivery and receipt.
5. *Efficient*: Reduction of waste in equipment, supplies, ideas, and energy.
6. *Equitable*: Care does not vary in quality regardless of any personal characteristics of the recipient of that care.

To ensure the best possible outcomes for patients, clinicians are expected to keep up to date with ongoing research in their fields. In this chapter, we highlight four specific examples of how research guides clinical practice for hospitalists and other specialist physicians. The ever-changing and growing body of evidence for practice over a few short years will be showcased through the effect research has on practice protocols (i.e., choice of investigation, drug use, and interventions) and practice outcomes as related to the six quality-of-care domains. The four research-guided practices presented are as follows:

1. Research as a driver for clinical decision-making pathways for safe, effective, timely, and efficient investigative decisions in suspected PE.
2. Research used to challenge the use or avoidance of medications based on previous poor evidence.
3. Research improving scientific understanding of clot retrieval to guide timely and effective management of a thrombotic ischemic stroke.
4. Research in the field of robotics paving a new clinical practice approach in the fields of perioperative care and surgery.

To Scan or Not to Scan? Research Probability Guiding Practice Investigations in Suspected PE

Hospital clinicians now have a multitude of diagnostic tests available to them. Not only are there a greater number of tests, but there are also increasing sensitivity and specificity in the tests. While it is good that there are resources to confirm a suspected pathological condition, without clinical guidelines, these diagnostic tests can easily become overused as a long list of unnecessary rule-out investigations. As a result, the number of incidental findings which lead to a cascade of additional tests has been increasing with no additional mortality benefit [4]. To reduce waste on resources, pre-test probability allows physicians to gauge how probable a diagnosis is prior to investigative confirmations. Pre-test probability is the likelihood of a suspected disease given the patient's presentation prior to testing. This is useful clinically as it helps physicians decide whether a diagnosis should be accepted, ruled out, or require further testing. This then reduces the number of false positive results and unwarranted investigations. One example of how research has continuously built upon evidence-based knowledge for pre-test probability and investigative pathways is the diagnosis of PE.

PE is common in patients presenting to hospital emergency departments or within the inpatient ward and perioperative care settings [5]. If left untreated, PE is associated with a high mortality rate [5]. Additionally, a delay in the diagnosis of PE often contributes to death and disability even if the patient was previously hemodynamically stable [6]. Thus, appropriate investigation and timely management are crucial in ensuring the best possible outcome.

Since PE often presents with non-specific symptoms, it was once thought that clinical diagnosis of PE was inaccurate with little added value [7, 8]. The Prospective Investigation of Pulmonary Embolism Diagnosis (PIOPED) clinical trial back in 1989, however, showed that experienced physicians were able to categorize patients with suspected PE based on clinical assessments into appropriate groups of low, moderate, and high probabilities [7]. Thus, the potential utility of a pre-test probability in the diagnosis of PE became widely researched with several new models created to help determine likelihoods of PE. The pre-test tools use a combination of patient history, clinical signs and symptoms, and clinician judgment. As noted in Table 20.1, some of the current validated clinical prediction tools commonly used for the pre-test probability of PE include the following:

- Well's criteria
- Simplified Well's criteria
- Revised Geneva Score
- Simplified Geneva Score

Table 20.1 Examples of criterion components within the Well's criteria and Simplified Geneva score for PE

Well's criteria for PE	Scoring points	Simplified Geneva criteria	Scoring points
Clinical signs and symptoms of DVT	3	Pain on deep palpation of lower limb and unilateral edema	1
PE as or more likely than an alternate diagnosis	3	Unilateral lower limb pain	1
Heart rate > 100 bpm	1.5	Heart rate 75–94 bpm	1
Immobilization or major surgery in previous 4 weeks	1.5	Surgery (under general anesthesia) or fracture (lower limbs) within 1 month	1
Previous, objectively diagnosed PE or DVT	1.5	Previous DVT or PE	1
Hemoptysis	1	Hemoptysis	1
Malignancy (ongoing treatment or treatment within the last 6 months, or palliative)	1	Active malignant condition (solid or hematologic) currently active or considered cured <1 year	1
		Age > 65 years old	1
		Heart rate ≥ 95 bpm	2
3 Levels pretest probability score: Low <2 Moderate 2–6 High >6		*3 Levels pretest probability score*: Low <2 Moderate 2–4 High ≥5	

Adapted from Penaloza et al. [9]

These prediction tools allow clinicians to decide whether or not they should obtain a D-dimer measurement or imaging in patients suspicious of having a PE. A D-dimer is a marker unique to fibrin degradation and is a sensitive measure in the exclusion of venous thromboembolisms; however, it is non-specific. Thus, D-dimer is use differently based on pre-test probabilities. For those with a low pre-test probability of PE, the Pulmonary Embolism Rule-Out Criteria (PERC) is applied (Table 20.2) [8]. D-dimer and imaging do not need to be obtained if the patient with a low pre-test probability also has negative PERC as this means that PE has been successfully ruled out with a risk of less than 2% [8, 10]. Investigations into other diagnoses should then follow.

Patients with low pre-test probability with a positive PERC, however, require a high sensitivity D-dimer measurement for initial diagnostic testing [8]. Patients with an intermediate pre-test probability should also have their D-dimer obtained, however, without having to go through PERC [8]. If the patient has a high pre-test probability for PE, computer tomography pulmonary angiography (CTPA) should be immediately obtained [8]. Ventilation-perfusion scans can be used as an alternative to CTPA if CTPA is not available or is contraindicated. A D-dimer is not warranted in patients with a high pre-test probability of PE [8].

In summary, these various pre-test probability tools help clinicians categorize patients into the most appropriate groups for different diagnostic strategies – those

Table 20.2 Pulmonary Embolism Rule-out Criteria (PERC)

PERC: +1 Score if the answer is yes
1. Is the patient older than 49 years old?
2. Is the pulse rate >99 beats per minute?
3. Is the patient saturating lower than 95% on pulse oximetry with room air?
4. Is there a history of hemoptysis?
5. Is the patient taking exogenous estrogen?
6. Does the patient have a prior diagnosis of venous thromboembolism?
7. Has the patient had recent surgery or trauma (requiring endotracheal intubation or hospitalization in the previous 4 weeks)?
8. Does the patient have unilateral leg swelling (visual observation of asymmetry of the calves)?

Adapted from Penaloza et al. [10]
Patients who do not satisfy any criteria are identified as negative PERC and PE is unlikely in low pretest probability groups

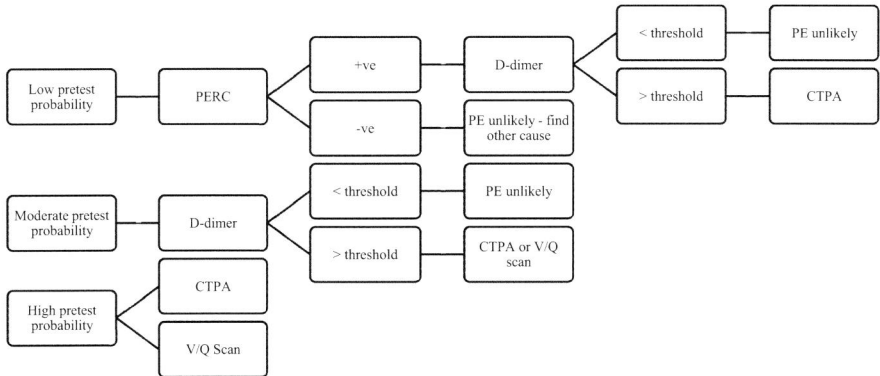

Fig. 20.1 Pre-test probability-guided investigation pathway for patients suspicious of PE. D-dimer thresholds should ideally be age-adjusted; however, 500 ng/mL is the generic cut off [8]

who require no further testing, those requiring further risk stratification with D-dimer, and those with high risk requiring immediate imaging (Fig. 20.1) [8]. All four validated pre-test probability tools in combination with a D-dimer result show similar performance for excluding acute PE or for indicating the need for further investigations [11]. When used correctly, physicians can choose any of the four validated pre-test probability tools to assist in evaluating the patient with a suspected PE [11].

This use of pre-test probability reduces unnecessary use of computed tomography (CT) scan, associated healthcare costs, and potential risks from radiation. Furthermore, these pre-test probabilities provide a standardized decision-making tool for physicians who may be less experienced with the presentation and management of PE. Research in this case has provided clinicians with a validated decision-making pathway that is safe, effective, timely, and equitable.

Black-Box Warning: What Is the Evidence? Research Guiding Risk-Benefit Analysis

Medical intervention often offers patient comfort despite additional side effects. Thus, when physicians decide on management plans, the risk and benefit of prescribing certain medications or conducting certain procedures has to be weighed. As part of the commonly known "prima facie" principle of medical ethics – at the forefront of risk-benefit analysis – physicians must consider the principles of beneficence and non-maleficence [12]. Research in this area provides evidence-based knowledge of how our current medical interventions work, how they benefit patients, and how they may cause unintended adverse reactions. The decision to then apply certain procedures and medications for patients, therefore, relies on sound research methods and results.

Before a medication can be approved, a rigorous process to ensure safety and efficacy must take place. This takes at least 8 years on average as well as a significant amount of money until the drug is available for use in patient care [13]. However, in cases of extreme urgency as seen with the development of the COVID-19 vaccination, fast-tracking is possible. Understanding the process of drug research development and approval, therefore, is important in guiding a physician's practice.

The process involves both pre-clinical and clinical testing for safety and is summarized in Table 20.3 [13]. This differs slightly between countries as each has their

Table 20.3 Typical pathway for drug development and approval in the United States

Step	Involvements	Purpose	Timeframe (Years)
Pre-clinical phase	Finding an agent through knowledge of disease, technology, pharmacology, chemistry lab, and animal studies	Identify potential agents and assess biological activity and safety	1–2
FDA application as an investigational new drug (IND)			
Clinical phase 1	20–100 healthy human volunteers	Determine safety and appropriate dosages	3
Clinical phase 2	100–300 patient volunteers	Evaluate effectiveness and monitor side effects	4–5
Clinical phase 3	1000–3000 patient volunteers	Verify effectiveness and monitor long-term adverse effects	6–8
NDA filing with FDA			
Post-marketing studies/ Clinical phase 4	Physician, patient, and manufacturer reports of any unfitting complications. Special reports for any serious and unexpected adverse reactions	To analyze the risks and benefits of the drug in different populations (i.e., high risk, pediatric, elderly). Long-term exposure side effects are reviewed	3

Adapted from Lipsky and Sharp [13]

own regulatory agency. In the United States, the process is filed for approval with the Food and Drug Administration (FDA); in Australia, the Therapeutic Goods Administration (TGA); and in the United Kingdom, the Medicines and Healthcare products Regulatory Agency (MHRA) [13].

For the most part, clinical trials are then split into four phases. Phase 1 focuses on safety and pharmacology, phase 2 ensures the compound is effective, phase 3 involves submitting a new drug application (NDA) with results from all phases thus far, and phase 4 involves a post-marketing study after product approval [13]. This process is sometimes referred to as translational research from "bench to bedside," where laboratory research leads to clinical research that can be practically applied in patient care settings.

Once a drug has been approved and used in the market, post-marketing studies in phase 4 can sometimes revise how a drug is labeled for use. The research process, thus, can be seen as a continuous process in risk-benefit analysis rather than a hurdle. Doubts and questioning of new findings or adverse effects of a drug should then be re-studied to rule out confounding factors. A good example of how research guides the process into evidence-based risk-benefit decision-making is in the research into the use of droperidol.

Droperidol is a drug commonly used as an antiemetic and antipsychotic approved for use in the United States since 1970 [14]. It has widespread use in many settings, from treating postoperative or chemotherapy nausea, tranquilizing violent patients, and treating acute migraine to many other critical care and emergency situations [14]. On December 5, 2001, the FDA issued a new black-box warning for serious adverse reactions that included QT prolongation, which may lead to torsades de pointes and death [14]. As droperidol had been so commonly used prior to the black-box warning, these changes came as a surprise to many physicians. Thus, widespread confusion for its place in medical therapy was brought into question.

Studies analyzing how the black-box warning came to be led back to post-marketing research surveillance by the FDA. The evidence which guided their decision looked at worldwide reported data on adverse reactions with the use of droperidol. These data included information from countries that routinely used droperidol at very high doses (50–100 mg) and administered orally instead of intramuscularly or intravenously as was common in the United States [14, 15]. Furthermore, evidence showing the drug's relationship to QT prolongation was based on only two non-randomized prospective studies, one observational cross-sectional survey, and 65 cases reported over 5 years through the FDA MedWatch system [14, 15]. That body of evidence was far from convincing and not based on strong data. Thus, substantial evidence in regard to adverse cardiac events that would warrant the black-box warning from peer review was lacking [15]. Available systematic reviews and analysis found that adverse events such as sedation, agitation, and extrapyramidal effects were common [14, 16–19]. However, none reported cardiac events such as QT prolongation and torsades de pointes as included in the black-box warning. Thus, in clinical uses, physicians rightly questioned both the FDA warning and whether droperidol used in the recommended doses and route was an independent cause of life-threatening cardiac events [14].

Subsequent research used an evidence-based system to determine cause-and-effect of droperidol and cardiac events through a specific criterion. This criterion was proposed by Sir Bradford Hill, an English epidemiologist who pioneered randomized clinical trials. The so-called Hill's criteria looks at whether or not the cause precedes a specific effect, if there is a dose-response relationship, if there are large relative risks, if results from different studies are consistent, if there are plausible biological explanation, and if an analogous relationship is present with comparable exposure [14]. From available data on droperidol, a review by Kao et al. [14] suggested that droperidol associations with prolonged QT intervals have no significant adverse cardiovascular reactions shown. This implies that in the clinical setting, the choice to use droperidol depends on the situation and the individual clinician's risk-benefit analysis preference.

The black-box warning in 2001 caused a significant reduction of droperidol use around the world despite increasing evidence of its safety and systematic research reviews showing minimal risk of QT prolongation [20]. In subsequent years, studies to assess for safety and efficacy of droperidol were published examining its use with differing doses, routes, and circumstances. Calver et al. [20] published a study on droperidol use in Australia for sedation in the acute care and emergency settings [20]. They investigated the use of droperidol (10 mg or more) across multiple emergency centers for acute behavioral disturbance showing that there was no evidence for increased QT prolongation risks or adverse cardiac reactions [20]. Furthermore, the study showed that droperidol is potentially safer and at least as effective as benzodiazepines for use in emergency settings to sedate patients [20]. Droperidol was, in the words of Boyer, "back" [21].

In 2020, a large observational cohort study at an academic emergency department in the United States further showed droperidol safety and effectiveness for analgesic, antiemetic, and sedative use [15]. This study built upon evidence from other research that showed low-dose droperidol in emergency use for treating acute migraine, agitation, or combination treatment for sedation is safe and effective [15, 22–24].

Thus, good clinical research in this case overrides poor evidence and supports the need for clinicians to follow the latest available data and critically appraise studies in their area of applied pharmacological use. As with the use of droperidol, research has helped weigh its risk-benefit with the most up-to-date and vigorously peer-reviewed evidence against pre-emptive warnings that it is safe to use after all.

What Is in the Clot? Research on Clot Retrieval and Components Guiding Practice Protocols

Acute ischemic stroke is the occlusion of a cerebral vessel by a thrombus, causing a loss of blood circulation to the affected area. This can result in the loss of neurologic function. Across the world, acute ischemic stroke is a leading cause of death, with reperfusion treatments constantly being investigated and updated [25]. As the medical field develops a better understanding of acute ischemic strokes and technological advances, evolution of treatment protocols follows. The standard of care for treatment has been the administration of IV thrombolysis using tissue plasminogen activator (tPA/alteplase). However, tPA has a short therapeutic window of 4.5 hours. Research into alternative treatments with a longer therapeutic window has continually been on the radar to improve the current standard of care; one such therapy is a device used for endovascular retrieval of clots [25].

History of Clot Retrieval Protocols

The use of mechanical devices to retrieve clots carries a reduced risk of intracranial hemorrhage as well as a longer therapeutic window [25]. However, these treatment options also carry the risk of trauma to the vasculature due to technical difficulty. The Mechanical Embolus Removal in Cerebral Ischemia (MERCI) trial in 2004 conducted across multiple sites in the United States was the first to evaluate a mechanical device in a randomized clinical trial [26]. The device was spring-like and could be used together with a balloon-guided catheter or microcatheter. Continued testing of the device led to improved safety and outcomes [27]. The next device was the Penumbra system, for which initial trials were published in 2008 [27]. This system used aspiration to remove clots and open vessels. A systematic review in 2008 conducted by Stead et al. evaluated a total of 298 patients over 23 studies [28]. They found that the clot was accessible in 86% of patients. Furthermore, using mechanical devices, a partial or complete recanalization of the vessel occurred in 73% of these patients. The next device to be trialed was a stent retriever, a self-expanding device deployed at the site of a blood clot to push it against vessel walls and re-establish blood flow. These stents then retrieve the clot to remove the thrombus. Overall, they showed recanalization rates up to 90%, higher than previously designed devices [25].

Despite these recanalization rates, clinical trials showed that endovascular mechanical retrieval devices were not superior to the standard care of IV thrombolysis. However, the American Heart Association's (AHA) 2013 guidelines recommended the use of endovascular revascularization within 6 hours as an option in patients with contraindications to IV thrombolysis (Table 20.4). Furthermore, they suggested that mechanical thrombectomy can be used in large-artery occlusions that have not responded to IV fibrinolysis [25].
The Multicenter Randomized Clinical Trial of Endovascular Treatment for Acute Ischemic Stroke in the Netherlands (MR CLEAN) trial conducted in the Netherlands was the first to show that mechanical thrombectomy should be used as first-line treatment for patients with anterior circulation strokes presenting within 6 hours [29]. This was then confirmed by the Extending the Time for Thrombolysis in Emergency Neurological Deficits – Intra-Arterial (EXTEND-IA) trial in 2015 [30]. Based on these trials, intra-arterial retrieval of clots is now increasingly used for patients presenting with ischemic stroke [29, 30].

Table 20.4 Absolute and relative contraindications of IV thrombolysis [31]

Absolute contraindications	Relative contraindications
Acute intracranial hemorrhage	Advanced age
History of intracranial hemorrhage	Mild or improving stroke symptoms
Severe uncontrolled hypertension	Severe stroke and coma
Serious head trauma or stroke in the last 3 months	Recent major surgery
	Arterial puncture of non-compressible vessel
Thrombocytopenia	Recent gastrointestinal or genitourinary hemorrhage
Coagulopathy	
Low molecular weight heparin	Seizure at onset
Direct thrombin inhibitors	Recent myocardial infarction
Factor Xa inhibitors	Central nervous system structural lesions
Severe hypoglycemia or hyperglycemia	Dementia
Early radiographic ischemic changes	

Effect of Clot Composition on Management

Following the results of the MR CLEAN and EXTEND-IA trials, mechanical thrombectomy became the treatment of choice for stroke patients. However, at this point, clot compositions were not readily considered in the decision-making of treatments. Thrombi consist of variable proportions of fibrin, platelets, red blood cells (RBCs), von Willebrand factor, and extracellular DNA [32]. As the thrombus forms over time, its composition and structure evolve. Some have suspected that changes in clot composition over time could affect the efficacy of mechanical thrombectomy. Thus, research into the composition and structure of clots may guide a more appropriate intervention.

In addition, a study done by Boeckh-Behrens et al. [33] found that a higher percentage of white blood cells was associated with higher recanalization times as well as less favorable recanalization and clinical outcomes [33]. They speculated that the number of white blood cells in a thrombus is an indication of the thrombus age. Increased age of a thrombus leads to greater stability and adherence to the vessel wall leading to increased difficulty of retrieval using mechanical thrombectomy.

A 2021 scoping review conducted by Jolugbo, Ariëns [32] investigated the impact of thrombus composition on the efficacy of mechanical thrombectomy and patient outcomes. The outcome of this review suggested fibrin-rich thrombi require more attempts with mechanical thrombectomy devices than RBC-rich thrombi [32]. This is suspected to be due to the increased stiffness and elasticity of a fibrin-rich clot [33–36] and a higher friction coefficient [37] compared to RBC-rich clots which are easily deformable [38].

Research in this area has impacted treatment choices in patients presenting with stroke. These discoveries led to an emerging area of research on techniques that can be used during endovascular clot retrieval based on clot composition [32]. The composition of a clot can also influence the long-term therapy of patients. For example, patients presenting with platelet-rich clots would likely benefit from antiplatelet therapy for the prevention of recurrent strokes [39].

Secondary Embolism

Mechanical thrombectomy carries a risk of fragmenting the thrombus during the procedure, which can lead to embolism at a downstream site [32]. Furthermore, it can result in incomplete recanalization. Therefore, research has been conducted in order to explore the best approach to decrease the risk of fragmentation.

It has been found that while fibrin-rich clots are difficult to retrieve using mechanical thrombectomy; they are less likely to fragment and result in secondary embolisms [40]. Multiple other studies have found that thrombi rich in RBCs are easier to fragment, and thus are more likely to cause secondary embolisms [41]. Techniques for reducing the risk of secondary embolisms include the following [40]:

- Addition of proximal balloon catheters to reduce anterograde blood flow
- Stent-retriever Assisted Vacuum-Locked Extraction (SAVE) technique: stent partially retrieved during thrombectomy for the embolus to be removed as a whole

When mechanical thrombectomy is the treatment of choice in an acute ischemic stroke, the use of researched techniques has helped to improve patient outcomes.

Prediction of Clot Composition

It has been suggested that pre-intervention imaging could be used to identify clot composition, enabling clinicians to make treatment decisions prior to attempting mechanical thrombectomy [41]. Presently, imaging markers are being investigated for their correlation with clot composition along with the use of machine learning software for the prediction of clot composition. These advancements in technology can aid in the selection of devices for each clot allowing for personalized thrombectomy strategies. Fitzgerald et al. investigated the use of Orbit Image Analysis to identify the components of clots compared to the gold standard of H&E staining [39]. Orbit Image Analysis is a software that assists in the quantifying of tissue content using machine learning. This is a promising development as it helps to eliminate human variation and errors in analysis, including the lack of reproducibility of results. This research will aid in decision-making for the short- and long-term treatment and management of clots.

Robots: Can Research and Practice Keep Up with Medical Technology?

The constant development of new technology leads to continued developments for the application of robotics in medicine. It is an area with a great deal of potential and a wide range of applications including surgery, rehabilitation, assistive technologies, and cellular level alterations through the use of micro-/nanorobotics. The focus of this section will be on robotics in surgery.

Evolution of Robotic Surgery

The use of robotics in the surgical field has been rapidly developing and has been widely accepted as a new standard of care. Initially developed with the intention for use in the military, it was not until later that its application for healthcare became recognized.

Initial systems that were developed were highly procedure-specific, e.g., prostate surgery and assisted systems in neurosurgery. The first fully functional multipurpose surgical robot was developed in the late 1900s in the United States [42]. Initial prototypes and systems were developed using virtual reality (VR) and manipulators which transmitted surgeon movements to the robotic instruments. These systems were originally developed for open surgeries before being further improved for laparoscopic procedures. The result of trials on anatomical models, ex vivo and in vivo animal models revealed that using these robotic systems increased the time of open surgeries. However, they were beneficial in decreasing operation time in laparoscopic and microsurgical procedures [42].

Despite a drive to develop technologies for robotics in surgery, the initial models trialed in humans were short-lived. This was due to increasing surgery time in some cases, increased costs of surgeries, and inferior care outcomes. At that time, progression of robotic surgery was limited by the technology available in hospitals to support its use. However, as technology continued to advance, further developments and refinements created new software and hardware suitable to run robotics programs. This has led to the use of robotics in surgery becoming increasingly accepted and utilized. At present, it has had benefits for visceral surgery, urology, and colorectal and gynecological procedures [43].

The current barriers to the use of robotic surgery includes the cost and, in some cases, the longer operation time [43]. An outline of the barriers and benefits of robotic surgery is presented in Table 20.5. The use of robotics in procedures comes with a learning curve for surgeons which varies between procedures, pathologies, and anatomical sites [44]. Further, this learning curve extends to anesthetists due to the differences of robotic surgery compared to traditional surgery.

Changes to Perioperative Care

Surgical interventions are often associated with perioperative complications that affect the care of patients post-surgery as well as their long-term prognosis [45]. Common complications of surgeries include risk of infections, cardiovascular and cerebrovascular events, deep vein thrombosis and/or pulmonary embolisms, and intensive care unit (ICU) admissions. These complications occur to varying degrees depending on the classification of the surgery as low, intermediate, or high risk. The development of technology and implementation of robotics in surgery not only come with changes within the operating theatre but also the care of patients perioperatively.

Table 20.5 Summary of the advantages, disadvantages, limitations, and barriers of robotic surgery

Advantages	Disadvantages	Limitations	Barriers
Shorter surgery times in some cases Decreased post-operative complications Potential for telesurgery	Higher costs Longer surgery times in some cases	Lack of standard operating protocols Lack of training programs specific to robotic surgeries Difficult acquiring equipment Development of a global network needed in order to establish connections between countries for collaborations of tele-surgeries Billing and funding issues Legal issues: crossing state and country borders	Cost of surgery Longer surgery times in some cases Learning curve of clinicians

Overall, research has indicated that robot-assisted procedures are associated with decreased rates of complications [42, 44, 46–48]. As with traditional surgeries, these rates vary depending on the procedure. In the majority of instances, patients who underwent robot-assisted surgeries had a decreased length of stay in the hospital compared to patients who underwent open or laparoscopic surgery. Loss of blood is one of the most common complications of surgery, potentially leading to a need for blood transfusions [46]. Robotic surgeries decrease the amount of blood loss that patients experience, thus reducing the need for blood transfusions. In addition, robot-assisted surgeries have been shown to have lower pain scores, fewer wound complications, and lower infection rates. The reduced rates of these complications lead to a decrease in the use of hospital resources and the patient's length of stay in the hospital [46]. The reduction in complications is associated with reduced systemic inflammatory and metabolic insult [44]. In robot-assisted prostatectomies, it has been found that patients need less help with hygiene and mobility following the procedure, as well as a shorter catheterization time [48].

The move toward robot-assisted surgeries changes the role of healthcare professionals during perioperative care. As the technology utilized in surgery continues to evolve, so will the care of patients perioperatively.

Future Applications

The future of robotic surgery is dependent on five core dimensions [44]:

1. *Technology*: application of advances in technology
2. *Evidence*: increasing evidence for the best robotic platforms
3. *Cost*: cost-effectiveness for individuals, institutions, and governments
4. *Awareness*: increased societal and patient awareness of robotic surgery
5. *Training*: new training for all healthcare professionals involved in robotic surgeries including surgeons, anesthetists, nurses, and allied health

Future directions of robotic surgery include allowing surgeons to have higher interface with robots through the development of new tools and integration with artificial intelligence [43]. One specific area of robotic surgery that has potential is the ability for surgeons to conduct telesurgery. Telesurgery is the utilization of wireless networking and robotic technology to undertake operations from a remote location [49]. This allows operations to be conducted despite geographical barriers and allows surgical collaborations between surgeons in multiple locations.

However, an issue in the development of telesurgery is latency time. This is the time delay that occurs when transferring auditory, visual, and tactile feedback from one location to another [49]. This could lead to longer operation times and more importantly, inaccuracy during a procedure – a concern for patient safety and recovery. This can be especially difficult if emergencies occur during surgery [50] as a sudden change in procedural approach may be required, e.g., the need for additional supplies. There may also be network delays adding additional layers to the complexities of emergency situations. Nevertheless, as internet speeds increase and technology advances, these complications will become less of an obstacle.

Research in the field of robotics thus provides advantages not just intraoperatively but also perioperatively. As medicine evolves with technology, research has provided a vehicle for bench science to be translated into safe, effective, and patient-centered clinical care. However, as there are still limitations to current evidence, research scientists will have to continue to configure the vast field of medicine.

Key Points
- It is essential for physicians to be familiar with research in order to ensure that patient care is rooted in the practice of "evidence-based medicine."
- Quality-of-care domains are useful as points of reference to confirm that patient care is optimal.
- Pre-test probability provides researched-backed evidence for improved practice. Thus, these algorithms should be followed when available.
- Knowing the approval pathways for pharmacological use is invaluable for risk-benefit analysis of a treatment.
- Research is an ongoing process; thus, hospital practice should also change based on ongoing research evidence.
- Translational research from bench to bedside is useful in taking pathophysiology – such as that of clot composition – to help guide practice and management of patients who present with differing risk factors for the same medical condition (e.g., stroke).
- Technology can outpace medical practice. However, utilizing and keeping up with what is available has immense benefits as shown through robotic surgery.

Research in medicine will continue to discover new evidence or re-examine old practices that will influence how physicians care for patients.

References

1. Oppel L. Allopathy – a term that diminishes the profession. B C Med J. 2010;52:91.
2. Montori VM, Guyatt GH. Progress in evidence-based medicine. JAMA. 2008;300(15):1814–6. https://doi.org/10.1001/jama.300.15.1814.
3. Institute of Medicine Committee on Quality of Health Care in A. In: Crossing the quality chasm: a new health system for the 21st century. Washington (DC): National Academies Press (US) Copyright 2001 by the National Academy of Sciences. All rights reserved; 2001. https://doi.org/10.17226/10027.
4. Smith-Bindman R. Use of advanced imaging tests and the not-so-incidental harms of incidental findings. JAMA Intern Med. 2017;178(2):227–8. https://doi.org/10.1001/jamainternmed.2017.7557.
5. Carson JL, Kelley MA, Duff A, Weg JG, Fulkerson WJ, Palevsky HI, Schwartz JS, Thompson BT, Popovich J, Hobbins TE, Spera MA, Alavi A, Terrin ML. The clinical course of pulmonary embolism. N Engl J Med. 1992;326(19):1240–5. https://doi.org/10.1056/NEJM199205073261902.
6. Kline JA, Webb WB, Jones AE, Hernandez-Nino J. Impact of a rapid rule-out protocol for pulmonary embolism on the rate of screening, missed cases, and pulmonary vascular imaging in an urban US emergency department. Ann Emerg Med. 2004;44(5):490–502. https://doi.org/10.1016/j.annemergmed.2004.03.018.
7. Wells PS, Anderson DR, Rodger M, Ginsberg JS, Kearon C, Gent M, Turpie AG, Bormanis J, Weitz J, Chamberlain M, Bowie D, Barnes D, Hirsh J. Derivation of a simple clinical model to categorize patients probability of pulmonary embolism: increasing the models utility with the SimpliRED D-dimer. Thromb Haemost. 2000;83(3):416–20.
8. Raja AS, Greenberg JO, Qaseem A, Denberg TD, Fitterman N, Schuur JD. Evaluation of patients with suspected acute pulmonary embolism: best practice advice from the Clinical Guidelines Committee of the American College of Physicians. Ann Intern Med. 2015;163(9):701–11. https://doi.org/10.7326/M14-1772.
9. Penaloza A, Melot C, Motte S. Comparison of the Wells score with the simplified revised Geneva score for assessing pretest probability of pulmonary embolism. Thromb Res. 2010;127(2):81–4. https://doi.org/10.1016/j.thromres.2010.10.026.
10. Penaloza A, Soulié C, Moumneh T, Delmez Q, Ghuysen A, El Kouri D, Brice C, Marjanovic NS, Bouget J, Moustafa F, Trinh-Duc A, Le Gall C, Imsaad L, Chrétien J-M, Gable B, Girard P, Sanchez O, Schmidt J, Le Gal G, Meyer G, Delvau N, Roy P-M. Pulmonary embolism rule-out criteria (PERC) rule in European patients with low implicit clinical probability (PERCEPIC): a multicentre, prospective, observational study. Lancet Haematol. 2017;4(12):e615–21. https://doi.org/10.1016/S2352-3026(17)30210-7.
11. Douma RA, Mos ICM, Erkens PMG, Nizet TAC, Durian MF, Hovens MM, van Houten AA, Hofstee HMA, Klok FA, ten Cate H, Ullmann EF, Büller HR, Kamphuisen PW, Huisman MV. Performance of 4 clinical decision rules in the diagnostic management of acute pulmonary embolism: a prospective cohort study. Ann Intern Med. 2011;154(11):709–18. https://doi.org/10.7326/0003-4819-154-11-201106070-00002.
12. Gillon R. Correction: defending the four principles approach as a good basis for good medical practice and therefore for good medical ethics. J Med Ethics. 2015;41(10):829. https://doi.org/10.1136/medethics-2015-102811corr1.
13. Lipsky MS, Sharp LK. From idea to market: the drug approval process. J Am Board Fam Pract. 2001;14(5):362–7.
14. Kao LW, Kirk MA, Evers SJ, Rosenfeld SH. Droperidol, QT prolongation, and sudden death: what is the evidence? Ann Emerg Med. 2003;41(4):546–58. https://doi.org/10.1067/mem.2003.110.
15. Gaw CM, Cabrera D, Bellolio F, Mattson AE, Lohse CM, Jeffery MM. Effectiveness and safety of droperidol in a United States emergency department. Am J Emerg Med. 2020;38(7):1310–4. https://doi.org/10.1016/j.ajem.2019.09.007.

16. Hirayama T, Ishii F, Yago K, Ogata H. Evaluation of the effective drugs for the prevention of nausea and vomiting induced by morphine used for postoperative pain: a quantitative systematic review. Yakugaku Zasshi. 2001;121(2):179–85. https://doi.org/10.1248/yakushi.121.179.
17. Henzi I, Sonderegger J, Tramèr MR. Efficacy, dose-response, and adverse effects of droperidol for prevention of postoperative nausea and vomiting. Can J Anaesth. 2000;47(6):537–51. https://doi.org/10.1007/BF03018945.
18. Hameer O, Collin K, Ensom MHH, Lomax S. Evaluation of droperidol in the acutely agitated child or adolescent. Can J Psychiatr. 2001;46(9):864–5. https://doi.org/10.1177/070674370104600922.
19. Eberhart LHJ, Morin AM, Bothner U, Georgieff M. Droperidol and 5-HT3-receptor antagonists, alone or in combination, for prophylaxis of postoperative nausea and vomiting. Acta Anaesthesiol Scand. 2000;44(10):1252–7. https://doi.org/10.1034/j.1399-6576.2000.441011.x.
20. Calver L, Page CBM, Downes MAM, Chan BMP, Kinnear FM, Wheatley LM, Spain DM, Isbister GKMDB. The safety and effectiveness of droperidol for sedation of acute behavioral disturbance in the emergency department. Ann Emerg Med. 2015;66(3):230–238.e231. https://doi.org/10.1016/j.annemergmed.2015.03.016.
21. Boyer E. Droperidol is back (and here's what you need to know). ACEP Now. 2019.
22. Perkins JMD, Ho JDMD, Vilke GMMD, DeMers GDODMPH. American Academy of Emergency Medicine Position statement: safety of droperidol use in the emergency department. J Emerg Med. 2015;49(1):91–7. https://doi.org/10.1016/j.jemermed.2014.12.024.
23. Taylor DMMDMPH, Yap CYLM, Knott JCMP, Taylor SEP, Phillips GAM, Karro JM, Chan EWBP, Kong DCMBP, Castle DJMD. Midazolam-droperidol, droperidol, or olanzapine for acute agitation: a randomized clinical trial. Ann Emerg Med. 2016;69(3):318–326.e311. https://doi.org/10.1016/j.annemergmed.2016.07.033.
24. Thomas MC, Musselman ME, Shewmaker J. Droperidol for the treatment of acute migraine headaches. Ann Pharmacother. 2015;49(2):233–40. https://doi.org/10.1177/1060028014554445.
25. Dorado L, Millan M, Davalos A. Reperfusion therapies for acute ischemic stroke: an update. Curr Cardiol Rev. 2014;10(4):327–35. https://doi.org/10.2174/1573403X10666140320144637.
26. Gobin YP, Starkman S, Duckwiler GR, Grobelny T, Kidwell CS, Jahan R, Pile-Spellman J, Segal A, Vinuela F, Saver JL. MERCI 1: a phase 1 study of mechanical embolus removal in cerebral ischemia. Stroke. 2004;35(12):2848–54. https://doi.org/10.1161/01.Str.0000147718.12954.60.
27. Bose A, Henkes H, Alfke K, Reith W, Mayer TE, Berlis A, Branca V, Sit SP. The Penumbra system: a mechanical device for the treatment of acute stroke due to thromboembolism. AJNR Am J Neuroradiol. 2008;29(7):1409–13. https://doi.org/10.3174/ajnr.A1110.
28. Stead LG, Gilmore RM, Bellolio MF, Rabinstein AA, Decker WW. Percutaneous clot removal devices in acute ischemic stroke: a systematic review and meta-analysis. Arch Neurol. 2008;65(8):1024–30. https://doi.org/10.1001/archneur.65.8.1024.
29. Berkhemer OA, Fransen PS, Beumer D, van den Berg LA, Lingsma HF, Yoo AJ, Schonewille WJ, Vos JA, Nederkoorn PJ, Wermer MJ, van Walderveen MA, Staals J, Hofmeijer J, van Oostayen JA, Lycklama à Nijeholt GJ, Boiten J, Brouwer PA, Emmer BJ, de Bruijn SF, van Dijk LC, Kappelle LJ, Lo RH, van Dijk EJ, de Vries J, de Kort PL, van Rooij WJ, van den Berg JS, van Hasselt BA, Aerden LA, Dallinga RJ, Visser MC, Bot JC, Vroomen PC, Eshghi O, Schreuder TH, Heijboer RJ, Keizer K, Tielbeek AV, den Hertog HM, Gerrits DG, van den Berg-Vos RM, Karas GB, Steyerberg EW, Flach HZ, Marquering HA, Sprengers ME, Jenniskens SF, Beenen LF, van den Berg R, Koudstaal PJ, van Zwam WH, Roos YB, van der Lugt A, van Oostenbrugge RJ, Majoie CB, Dippel DW. A randomized trial of intraarterial treatment for acute ischemic stroke. N Engl J Med. 2015;372(1):11–20. https://doi.org/10.1056/NEJMoa1411587.
30. Campbell BCV, Mitchell PJ, Kleinig TJ, Dewey HM, Churilov L, Yassi N, Yan B, Dowling RJ, Parsons MW, Oxley TJ, Wu TY, Brooks M, Simpson MA, Miteff F, Levi CR, Krause

M, Harrington TJ, Faulder KC, Steinfort BS, Priglinger M, Ang T, Scroop R, Barber PA, McGuinness B, Wijeratne T, Phan TG, Chong W, Chandra RV, Bladin CF, Badve M, Rice H, de Villiers L, Ma H, Desmond PM, Donnan GA, Davis SM. Endovascular therapy for ischemic stroke with perfusion-imaging selection. N Engl J Med. 2015;372(11):1009–18. https://doi.org/10.1056/NEJMoa1414792.
31. Fugate JE, Rabinstein AA. Absolute and relative contraindications to IV rt-PA for acute ischemic stroke. Neurohospitalist. 2015;5(3):110–21. https://doi.org/10.1177/1941874415578532.
32. Jolugbo P, Ariëns RAS. Thrombus composition and efficacy of thrombolysis and thrombectomy in acute ischemic stroke. Stroke. 2021;52(3):1131–42. https://doi.org/10.1161/STROKEAHA.120.032810.
33. Boeckh-Behrens T, Schubert M, Förschler A, Prothmann S, Kreiser K, Zimmer C, Riegger J, Bauer J, Neff F, Kehl V, Pelisek J, Schirmer L, Mehr M, Poppert H. The impact of histological clot composition in embolic stroke. Clin Neuroradiol. 2016;26(2):189–97. https://doi.org/10.1007/s00062-014-0347-x.
34. Yuki I, Kan I, Vinters HV, Kim RH, Golshan A, Vinuela FA, Sayre JW, Murayama Y, Vinuela F. The impact of thromboemboli histology on the performance of a mechanical thrombectomy device. AJNR Am J Neuroradiol. 2012;33(4):643–8. https://doi.org/10.3174/ajnr.A2842.
35. Chueh JY, Wakhloo AK, Hendricks GH, Silva CF, Weaver JP, Gounis MJ. Mechanical characterization of thromboemboli in acute ischemic stroke and laboratory embolus analogs. AJNR Am J Neuroradiol. 2011;32(7):1237–44. https://doi.org/10.3174/ajnr.A2485.
36. Kaesmacher XJ, Boeckh-Behrens T, Simon S, Maegerlein C, Kleine JF, Zimmer C, Schirmer L, Poppert H, Huber T. Risk of thrombus fragmentation during endovascular stroke treatment. AJNR Am J Neuroradiol. 2017;38(5):991–8. https://doi.org/10.3174/ajnr.A5105.
37. Gunning GM, McArdle K, Mirza M, Duffy S, Gilvarry M, Brouwer PA. Clot friction variation with fibrin content; implications for resistance to thrombectomy. J Neurointerv Surg. 2018;10(1):34–8. https://doi.org/10.1136/neurintsurg-2016-012721.
38. Sporns Peter B, Hanning U, Schwindt W, Velasco A, Buerke B, Cnyrim C, Minnerup J, Heindel W, Jeibmann A, Niederstadt T. Ischemic stroke: histological thrombus composition and pre-interventional CT attenuation are associated with intervention time and rate of secondary embolism. Cerebrovasc Dis. 2017;44(5–6):344–50. https://doi.org/10.1159/000481578.
39. Fitzgerald S, Wang S, Dai D, Murphree DH, Pandit A, Douglas A, Rizvi A, Kadirvel R, Gilvarry M, McCarthy R, Stritt M, Gounis MJ, Brinjikji W, Kallmes DF, Doyle KM. Orbit image analysis machine learning software can be used for the histological quantification of acute ischemic stroke blood clots. PLoS One. 2019;14(12):e0225841. https://doi.org/10.1371/journal.pone.0225841.
40. Sporns PB, Jeibmann A, Minnerup J, Broocks G, Nawabi J, Schön G, Fiehler J, Wildgruber M, Heindel W, Kemmling A, Hanning U. Histological clot composition is associated with preinterventional clot migration in acute stroke patients. Stroke. 2019;50(8):2065–71. https://doi.org/10.1161/STROKEAHA.118.023314.
41. Ye G, Qi P, Chen K, Tan T, Cao R, Chen J, Lu J, Wang D. Risk of secondary embolism events during mechanical thrombectomy for acute ischemic stroke: a single-center study based on histological analysis. Clin Neurol Neurosurg. 2020;193:105749. https://doi.org/10.1016/j.clineuro.2020.105749.
42. George EI, Brand TC, LaPorta A, Marescaux J, Satava RM. Origins of robotic surgery: from skepticism to standard of care. JSLS. 2018;22(4):e2018.00039. https://doi.org/10.4293/JSLS.2018.00039.
43. Morrell ALG, Morrell-Junior AC, Morrell AG, Mendes JMF, Tustumi F, DE-Oliveira-E-Silva LG, Morrell A. The history of robotic surgery and its evolution: when illusion becomes reality. Rev Col Bras Cir. 2021;48:e20202798. https://doi.org/10.1590/0100-6991e-20202798.
44. Ashrafian H, Clancy O, Grover V, Darzi A. The evolution of robotic surgery: surgical and anaesthetic aspects. Br J Anaesth. 2017;119(Suppl_1):i72–84. https://doi.org/10.1093/bja/aex383.

45. Tjeertes EKM, Ultee KHJ, Stolker RJ, Verhagen HJM, Bastos Gonçalves FM, Hoofwijk AGM, Hoeks SE. Perioperative complications are associated with adverse long-term prognosis and affect the cause of death after general surgery. World J Surg. 2016;40(11):2581–90. https://doi.org/10.1007/s00268-016-3600-4.
46. Schulster ML, Sidhom DA, Sturgeon K, Borin JF, Bjurlin MA. Outcomes and peri-operative complications of robotic pyelolithotomy. J Robot Surg. 2020;14(3):401–7. https://doi.org/10.1007/s11701-019-01004-2.
47. Stewart C, Wong P, Warner S, Raoof M, Singh G, Fong Y, Melstrom L. Robotic minor hepatectomy: optimizing outcomes and cost of care. HPB (Oxford). 2020. https://doi.org/10.1016/j.hpb.2020.09.005.
48. Uvin P, de Meyer JM, Van Holderbeke G. A comparison of the peri-operative data after open radical retropubic prostatectomy or robotic-assisted laparoscopic prostatectomy. Acta Chir Belg. 2010;110(3):313–6. https://doi.org/10.1080/00015458.2010.11680623.
49. Choi PJ, Oskouian RJ, Tubbs RS. Telesurgery: past, present, and future. Cureus. 2018;10(5):e2716. https://doi.org/10.7759/cureus.2716.
50. Xia SB, Lu QS. Development status of telesurgery robotic system. Chin J Traumatol. 2021. https://doi.org/10.1016/j.cjtee.2021.03.001.

Chapter 21
Sustainability and Healthcare: Expanding the Scope of "Do No Harm" Models of Success

Kevin Conrad and Margaret Conrad

The dictum of "primum non nocere" has been the cornerstone of medical ethics for a millennia [1]. Each generation views it in a different light, often guided by the circumstances of the times. At some point, most healthcare providers find themselves asking what encompasses harm and how will that translate to their responsibility as an individual practitioner and at the institutions where they work. While it is obvious that first do no harm applies to clinical practice, which we as providers have some control over, it also can apply to behavior and the unintended consequences of providing healthcare.

A growing concern is how the energy-intensive practice of modern medicine is impacting the environment and how we as providers are accountable for that impact. Climate change and the delivery of healthcare are no longer separate issues. A possible relationship between the two is no longer abstract. The environmental impact of practicing medicine is measurable.

In addition, what is our responsibility to promote sustainable practices among all industries that potentially lowers the risk of environmentally induced disease. Now more than ever, it has become obvious that the changing environment is having a direct and increasing impact on our health.

Our first priority should be to determine and mitigate our own impact on the environment. Hospitals operate 24 hours per day, 7 days a week. Much of its operation is energy intensive and require carbon fuel as to run critical systems. The World's Healthcare systems produce as much CO_2 as the seventh largest country.

K. Conrad (✉)
Ochsner Health, New Orleans, LA, USA
e-mail: kconrad@ochsner.org

M. Conrad
Louisiana State University School of Medicine, New Orleans, LA, USA

© The Author(s), under exclusive license to Springer Nature Switzerland AG 2022
K. Conrad (ed.), *Clinical Approaches to Hospital Medicine*,
https://doi.org/10.1007/978-3-030-95164-1_21

It is understandable that a generation of healthcare providers, raised in the context of severe climate change warnings and events, would be eager to incorporate sustainability not only in their personal lives but into their practices as well.

"Sustainable healthcare" refers to the goal of providing high quality care while having minimal or no environmental impact. This goal is achieved primarily through decreasing energy use reducing various types of waste and procuring clean energy. This includes all of the many downstream aspects of healthcare such as transportation, food production, and waste disposal. Healthcare is reliant upon a large and diverse infrastructure. Sustainable healthcare also considers healthcare's facilities immediate impact on the local community, such as in its impact on local air quality.

The medical industry and its support systems in the United States are responsible for approximately 10% of the world's carbon emissions [2]. In addition, a significant amount of local air pollution, primarily due to transportation can be attributed to healthcare operations. While many industries, such as the automotive, have made great strides in transitioning to sustainable practices, healthcare has ironically lagged behind. Market forces have not particularly pushed healthcare in that direction.

The most obvious hurdle to converting hospital systems to a sustainable framework is the initial financial cost, and making the argument that it is a cost-effective endeavor. There is an increasing body of literature that demonstrates this.

Guidelines for sustainable healthcare are just beginning to emerge. The World Health Organization has set parameters for creating healthcare systems that are environmentally sustainable while ensuring greater affordability [3]. The areas defined for interventions include workforce development, water use, sanitation, hygiene, waste management, sustainable energy, infrastructure, technology, and product procurement [3]. This document serves as one of the first to provide a major overview of the issues by an international organization. It sets out to define the healthcare industry's impact on the environment and gives advice on how to achieve remediation in each area.

At times, the healthcare industry has been slow to change and driven by custom and tradition. For this reason, sustainable healthcare is searching for inspirational solutions to foster a new way for health systems to operate. The new mantra of healthcare, one that does transform the traditional delivery of healthcare, is to meet the patient's needs where they live work and play. Addressing sustainability is key to this concept.

It is easy to point out concerns regarding sustainability in a medical setting, but it is hard to discover solutions that can be easily implemented with rapidly definable metrics. The road forward will require extensive research and an honest evaluation of our efforts, but the preliminary results are already promising. For example, investing in sustainable upgrades to a single operating room can save up to $56,000 annually [4]. Startup costs can be extensive, but this one example demonstrates that the financial best interest of the healthcare industry can be to move toward sustainability, even in short term.

As in other industries, sustainable initiatives have financial benefits in the long run due to decreasing energy, reducing waste, and minimizing transportation costs.

An obvious added component is the goodwill that is generated among patients and employs with these initiatives. Much of this can be translated into improved patient satisfaction and enhanced employee retention. Increasingly, employees have the expectation of a workplace that support sustainability. In a time of increasing climate change-related weather events, this can be reassuring.

In the United States, many hospital systems are taking formal steps toward increasing sustainability. Some have fully employed sustainability directors that report directly to the CEO. This position has become the norm for most other industries, and it is being seen in many of the major healthcare systems. The following are three examples of efforts of various sizes that have formalized their sustainability efforts.

Kaiser Permanente: An Innovator of Sustainability Efforts in the Healthcare Industry

The United States's largest integrated healthcare system, Kaiser Permanente, has made significant strides toward sustainable healthcare. They are often viewed as the pioneer and leaders is this field, with a long history of innovation. Starting with limited goals, employees in 1970 at Kaiser Permanente Santa Clara Medical Center created an "Ecology Committee" to teach other employees about common ecology [5].

Kaiser Permanente has not only utilized but has invested in solar energy projects and infrastructure. It has a long history as one of the first adopters of solar energy on a large scale. In 1977, Kaiser Permanente Redwood City Medical Center began using solar energy for water heating. At the time, this was one of the first and largest solar projects at a US medical facility. Solar power was expanded in 1980 at Kaiser Permanente with the development of a solar thermal project in Silicon Valley at Santa Clara Medical Center [5]. Since that time, solar utilization has continued its expansion.

Hospitals require large amounts of produce and are one of the major purchasers in a given region. Many sustainability goals can be achieved by local sourcing. Kaiser Permanente Oakland Medical Center began the first farmers market at a United States hospital. This initiative has spread to over 50 farmers markets at hospitals associated with Kaiser Permanente [5].

In addition to developing sustainable energy sources, in 2010, Kaiser Permanente began evaluating all suppliers' environmental impact. This involves a scorecard that provides information on supplier's use of harmful chemicals and recycling policies. The goal of this endeavor is both to analyze the environmental impact of items purchased and to encourage suppliers to utilize more environmentally friendly ways of creating and sourcing products [5]. These initiatives all are developed with short-term achievable metrics.

More recently, Kaiser Permanente has set more aggressive goals and long-term initiatives. In 2010, Kaiser Permanente committed to reducing greenhouse gas emissions 30% by 2020. This goal was based off of the emissions recorded in 2008 [5]. A large step toward this goal involved investing in the construction and operation of wind and solar energy farms. By investing in these renewable energy projects, Kaiser Permanente generated 590 million kilowatt hours of power in a year. This is equivalent to the electricity used by 82,000 average American homes in a year.

Another major goal was set in 2016 when Kaiser announced it would be carbon neutral by 2020 [5]. This involved a more aggressive effort in investing in clean energy projects to reduce greenhouse gas usage, committing to recycling, reusing, and composting all non-hazardous waste, and acquiring all food from local farmers. The success of these initiatives shows the potential for a hospital institution to enact large-scale change. Kaiser's success demonstrates the abilities of healthcare systems not only achieve sustainability but to drive the green industry as a whole.

Kaiser Permanente has been officially recognized multiple times for their environmental endeavors. In San Diego, Kaiser Permanente opened the first LEED Platinum certified hospital [5]. This hospital produces its own electricity, cooling, and heating. The design reduces water usage and overall energy consumption. By 2020, 40 Kaiser Permanente building were LEED certified. The EPA awarded Kaiser Permanente the Green power Leadership Award in 2019 for their use of renewable energy. Kaiser Permanente achieved their goal of being the first carbon-neutral hospital system in the United States in 2020. Their work toward sustainability has been recognized on a national scale. Since 2002, Kaiser Permanente has received over 300 awards from the organization Practice Greenhealth for their environmental achievements.

Future goals remain ambitious as well. Having achieved success in their previous environmental initiatives, Kaiser is looking to the future to improve their facilities. By 2025, Kaiser Permanente plans to become carbon net positive, purchase all food locally, recycle 100% of non-hazardous waste, reduce water use by 25%, and collaborate with local organizations to reduce environmental impact on local communities [6]. The motivation behind this initiative stems from a concern for the rising impact of the environment on health and the disproportionate effects of climate change on marginalized communities. There is also a financial incentive to transition toward sustainability. Compared to their usage and cost of water and energy in 2013, Kaiser Permanente annually saves an estimated $19.6 million on energy and $2.8 million on water usage. The state of California has encouraged industries to become more sustainable and certainly much of its workforce has set that as an expectation for employment, but Kaiser has exceeded that expectation. Kaiser Permanente is the prime example of how a large hospital system with the urging of its workforce and cooperation of its administration can achieve sustainability, financial benefit, and an improved local environment.

Kaiser has a well-developed infrastructure to promote its sustainability operations. It has created and empowered the position of chief environmental officer. This position goes beyond sustainability issues, to examine healthcare's overall interaction and influence with the environment: a concept that is increasingly being recognized as essential to the future of healthcare.

Boston Green Ribbon Healthcare Working Group: Cooperation and Competition Among Healthcare Systems

In contrast to the example of Kaiser Permanente, which is one hospital system, the Boston Green Ribbon Healthcare Working Group unites multiple hospitals in a mutual goal of pursuing sustainability. This group is part of Boston Green Ribbon Commission which is composed of business, institutional, and civic leaders in the city of Boston, MA, working in coordination with the City's Climate Action Plan to fight climate change and achieve city-wide carbon neutrality by 2050 [7]. By working with a variety of hospitals in Boston, they have reduced greenhouse gas emission by 33% in 2020. An impressive goal as the average US hospital has increased emissions by 1.5% yearly [7]. This was achieved through smaller changes made in coordination with the individual hospitals as well as by purchasing renewable energy options. This achievement came with corresponding financial savings. This initiative benefitted from close ties to the city government which controlled and regulated much of the energy industry. No one system in Boston is as large as Kaiser and thus does not have the ability to develop large-scale energy projects on its own. Also eliminated was much of the competition and individual bargaining for energy resources among healthcare systems.

These goals were achieved predominantly by initiatives and limited beneficial competition among individual hospitals, which often set goals that could be rewarded. For example, Beth Israel Deaconess Medical Center was converted to energy-efficient labs which lowered greenhouse gas emissions by 38% in one building. This achievement earned the medical center an award that funded an energy-efficient freezer program [7]. Area hospitals often utilized the expertise and enthusiasm of local academic institutions. Boston Medical Center constructed a 60-megawatt solar farm with MIT in North Carolina. By purchasing 26% of the power, Boston Medical Center moved to carbon neutrality in 2020 [7]. Similarly, by 2018, 80% of Partners HealthCare's energy came from zero-emission generators and the entire facility will be carbon positive by 2025.

In addition to reducing the environmental impact of hospitals, the Healthcare Working Group aims to assess current environmental threats and help hospitals prepare for a potential environmentally driven crisis [7]. This was achieved through an assessment of the impact of an environmental crisis would have on healthcare with an emphasis on unexpected conditions arising from climate change. The goal of this assessment was to define areas of need to ensure socially equitable improvements to community health [7]. This initiative represents the potential of sustainable medicine to support community health in high-risk areas. Another part of this goal is to prepare the infrastructure of hospitals for potential environmental catastrophes such as storms, heavy wind, and storm surge. The waterfront Spaulding Rehabilitation Hospital, part of Partners HealthCare, was designed with this in mind. The rehabilitation gardens double as storm surge barriers protect the raised ground floor. Additionally, mechanical and power systems are placed on rooftops to protect against potential flooding. Functional windows allow for ventilation and storm surge water is captured and reused [7]. Not only do these initiatives reduce waste, but they ensure the facility will be functional in the event of a large storm.

While most of these initiatives have long-term energy savings, start-up costs were considerable. Boston's Newton-Wellesley Hospital spent $50 million for a mechanical, electrical, and plumbing upgrade that included cooling towers and automated building controls. This reduced electric consumption by 44%, reduced demand by 51%, and reduced natural gas consumption by 40% [7]. Much of this expenditure was justified to administration by having the technical support of the Green Ribbon Commission Healthcare Working Group. The group also connected hospitals with unique funding options. This collaboration of hospitals has proven to be a great success. Many of the issues of sustainability require the coordination of many civil and private entities. This along with some friendly competition has been the path forward in Boston.

Cleveland Clinic

Kaiser Permanente operates in many different cities in California and neighboring states. The Boston Green Ribbon Healthcare Working Group guides potentially all of Boston's hospital systems. In contrast, the Cleveland Clinic provides an example of how a single system, albeit large, can make sustainability an essential part of their mission.

The Cleveland Clinic's Office for a Healthy Environment stated its focus is on limiting the impact of climate change and its corresponding effects on human health [8]. Their green initiatives focus on four categories: buildings, operations, buying, and involvement.

The design of Cleveland Clinic Buildings is influenced by the United States Green Building Council's Leadership in Energy and Environmental Design (LEED) system. Thirteen of Cleveland Clinic's projects have been LEED certified, and all new major construction projects aim for certification as a minimum and silver certification as a larger goal [8]. Additionally, the "Operations" aspect of their environmental initiative aims to combat sustainability issues related to waste, transportation, energy, food, toxics, climate, and water. By working with supply chains, Cleveland Clinic hospital's landfill diversion rate was above 30% in 2010 [8]. Much of the landfill diversion comes from changes made in their operating room. Cleveland Clinic has standardized their operating room recycling program and offers it to hospitals across the nation. Unable to find an existing way to recycle operating room waste, Cleveland Clinic found a market for recycling operating room packaging and connected their waste hauler to this market in a way that ensured safety from contamination. To combat waste from transportation, Cleveland Clinic has invested in alternative fuel vehicles and instituted a "No Idle Zone" in their parking areas.

They have also addressed the significant carbon footprint of employee transportation. They offer a carpooling match program for employees with preferred parking for carpoolers and discounted parking for low-emission vehicles. They have also addressed small issues where they can be found, for example, switching from a badge swipe to an automated sensor in parking.

Direct energy consumption use accounted for 80% of Cleveland Clinic's carbon emissions in 2008 [8]. They were instrumental in the development of Ohio Cooperative Solar, now called Evergreen Energy Solutions, by investing in solar panels in 2010 that provided 9% of their Main Campus hospital energy needs: an example of how healthcare can drive green industry.

To reduce waste from food production, Cleveland Clinic utilizes farmers markets and hospital kitchen gardens and aims to procure food within 200 miles of Cleveland. This involves working with local farmers and is celebrated with a mark on the food signs in the cafeteria indicating how far the food travelled. To reduce toxicity exposure and make environmentally friendly changes, Cleveland Clinic uses Green Seal-certified cleaning products, maintains a mercury-free environment, and reduces plastic to food.

Practice Greenhealth

A study by the *Commonwealth Fund* found that despite the initial cost of moving toward sustainable initiatives, healthcare institutions through green initiatives could save up to $5.4 billion in 5 years and $15 billion in 10 years [9].

There is no one way for healthcare systems to move toward sustainability and different institutions will take different routes. One of the greatest challenges is quantifying sources of waste and finding scalable solutions that fits the financial resources of the institution. Some may pursue local solutions while others may go as far as investing in energy generation plants, such as solar and wind farms. Globally, there are several organizations of various sizes that can serve as guides for converting to sustainable healthcare.

In the United States, *Practice Greenhealth* provides the framework for health systems aiming to transition toward sustainability. They offer achievable goals and guidelines that can apply to institutions of any size and financial ability. *Practice Greenhealth* aims to work with hospital systems by disseminating solutions to the many challenges of greening the healthcare system while maintaining public health standards [10]. For example, through their Greening the Operating Room initiative, *Practice Greenhealth* will assess operating rooms, identify short-term and long-term sources of waste reduction, and provide a financial assessment of these changes. Operating rooms are a source of opportunity because a typical one consumes more energy per square foot than any other part of a hospital and can produce up to 33% of a facility's waste [4]. Cleveland Clinic and *Practice Greenhealth* have worked together to "green the OR" in Cleveland and have marketed this initiative to other hospitals.

On a global scale, the organization *Healthcare Without Harm* advocates for sustainable healthcare. A promotional video created by *Healthcare Without Harm* outlines the argument that it is hypocritical of a healthcare system to be the cause of the health issues that it aims to cure. Sustainable medicine is a form of preventative care and has the potential for a substantial impact on slowing or reversing climate change [11].

Conclusion

In our challenge to mitigate the effects climate change, time is limited. I believe the previous described efforts represent some of our best efforts so far and can serve as guide to jump start efforts. This statement by Dr. Dana Hanson, president of the World Medical Association summarizes the effects of climate change on the delivery of healthcare:

"Climate change represents an inevitable massive threat to global health that will likely eclipse the major pandemics as a leading cause of death in the 21st century." In the midst of the current suffering endured during the current pandemic, it is difficult to comprehend those consequences that climate change may bring.

The healthcare system is transitioning. It strives to provide care patients where they live, work, and play. A key component of this will be addressing our environmental impact on the communities we serve and that impact is measurable and considerable.

We are at an inflection point on our efforts to reduce carbon emissions and that is good. There is an almost a universal consensus that action is needed now. But time has become our enemy. According to the authors of the landmark report by the UN Intergovernmental Panel on Climate Change released in October of 2018, 10 years is what we have to reverse carbon emissions to prevent significant environmental-driven emergencies. The report states urgent and unprecedented changes are needed to limit temperature elevations 1.5C and 2C, as compared to the pre-industrial era. Exceeding a 2C elevation will lead to global adverse events at an unprecedented level [12].

I am optimistic and believe this will be the decade of action. If anything can be said positive about the current COVID-19 pandemic is that we have collectively come to realize how fragile our existence is. A new awareness has developed that better understands humankind's interaction with the environment. Our challenge is to convert this opportunity into action.

Carbon neutrality as demonstrated by Kaiser Permanente is achievable in the healthcare sector and should be our immediate goal. It can drive economic development locally by its implementation, and it can engage the community in environmental stewardship efforts to a level not yet seen. But time is of the essence, and worldwide leaders of these efforts are needed now. We have passed the time when our actions are concentrated on convincing stakeholders of the problems. We must transition to practical, meaningful, and rapidly developed solutions.

Healthcare is one of the few industries that has the economic size, the scientific background, community engagement, and perhaps most importantly the motivations to "first do no harm" that could lead a national if not a global transformation in environmental stewardship among all industries. It is our duty to be leaders in these efforts and make it one, if not our most important priority.

References

1. Hippocrates. Hippocratic Oath. 275 CE.
2. Cummings. Healthcare industry is a major source of harmful emissions. Yale; 2019. https://news.yale.edu/2019/08/02/healthcare-industry-major-source-harmful-emissions.
3. WHO Guidance for climate resilient and environmentally sustainable health care facilities. https://www.who.int/publications-detail-redirect/climate-resilient-and-environmentally-sustainable-health-care-facilities. Accessed 9 Feb 2021.
4. Greening the OR | Practice Greenhealth. https://practicegreenhealth.org/topics/greening-operating-room/greening-or. Accessed 9 Mar 2021.
5. The road to carbon neutral. https://about.kaiserpermanente.org/community-health/improving-community-conditions/environmental-stewardship/the-road-to-carbon-neutral.
6. Pledging bold environmental performance by 2025. https://about.kaiserpermanente.org/community-health/news/kaiser-permanente-pledges-bold-2025-environmental-performance-to. Accessed 9 Feb 2021.
7. Health Care Working Group. Boston Green Ribbon Commission, https://www.greenribboncommission.org/work/health-care-working-group/. Accessed 22 Mar 2021.
8. About The Office for a Healthy Environment. Cleveland Clinic, https://my.clevelandclinic.org/about/community/sustainability/about. Accessed 24 Mar 2021.
9. Sustainability efforts could save healthcare industry $15B over 10 years. Healthcare Finance News, https://www.healthcarefinancenews.com/news/sustainability-efforts-could-save-healthcare-industry-15b-over-10-years. Accessed 9 Feb 2021.
10. Topics | Practice Greenhealth. https://practicegreenhealth.org/topics. Accessed 9 Feb 2021.
11. Home | First, Do No Harm. https://healthforclimate.org/. Accessed 9 Feb 2021.
12. Special report on global warming of 1.5°C (Report). Incheon: Intergovernmental Panel on Climate Change (IPCC); 2018. Retrieved 7 Oct 2018.

Chapter 22
The Evolution of International Health: Lessons to Be Learned

Rajasekaran Warrier, Haripriya Madabushi, Santoshi M. Kandalam, Ahmed Noreddin, and Carl Kim

The Ultimate Question

The coronavirus disease of 2019 (COVID-19) pandemic, if anything, has proven the interconnectedness of the world, showing how certain health diseases can directly affect those in other countries, bringing the need to understand global health to the forefront of medicine. For a while now, the global health community has been using international comparisons of healthcare systems to evaluate and improve healthcare delivery. These metrics helped countries evaluate their response to COVID-19 [1]. Despite the United States' unique delivery of healthcare and status as a place of discovery and cutting-edge science, overall life expectancy is actually lower than that of other countries with similar per capita income [2]. The United States is also known to be the largest spender within healthcare as compared with any other country in the world [2]. In comparison, developing countries around the world are utilizing innovative tactics to provide care to large amounts of people in a cost-effective way [3]. These tactics may be a stepping stone in making the United States' healthcare system more sustainable.

Taking the time to learn the perspectives of global citizens can be an extremely powerful experience [4]. Understanding health and healthcare systems in communities across the world not only provides insight into different models of care that could be utilized to improve our own systems but also better prepares physicians in

R. Warrier (✉) · A. Noreddin · C. Kim
The University of Queensland-Ochsner Clinical School, New Orleans, LA, USA
e-mail: rwarrier@ochsner.org

H. Madabushi
Jawaharlal Nehru Medical College, Belgaum, India

S. M. Kandalam
University of Queensland, Faculty of Medicine, QLD, Australia

© The Author(s), under exclusive license to Springer Nature Switzerland AG 2022
K. Conrad (ed.), *Clinical Approaches to Hospital Medicine*,
https://doi.org/10.1007/978-3-030-95164-1_22

the United States care for patients of all diverse backgrounds. Many medical professionals and trainees in the United States have taken a keen interest in global health, eager to share innovative research and cures with other areas of the world. Many physicians are motivated to participate in global health because they believe that one's country should not determine their access to good quality healthcare [5].

The ultimate question is how do we achieve the "best of both worlds" scenario where we continue to provide specialized care, encourage cutting-edge research that significantly improves mortality of certain diseases, while getting better at managing noncommunicable diseases and reducing costs to make healthcare sustainable? This chapter certainly does not contain all the answers to the betterment of health around the world, but it does aim to discuss certain parameters that help evaluate and understand the current state of healthcare in different countries as it applies to hospitalists in the United States.

Evolution

Globally, life expectancy has increased more in the past 50 years than in the preceding 5000 years combined [6]. There is no argument that modern medicine now has the tools to accomplish a variety of seemingly impossible feats; however, it is the more subtle advances, the ones that are able to be implemented around the globe that have contributed most to increased life expectancy [6]. The medical conditions that broadly affect most nations tend to be the most pressing issues. This is why global health timelines often highlight the major pandemics that have spread throughout the world. In 2009, The Lancet published a more unifying definition of global health:

> Global health is an area for study, research, and practice that places a priority on improving health and achieving equity in health for all people worldwide. Global health emphasizes transnational health issues, determinants, and solutions; involves many disciplines within and beyond the health sciences and promotes interdisciplinary collaboration; and is a synthesis of population-based prevention with individual-level clinical care. Although global health places greater priority on prevention, it also embraces curative, rehabilitative, and other aspects of clinical medicine and the study of basic sciences [7].

The understanding of global health is still largely variable: some see it as a means to help those who are perceived to be in more dire situations, some believe strongly that an advancement in the medical field should be equally accessible to all citizens of the world, others believe it will help their own countries' interests to learn about global health, and most believe in a combination of these things. Although the perspective that other countries do not have similar access to resources as the United States motivates people to be more charitable, it can also cause people to partake in medical voluntourism, which can be dangerous.

The origin of medical mission trips started with religious missions and colonization efforts. Medical services have been offered to sway people both toward and away from political and religious ideologies. Medical surgeries were offered by Christian missionaries to gain trust and encourage conversions to their faith [8]. Dr. Bethune, a trauma surgeon and early proponent of universal healthcare, provided surgeries during the Spanish Civil War in China while promoting communism [9]. Though certain faith-based medical mission trips still exist, the majority of current global health trips originate from nonprofit organizations such as the WHO, Red Cross, and Doctors without Borders.

A major stepping stone for the development of global health was the formation of Médecins Sans Frontières (MSF), also known as Doctors without Borders, in May 1968. The Red Cross, one of the earlier organizations established to care for victims of unfortunate catastrophes; however, it consisted largely of nonmedical personnel. A group of young French doctors, on a Red Cross mission to treat the wounded during a Nigerian conflict, saw the need for a doctor-run association; thus, MSF was born. Today many more doctor-run nonprofit, organizations cater to patients globally. As of 2021, Doctors Without Borders is established in 28 countries, serving over a hundred million patients and counting [10].

Though the term Global Health was used in scientific journals and articles since the 1940s, as well as by organizations like MSF and WHO, it was not until the 1990s that the concept garnered worldwide attention. President Barack Obama made global health a key part of his international policy by signing *The Global Health Initiative*. This act worked with countries around the world to push funding for out-reach programs, development aids, education and awareness campaigns, and scientific research. Nonprofit organizations and funds started by private citizens like the Bill and Melinda Gates Foundation also play a huge role in improving global health. These nonprofits often make significant positive impacts by targeting specific conditions and locations; examples include AIDS and malaria treatments in Africa by the Gates foundation and the Sankara Eye Foundation focusing on eye health and vision impairment in India. These organizations managed to change global health to a secularly driven humanitarian efforts with noble mission statements and values [11].

Physicians in these organizations have had the chance to participate in incredible work, so there is no surprise that trainees and students are becoming increasingly interested in global health experiences [12]. Currently, short-term global health experiences are organized by a myriad of different institutions with varying degrees of regulation. Many of these organizations and initiatives are well-intentioned; however, the lack of regulated structure endangers lives that are dependent on certain initiatives [13]. Global health initiatives can be detrimental in a variety of ways: increased dependency on volunteer groups, disruption to local cultural practices and values, medical errors in the setting of low consequences, etc.

In 2016, a perspective titled: Beyond Medical "Missions" to Impact Driven Short-Term Experiences in Global Health (STEGHs): Ethical Principles to Optimize Community Benefit and Learner Experience shared guidelines with the aim of correcting unintended negative consequences of certain short-term experiences in global health. The four principles are listed as follows:

1. *Principle 1: Skills building in cross-cultural effectiveness and cultural humility are critical components of successful STEGHs.*
2. *Principle 2: STEGHs must foster bidirectional participatory relationships.*
3. *Principle 3: STEGHs should be a part of longitudinal engagement that promotes sustainable local capacity building and health system strengthening.*
4. *Principle 4: STEGHs must be embedded within established, community-led efforts focused on sustainable development and measurable community health gains* [14].

These principles focus on sustainability, which is incredibly important when initiating any health intervention. For example, a one-time donation of glucose monitors to members of a small village is not likely to achieve the goal of decreasing uncontrolled diabetes within that area. Combining the donation with education, places to refill supplies, and partnerships with local nonprofits are some ways to ensure that there are lasting results for the initiative. Another misconception is assuming that lower quality care is acceptable because those receiving the care would not have been able to afford any regardless. Though there are laws that prohibit students, trainees, and others from participating in tasks they are not qualified to do, these laws are poorly enforced. An expert consensus written in 2019 highlights a few incidents where patients being managed by unqualified trainees have faced dire consequences [15]. This paper also calls for a more stringent oversight of STEGHs, stating that we should hold similar standards for all health initiatives geared toward patient care regardless of how underprivileged patients are. Since then, there has been a huge push to educate and train students to understand the importance of local partnerships and sustainability to maintain the principles outlined above.

During the COVID-19 pandemic, there was a transition of resources away from commonly run initiatives, which traditionally are disease-specific and privately funded. This highlighted the dependence that lower-income countries have on donors and organizations most often from citizens in higher-income countries [16]. These transactions are often unregulated, so in times of emergencies there is not a contingency plan. The lack of a plan, combined with the inability to travel and the decreased ability to fundraise for non-COVID initiatives, exacerbated the negative consequences of the one-way partnerships. The STEGHs listed above encourage responsible global health practices to help avoid this dependency; however, these are merely suggestions, far from being enforced.

Investing in education and incorporating local medical professionals are key to ensuring that initiatives are sustainable, especially in unpredictable times. This is not a possibility in all areas of the world. There are communities that will continue to be dependent on humanitarian aid and resources. Addressing these concerns is difficult for a multitude of reasons, one the biggest being the barriers to education. Medical education often takes time, money, and a certain amount of privilege, higher than most average world citizens. Even if students from low-income countries are able to receive medical education, the opportunities to pursue research and specializations are significantly limited, perpetuating the dependence that low-income countries have on wealthier countries [17]. Although there are many theories as to why people lack access to medical education, there is little debate that change must be made.

The medical community has started to make large efforts to increase access to medical education. A growing number of programs in the United States are understanding the value of offering specialized mentorship programs and jobs in partnered clinics overseas [18]. Though there is increasing interest in global health, there are not nearly enough physicians to attain adequate access in the United States, let alone the globe. For this reason, it is important for the medical community to utilize innovative approaches that are sustainable when addressing global health.

Understanding Global Systems of Health

The metrics that global health scholars used to measure a population's health and adequacy of healthcare systems has changed over the last couple decades. Mortality, life expectancy, quality of life, costs, and work status were commonly used to compare countries in the early 2000s [19].Taking into account the significance of education and innovation, current metrics include health IT infrastructure, policies, and access to education [20]. This transition from morbidity and mortality allowed us to use more than just outcomes to define the success of healthcare received by a certain population. These newer metrics provide a deeper understanding of the social determinants of health, yet another campaign that has gained popularity in this decade [21].

The Lancet, a family of accredited medical journals, has a dedicated global health journal, several commissions, and series that work together to highlight the work being done internationally and create plans with recommendations that help further the eradication of preventable or curable diseases across the globe. The Lancet has recently created a commission on High Quality Health Systems (HQSS), focused on preventing deaths due to low quality care in middle- and low-income communities around the world [22].

Started over two decades ago, the Lancet Commission on Global Eye Health is also well known for their impact on global health and economies. The commission has published several reviews on the work that they have done. They also continue to advocate for the global health community to come together to treat preventable blindness, emphasizing that 90% of vision impairment can be prevented and/or treated with cost-effective treatments. These treatments would make a huge impact at the individual level but also cause significant communal change, increasing the number of people able to contribute to different economies [23]. The Lancet commissions also ensure to continually review and reassess the work being done, keeping in mind both quality and the economic impact global health undoubtedly has. Other Commissions focus on Culture, Reproductive Health, Infectious Disease, Nutrition, and other key health areas that are often used as metrics to evaluate the health of nations.

Community health is impacted largely by a population's culture, religion, economics, prevalence of alternative medicine, and attitude toward healthcare. Different countries around the world differ enormously on these factors [4]. A few countries with drastically different healthcare systems and populations are discussed and compared to the United States within this chapter. The aim is to understand how different communities around the globe address different challenges in the hopes that it will help us understand how to improve the delivery of healthcare equitably to the diverse population of the United States.

Mortality and Life Expectancy

As stated earlier in this chapter these last few decades have improved life expectancy significantly, referred to as a golden age for health [22]. However, it is important to remember that we have not improved the prevalence of, or treatment for, all conditions. While largely government-led initiatives like access to clean water and vaccinations led to averting millions of deaths from communicable diseases, we, as a global community, have struggled with preventing deaths from noncommunicable diseases [24, 25].

The United States has a life expectancy of 77.4 years, with an increase from 2000 of 1.8 years. From the same data sheet, Qatar, a country with much lower per capita income, is shown to have an average life expectancy of 77.2 years, surprisingly similar to the United States; however, Qatar does have a substantially larger change in life expectancy over the last 20 years – 5.9 years. Qatar is also one of the few countries where males have a slightly increased life expectancy of about 1 year to females. There is conflicting evidence about the life expectancy of women being less than the life expectancy of men in the GCC. Some believe it could be related to the increased prevalence of obesity in women; however, it is important to note that while obesity is generally more common in women worldwide, females still tend to have higher life expectancies [26].

Another country with a significant improvement in life expectancy since the year 2000 is India, with a change of 8.7 years, bringing the current average life expectancy to 70.8. The increase in life expectancy in both of these countries, India and Qatar, is thought to be due to their economic gains. Though the United States has a higher life expectancy than most countries in the world, when adjusted for income and wealth, the United States predicted life expectancy is lower by approximately 3 years [27]. In comparison, other countries like Brazil and Ethiopia have significantly higher than predicted life expectancies [27].

One country that was able to continue a steep rate of improvement in life expectancy, while already having a high life expectancy in the year 2000, is South Korea. South Korea's current average life expectancy is one of the highest in the world at 83.3 years, after an increase of 7.1 years from the year 2000. None of the other members in the top 20 countries for life expectancy have a rate of increase close to that high. These statistics show both a need and possibility for the United States to improve its healthcare system as a whole. Understanding the underlying factors influencing shifts in life expectancy around the world can help guide policy here in the United States [26].

So What Changed? Economies and Healthcare

The major contributor to an increase in health in many countries is income. The graph depicting the positive correlation between health and income per capita is one of the best known relations in global health. Wealth and health are intertwined; healthier populations are more productive and have the ability to invest in future generations [28].

Although the positive correlation between health and income per capita is a well-established phenomenon, rapid economic development may have some negative impacts. The discovery of oil in the gulf region of the Middle East in the early twentieth century was a catalyst for dramatic changes in lifestyle changes of the population leading to an increase in the prevalence of lifestyle diseases. Initially, the inhabitants of the GCC (Gulf Cooperation Council) region led a nomadic lifestyle consisting of simple diets, large expenditures of energy compared to the regional population of today. The socioeconomic development of the GCC resulted in an epidemiological transition with chronic disease such diabetes and cardiovascular disease becoming the leading cause of morbidity and mortality. The extent of this epidemiological transition is alarming as all 6 countries in the region are ranked in the top 10 in the world for diabetes prevalence, as well as non-communicable diseases accounting for 70% of all deaths in the GCC [29].

This rapid increase in national wealth contributed to an unprecedented population growth of nearly doubling between 2000 and 2017 [30]. A lack of health system infrastructure and dependence on expatriate (migrant) medical professionals has left the GCC region without the necessary resources to accommodate this rapidly growing population. Sixty percent of medical professionals are expatriates with a 20–25% loss of trained health workforce personnel per-year [30]. A targeted solution has included strategic collaborations with foreign hospitals and medical schools such as the Cleveland Clinic in the United Arab Emirates (UAE). These collaborations have successfully expanded the US-based model of care to the GCC to help evolve human capital and infrastructural needs while building long-term health system capacity. Many other joint ventures have been established including John Hopkins Aramco in Saudi Arabia and Cornell Medical College in Qatar [31]. These establishments are mutually beneficial and are prime examples of the crucial role the United States plays in promoting the evolution of hospital medicine.

Building infrastructure in countries does not automatically result in better health outcomes. Though lack of access to infrastructure does play a role in decreasing mortality, it is only a part of the solution. For example, a program aimed to reduce infant mortality in India distributed cash incentives for women who gave birth at facilities found that increased facility delivery did not improve newborn or maternal mortality [32]. The HQSS, one of the Lancet commissions, was created to evaluate and understand this gap. The commission members develop frameworks and guidelines for implementing global health initiatives that go beyond donating resources. Their framework involves incorporating high quality, value-based care, in conjunction with providing the capital needed to improve healthcare [22].

Access and Reverse Innovation

Access to healthcare, whether it is rural Minnesota or villages in India, is another major contributor to the health of a population [22]. There are multiple contributing factors for a lack of access: education, geography, wealth, but most importantly a healthcare system that is not made in the best interests of the population. A healthcare systems' efficiency is limited by more than just the wealth of nations. The Organization for Economic Co-operation and Development contains countries with relatively high income and high life expectancy. The United States ranks lowest in life expectancy among the OECD countries, despite the amount of wealth the nation has [26]. This indicates an inefficient healthcare system that is not built in the best interests of the population as a whole. A comparison of nine OECD countries found that healthcare systems' efficiency is improved when countries focus on population behavior and welfare instead of highly specialized treatments affecting the minority of the population [33]. The proposed solution is a transition to a value-based system with increased focus on primary care [34]. Despite this push, we have yet to see health outcomes improve in the United States [26]. An alternative to large-scale policies is the implementation of smaller-scale, innovative projects that address population health at a local level.

A book written by Vijay Govindararajan titled *Reverse Innovation in Health Care: How to make Value-Based Delivery Work* discusses how the US healthcare system can learn about and improve upon innovative strategies that have worked in India [3].

India, a relatively young, developing country, has a unique way of catering to the healthcare of their large population. Initial hospitals were built by the British East-India Company and then taken over by the government. Modernization, the growing economy, and the global exchange of knowledge led to privatization. Presently, hospitals with the best infrastructure, updated techniques, and medical education are predominantly private. Though large multiple-specialty hospitals with around 2000–6000-bed capacity are numerous, smaller clinics are just as popular [35].

The concept of a Primary Health Center was suggested by the Bhore Committee (under the leadership of Sir Joseph Bhore) in 1946, and the first functional PHC was established in 1953 by the government. Since then, many hospitals have set up PHCs as smaller branches. The Primary Health Center (PHCs) are used as extensions of the hospital system to administer medical care as well as spread awareness about endemic diseases, to the urban and rural areas where healthcare is lacking [36]. A hub-and-spoke model allowed India to cut costs and increase quality by concentrating specialized care and spreading primary care [3]. Dr. Henderson, referred to as a visionary in the book, created a telemedicine network, with a similar hub-and-spoke model at the University of Mississippi. The network allowed rural hospitals to provide better care by involving specialists when needed, resulting in decreased costs and increased access to high-quality care [37]. The network is believed to have saved several hospitals that were headed toward closure by addressing challenges that many rural hospitals in the United States are facing: inability to staff physicians for specialized care, decreased admissions, and transfers to larger centers [38]. According to the North Carolina Rural Health Research program, from January of 2005 to December of 2015, 105 rural hospitals were closed down [39]. This trend highlights one of the core problems with the US hospital system – unsustainable costs leading to decreased access for low-income and rural members of society [38]. It is vital for all practicing physicians in the United States to understand the dynamics between costs and access. A qualitative study done in 2019 analyzing US physicians' takeaways regarding global health had a majority of respondents agree that a global health experience increased their awareness of excessive spending in the United States [5]. Although there are many things that the United States can learn from other countries to improve its own healthcare, the differences in culture and attitudes toward healthcare make certain initiatives difficult to generalize [22].

Cultural Competence

Finding a definition for culture that is both inclusive and accurate has puzzled scholars for decades; however, understanding the impact of culture on health is clear. The idea of cultural competence, how people communicate across cultural divides, began with a UNESCO-commissioned study to ensure that ethnocentrism did not gain popularity. World War II brought the discussion of racism and its impact to the forefront of discussions involving culture. UNESCO's study directly rejected the idea of colonialism and ethnocentrism, emphasizing the value of social diversity. This was the initial push to make health rights more applicable to those of all cultural backgrounds and laid the foundation for what we now discuss in medicine as cultural competence [4].

Another challenge regarding defining culture is the fact that the definition differs from person to person, perhaps an easier way to understand culture is the sum of things that bring value to a human being's life. Some have characterized culture as what separates human beings from other living animals. Taking this definition into account, in order to provide culturally competent care, it must be individualized. Value in healthcare is currently defined as outcomes over costs; this does not always directly align with an individual's definition of value. Cultural competence is understanding the divide and closing the gap between the value of healthcare and the value that an individual defines for themselves.

Closing the gap, especially in the setting of global health, is not easy. This challenge is commonly faced by expatriate healthcare workers in the GCC. The majority of all healthcare workers in the GCC come from countries that have very different cultural norms to those who live in the GCC region. These barriers play a significant role in the patient-physician relationship, particularly between members of the opposite gender. One of the unique cultural traditions is the refusal for a patient to be touched, maintain eye contact, or speak directly to a member of the opposite gender. This is very different from the norms seen in most Western cultures. It is impossible to generate positive health outcomes without accepting the sociocultural norms that people have chosen to live by [4]. Acknowledging this motivates, many institutions in the United States train and employ physicians that represent the populations they are serving. Developing countries that do not have the resources to educate local populations are at disadvantage. Increasing local training in the GCC may help address some of the health disparities unique to the country, for exampe, decreased life expectancy in women compared to men.

The understanding that health outcomes are significantly worse when cultural differences are not addressed is probably most emphasized when looking at the health of indigenous populations in wealthy countries, like Australia and the United States. Native Americans and Aboriginals have significantly worse health outcomes than the rest of the citizens in their respective countries. Aboriginal men in Australia are reported to have some of the worst health outcomes. They have also been shown to significantly underutilize health centers [40, 41]. As discussed earlier, increasing access does not always translate to improved health outcomes. Often our assumptions of why certain populations have worse outcomes paint the community with broad strokes – assuming certain populations would rather rely on traditional medicine or assuming that there is a significant lack of trust in the system. A qualitative study done in 2018 found that aboriginal men are motivated to improve their health. They also concluded from interviews that understanding the heterogeneity of their thoughts was essential. A one-size-fits all approach did not serve this population well [42]. When considering native populations, it is also important to have an understanding of alternative medicine.

Alternative Medicine and Religion

Yet another interesting aspect of culture and medicine is religion. Most individuals in this world, consider religion to be part of their culture, effectively stating that religious beliefs add value to their life [43]. Thus, religion plays a large role in healthcare. Medicine has long been thought of as a part of the Hindu and Buddhist religions. Whereas the relationship between religion and health has gained popularity relatively recently in the west. A systematic review looking at the relationship between religion and health published between 1975 and 2017 showed a significant increase in publications after 2009 [44]. This increase in publications shows the United States' interest toward broadening the understanding of culture and religion within healthcare. In many studies, religion is shown to have a positive effect on health outcomes and often informs attitudes toward healthcare.

Interestingly, both evidence-based medicine and alternative medicine have been gaining popularity across the globe. Ayurvedic medicine (originating in India), Unani medicine, Chinese Medicine, and Homeopathic medicine (originating in Germany) are all well-known alternatives to allopathic medicine. The medicinal ingredients used in alternative treatment come from natural ingredients: herbs, seeds, oils, etc. This, relatively, reduces the risk of drug-induced side effects that are commonly seen in allopathic drugs. In 1999, *To Err is Human*, a book discussing the magnitude of medical errors in hospitals leading to deaths was published. Though many institutions have pushed for quality improvement, a systematic review done in 2019 found the average rate of drug-related hospital admissions is still high, around 15.4% [45]. The increased transparency of medical errors and side effects of medicine since the 1990s are motivating factors for US citizens to seek out alternatives to allopathic medicines.

Other common subsets of patients that use alternative medicine are patients with chronic lifestyle conditions and terminal diseases. The current medical system in the United States is best fit to manage acute and correctable diseases, due to our investment in cutting-edge technology and pharmaceuticals. Though advances have been made to prevent and better manage chronic diseases, advances in education and awareness are still lacking [46]. Patients in the previously stated subsets, often hope alternative medicine will contain a cure or a better treatment regimen. Alternative medicine is extremely popular among cancer patients: 83% of 453 cancer patients in a National Cancer Institute study reported trying alternative medicine as a part of their treatment [47].

In Eastern culture, alternative medicine has always been prevalent; this is likely due to the significantly different perspective on the role of healthcare in one's life. Oral traditions in these communities play a powerful role in instructing and educating people about health. Medical education is passed down differently than in the Western world. The older members of the family serve as initial triage, providing medicinal remedies for mild, commonly occurring illnesses [48]. For example, in India, most grandmothers in villages, some who have not even had the chance to complete basic schooling, are taught to aid women in childbirth. Their medical knowledge is impressive, often guiding mothers through prenatal care and understanding their child's development.

One anecdotal story shared by an immigrant from India is the idea of using buttermilk to treat vaginal yeast infections. Though there are no published RCTs evaluating the effectiveness of douching with buttermilk to cure vaginal yeast infections, a systematic review looking at alternative treatments concurred that lactobacillus recolonization with yogurt capsules may have some promise [49]. Yeast infections are thought to be caused by an overgrowth of candida due to disruption of normal growth flora. Normal flora of the vagina is lactobacillus, often found in buttermilk. Though the pathophysiology is understood, studies show that there is a negligible amount of lactobacillus in commercially developed yogurts [50]. The draw of alternative medicine is the decreased risk of harm. The harm of douching with buttermilk is lower than the harm of antifungal creams and oral antifungal medications. Antifungals can contribute to the development of drug-resistant yeast infections, which can turn fatal [51].

This tradition of relying on oral traditions and family members for medical knowledge makes a huge difference in hospital medicine culture and dependency on hospitals. Though there are economic benefits to decreased dependency, there is also a downside: decreased primary preventative interventions. With globalization, illnesses now plaguing developing countries are changing, increasing the dependence of countries on allopathic medicine. Increased medical education about newly emerging conditions in addition to more research investigating old age cures is needed to achieve the best health outcomes [52].

The medical system in the United States has evolved to accept possible benefits of alternative medicine practices, investing nearly 366 million dollars in research in 2016. In 2013, a clinical trial was conducted in which an ayurvedic formulation (a plant extract against natural glucosamine sulphate) and the NSAID Celecoxib were compared for ability to reduce pain. The trial was conducted with 440 patients suffering from knee osteoarthritis. Both drugs showed similar effects in pain reduction with rise in SGPT but otherwise functioning liver [53]. Currently, more and more therapies from other countries are being adopted into the US healthcare system. Turmeric is one of the more well-known herbal therapies that has been widely accepted [54]. Though there is still a long way to go in terms of researching ayurvedic treatments, physicians across the globe have hope that it may provide aid in resolving some of the biggest healthcare challenges of our time [55].

COVID-19

The coronavirus, one of the biggest healthcare challenges we have faced in this century, exaggerated cultural and regional differences not only between different countries but between different states and even more specific communities within states. The different approaches taken by countries to manage a pandemic in the modern, globalized world allowed us to compare and analyze the effectiveness of different healthcare systems.

South Korea was a relative success story. In 2015, South Korea went through a devastating epidemic caused by the Middle East Respiratory Syndrome Coronavirus resulting in 186 cases and 38 deaths. The South Korean government swiftly identified potholes within the healthcare system and passed approximately 48 reforms to address the concerns of not having enough physicians, infrastructure, and communication between important government institutions.

They identified the potholes within the healthcare [56]. The first case of Severe Acute Respiratory Syndrome Coronavirus 2 (SARS-CoV-2) was confirmed on January 20, 2020, and by the end of February, the country was reporting up to 909 cases. The government immediately mandated masking, quarantining, and social distancing. The compliance rate in South Korea was thought to be high because

South Koreans were already accustomed to wearing masks due to pollution [57]. The government also enforced high-tech, vigorous, rapid contact tracing. By April 30, 2020, they were able to flatten the curve, and a downward trend in incidence was seen. The response to the initial wave of the pandemic was better than most other countries [58]. Though there has been much discussion about how the culture of South Koreans and the willingness to comply was the reason the country was so successful, they may not have been if the reforms in the healthcare system had not taken place.

In the United States, there is much debate about how culture and individual choice is impacting the response to this pandemic. There is a definite divide between the perspective of physicians in the United States and the majority of individuals in the United States. This is unsurprising as the demographics of physicians are extremely different to those of individuals living in the United States. There are significant differences in race, average salary, access to education, and location [59–61]. These differences contribute to the divide that has recently been exaggerated by the coronavirus. Other wealthy countries do not have as large of a demographic gap between practicing physicians and the populations they serve. Taking an approach similar to how doctors practice globally may improve the US healthcare system. Understanding the heterogeneity of the population, utilizing innovative methods to improve access to care, and catering care toward the best interests of an individual are all tools recommended by global health scholars that may bridge this gap [4, 62].

Conclusion

The Lancet Global Health Commission endorses four vital actions to consider when addressing global healthcare systems that lay the foundation for a good healthcare system: have a shared, clear, vision of quality care with strong regulations, focus on health outcomes rather than limiting systems to focusing on access, increase participation and competency in clinical education, and empower citizens to understand their healthcare and keep their governing bodies in check [22]. As medical professionals, it is extremely important to remember the assertion that providing services without quality is ineffective, wasteful, and unethical both in our own country and globally. Global health can be extremely rewarding, not only because of the satisfaction of helping those in need but also because the experiences generally empower physicians to be better in a multitude of ways. A survey done asking medical professionals about the impact that global health had on their careers was overwhelmingly positive. Around 85% of respondents agreed that global health activities enhanced the quality of their domestic work and increased their level of involvement with vulnerable populations, health policy advocacy, or research on social determinants of health [63]. The United States has its own share of complex problems within its healthcare system, and the solutions may come from practices employed in different countries. The answer to the ultimate question asked above may be as difficult to understand as culture is to define; however, educating communities of the evolution of health globally can undoubtedly help us create a more culturally aware, sustainable, healthcare system in the future.

References

1. Rudnicka L, Gupta M, Kassir M, Jafferany M, Lotti T, Sadoughifar R, Goldust M. Priorities for global health community in COVID-19 pandemic. Dermatol Ther. 2020;33(4):e13361. https://doi.org/10.1111/dth.13361.
2. Montez JK, Beckfield J, Cooney JK, Grumbach JM, Hayward MD, Koytak HZ, Woolf SH, Zajacova A. US state policies, politics, and life expectancy. Milbank Q. 2020;98(3):668–99. https://doi.org/10.1111/1468-0009.12469.
3. Govindarajan V. Reverse innovation in health care: how to make value-based delivery work ^ 10155. 1st ed. Harvard Business Review Press; 2018.
4. Napier AD, Ancarno C, Butler B, Calabrese J, Chater A, Chatterjee H, Guesnet F, Horne R, Jacyna S, Jadhav S, Macdonald A, Neuendorf U, Parkhurst A, Reynolds R, Scambler G, Shamdasani S, Smith SZ, Stougaard-Nielsen J, Thomson L, Tyler N, Volkmann AM, Walker T, Watson J, Williams AC, Willott C, Wilson J, Woolf K. Culture and health. Lancet (London, England). 2014;384(9954):1607–39. https://doi.org/10.1016/s0140-6736(14)61603-2.
5. Matthews-Trigg N, Citrin D, Halliday S, Acharya B, Maru S, Bezruchka S, Maru D. Understanding perceptions of global healthcare experiences on provider values and practices in the USA: a qualitative study among global health physicians and program directors. BMJ Open. 2019;9(4). https://doi.org/10.1136/bmjopen-2018-026020.
6. Laxminarayan R, Mills AJ, Breman JG, Measham AR, Alleyne G, Claeson M, Jha P, Musgrove P, Chow J, Shahid-Salles S, Jamison DT. Advancement of global health: key messages from the Disease Control Priorities Project. Lancet (London, England). 2006;367(9517):1193–208. https://doi.org/10.1016/s0140-6736(06)68440-7.
7. Koplan JP, Bond TC, Merson MH, Reddy KS, Rodriguez MH, Sewankambo NK, Wasserheit JN. Towards a common definition of global health. Lancet (London, England). 2009;373(9679):1993–5. https://doi.org/10.1016/s0140-6736(09)60332-9.
8. Loewenberg S. Medical missionaries deliver faith and health care in Africa. Lancet (London, England). 2009;373(9666):795–6. https://doi.org/10.1016/s0140-6736(09)60462-1.
9. Lynteris C. The spirit of selflessness in Maoist China: socialist medicine and the new man introduction. In: Spirit of selflessness in Maoist China. Socialist medicine and the new man. UK: Macmillan. 2013. p. 1–11.
10. Fox RC. Medical humanitarianism and human rights: reflections on doctors without borders and doctors of the world. Soc Sci Med. 1995;41(12):1607–16. https://doi.org/10.1016/0277-9536(95)00144-V.
11. Harman S. The Bill and Melinda Gates Foundation and legitimacy in global health governance. Glob Gov. 2016;22(3):349–68. https://doi.org/10.1163/19426720-02203004.
12. Cox JT, Kironji AG, Edwardson J, Moran D, Aluri J, Carroll B, Warren N, Chen CCG. Global health career interest among medical and nursing students: survey and analysis. Ann Glob Health. 2017;83(3–4):588–95. https://doi.org/10.1016/j.aogh.2017.07.002.
13. Gautier L, Sieleunou I, Kalolo A. Deconstructing the notion of "global health research partnerships" across Northern and African contexts. BMC Med Ethics. 2018;19. https://doi.org/10.1186/s12910-018-0280-7.
14. Melby MK, Loh LC, Evert J, Prater C, Lin H, Khan OA. Beyond medical "missions" to impact-driven short-term experiences in global health (STEGHs): ethical principles to optimize community benefit and learner experience. Acad Med. 2016;91(5):633–8. https://doi.org/10.1097/acm.0000000000001009.

15. Rowthorn V, Loh L, Evert J, Chung E, Lasker J. Not above the law: a legal and ethical analysis of short-term experiences in global health. Ann Glob Health. 2019;85(1). https://doi.org/10.5334/aogh.2451.
16. Birn AE. Backstage: the relationship between the Rockefeller Foundation and the World Health Organization, Part I: 1940s–1960s. Public Health. 2014;128(2):129–40. https://doi.org/10.1016/j.puhe.2013.11.010.
17. Boum Y, Burns BF, Siedner M, Mburu Y, Bukusi E, Haberer JE. Advancing equitable global health research partnerships in Africa. BMJ Glob Health. 2018;3(4). https://doi.org/10.1136/bmjgh-2018-000868.
18. Katz F, Glass RI. Mentorship training is essential to advancing global health research. Am J Trop Med Hyg. 2019;100(1_Suppl):1–2. https://doi.org/10.4269/ajtmh.18-0694.
19. Nurminen M. Working population health metrics. Scand J Work Environ Health. 2004;30(5):339–49. https://doi.org/10.5271/sjweh.821.
20. Hatef E, Lasser EC, Kharrazi HHK, Perman C, Montgomery R, Weiner JP. A population health measurement framework: evidence-based metrics for assessing community-level population health in the global budget context. Popul Health Manag. 2018;21(4):261–70. https://doi.org/10.1089/pop.2017.0112.
21. Fosse E, Helgesen MK, Hagen S, Torp S. Addressing the social determinants of health at the local level: opportunities and challenges. Scand J Public Health. 2018;46:47–52. https://doi.org/10.1177/1403494817743896.
22. Kruk ME, Pate M, Mullan Z. Introducing the lancet global health commission on high-quality health systems in the SDG era. Lancet Glob Health. 2017;5(5):E480–1. https://doi.org/10.1016/s2214-109x(17)30101-8.
23. Burton MJ, Ramke J, Marques AP, Bourne RRA, Congdon N, Jones I, Tong B, Arunga S, Bachani D, Bascaran C, Bastawrous A, Blanchet K, Braithwaite T, Buchan JC, Cairns J, Cama A, Chagunda M, Chuluunkhuu C, Cooper A, Crofts-Lawrence J, Dean WH, Denniston AK, Ehrlich JR, Emerson PM, Evans JR, Frick KD, Friedman DS, Furtado JM, Gichangi MM, Gichuhi S, Gilbert SS, Gurung R, Habtamu E, Holland P, Jonas JB, Keane PA, Keay L, Khanna RC, Khaw PT, Kuper H, Kyari F, Lansingh VC, Mactaggart I, Mafwiri MM, Mathenge W, McCormick I, Morjaria P, Mowatt L, Muirhead D, Murthy GVS, Mwangi N, Patel DB, Peto T, Qureshi BM, Salomao SR, Sarah V, Shilio BR, Solomon AW, Swenor BK, Taylor HR, Wang NL, Webson A, West SK, Wong TY, Wormald R, Yasmin S, Yusufu M, Silva JC, Resnikoff S, Ravilla T, Gilbert CE, Foster A, Faal HB. The Lancet Global Health Commission on Global Eye Health: vision beyond 2020. Lancet Glob Health. 2021;9(4):E489–551. https://doi.org/10.1016/s2214-109x(20)30488-5.
24. Tessema GA, Laurence CO, Melaku YA, Misganaw A, Woldie SA, Hiruye A, Amare AT, Lakew Y, Zeleke BM, Deribew A. Trends and causes of maternal mortality in Ethiopia during 1990–2013: findings from the Global Burden of Diseases study 2013. BMC Public Health. 2017;17. https://doi.org/10.1186/s12889-017-4071-8.
25. Lozano R, Naghavi M, Foreman K, Lim S, Shibuya K, Aboyans V, Abraham J, Adair T, Aggarwal R, Ahn SY, Alvarado M, Anderson HR, Anderson LM, Andrews KG, Atkinson C, Baddour LM, Barker-Collo S, Bartels DH, Bell ML, Benjamin EJ, Bennett D, Bhalla K, Bikbov B, Bin Abdulhak A, Birbeck G, Blyth F, Bolliger I, Boufous SA, Bucello C, Burch M, Burney P, Carapetis J, Chen HL, Chou D, Chugh SS, Coffeng LE, Colan SD, Colquhoun S, Colson KE, Condon J, Connor MD, Cooper LT, Corriere M, Cortinovis M, de Vaccaro KC, Couser W, Cowie BC, Criqui MH, Cross M, Dabhadkar KC, Dahodwala N, De Leo D, Degenhardt L, Delossantos A, Denenberg J, Des Jarlais DC, Dharmaratne SD, Dorsey ER, Driscoll T, Duber H, Ebel B, Erwin PJ, Espindola P, Ezzati M, Feigin V, Flaxman AD, Forouzanfar MH, Fowkes FGR, Franklin R, Fransen M, Freeman MK, Gabriel SE, Gakidou E, Gaspari F, Gillum RF, Gonzalez-Medina D, Halasa YA, Haring D, Harrison JE, Havmoeller R, Hay RJ, Hoen B, Hotez PJ, Hoy D, Jacobsen KH, James SL, Jasrasaria R, Jayaraman S, Johns N, Karthikeyan G, Kassebaum N, Keren A, Khoo JP, Knowlton LM, Kobusingye O, Koranteng A, Krishnamurthi R, Lipnick M, Lipshultz SE, Ohno SL, Mabweijano J, MacIntyre

MF, Mallinger L, March L, Marks GB, Marks R, Matsumori A, Matzopoulos R, Mayosi BM, McAnulty JH, McDermott MM, McGrath J, Mensah GA, Merriman TR, Michaud C, Miller M, Miller TR, Mock C, Mocumbi AO, Mokdad AA, Moran A, Mulholland K, Nair MN, Naldi L, Narayan KMV, Nasseri K, Norman P, O'Donnell M, Omer SB, Ortblad K, Osborne R, Ozgediz D, Pahari B, Pandian JD, Rivero AP, Padilla RP, Perez-Ruiz F, Perico N, Phillips D, Pierce K, Pope CA, Porrini E, Pourmalek F, Raju M, Ranganathan D, Rehm JT, Rein DB, Remuzzi G, Rivara FP, Roberts T, De Leon FR, Rosenfeld LC, Rushton L, Sacco RL, Salomon JA, Sampson U, Sanman E, Schwebel DC, Segui-Gomez M, Shepard DS, Singh D, Singleton J, Sliwa K, Smith E, Steer A, Taylor JA, Thomas B, Tleyjeh IM, Towbin JA, Truelsen T, Undurraga EA, Venketasubramanian N, Vijayakumar L, Vos T, Wagner GR, Wang MR, Wang WZ, Watt K, Weinstock MA, Weintraub R, Wilkinson JD, Woolf AD, Wulf S, Yeh PH, Yip P, Zabetian A, Zheng ZJ, Lopez AD, Murray CJL. Global and regional mortality from 235 causes of death for 20 age groups in 1990 and 2010: a systematic analysis for the Global Burden of Disease Study 2010. Lancet (London, England). 2012;380(9859):2095–128. https://doi.org/10.1016/s0140-6736(12)61728-0.
26. World Health O. World health statistics 2020: monitoring health for the SDGs, sustainable development goals. Geneva: World Health Organization; 2020.
27. Freeman T, Gesesew HA, Bambra C, Giugliani ERJ, Popay J, Sanders D, Macinko J, Musolino C, Baum F. Why do some countries do better or worse in life expectancy relative to income? An analysis of Brazil, Ethiopia, and the United States of America. Int J Equity Health. 2020;19(1):202. https://doi.org/10.1186/s12939-020-01315-z.
28. Bloom DE, Canning D. The health and wealth of nations. Science. 2000;287(5456):1207. https://doi.org/10.1126/science.287.5456.1207.
29. Khalil AB, Beshyah SA, Abdella N, Afandi B, Al-Arouj MM, Al-Awadi F, Benbarka M, Ben Nakhi A, Fiad TM, Al Futaisi A, Hassoun AA, Hussein W, Kaddaha G, Ksseiry I, Al Lamki M, Madani AA, Saber FA, Abdel Aal Z, Morcos B, Saadi H. Diabesity in the Arabian Gulf: challenges and opportunities. Oman Med J. 2018;33(4):273–82. (1999-768X (Print)).
30. Khoja T, Rawaf S, Qidwai W, Rawaf D, Nanji K, Hamad A. Health care in Gulf Cooperation Council countries: a review of challenges and opportunities. Cureus. 2017;9(8):e1586. https://doi.org/10.7759/cureus.1586.
31. Kisuule F, Howell E. Hospital medicine beyond the United States. Int J Gen Med. 2018;11:65–71. https://doi.org/10.2147/IJGM.S151275.
32. Ng M, Misra A, Diwan V, Agnani M, Levin-Rector A, De Costa A. An assessment of the impact of the JSY cash transfer program on maternal mortality reduction in Madhya Pradesh, India. Glob Health Action. 2014;7. https://doi.org/10.3402/gha.v7.24939.
33. Hadad S, Hadad Y, Simon-Tuval T. Determinants of healthcare system's efficiency in OECD countries. Eur J Health Econ. 2013;14(2):253–65. https://doi.org/10.1007/s10198-011-0366-3.
34. Ray JC, Kusumoto F. The transition to value-based care. J Interv Card Electrophysiol. 2016;47(1):61–8. https://doi.org/10.1007/s10840-016-0166-x.
35. Sodhi C, Singh P. Health service system in transition an assessment of the influence of the British and US healthcare systems on the evolution of health services in India. Int J Health Gov. 2016;21(4):204–21. https://doi.org/10.1108/ijhg-03-2016-0020.
36. Bajpai V, Saraya A. For a realistic assessment: a social, political and public health analysis of Bhore Committee. Social Change. 2011;41(2):215–31. https://doi.org/10.1177/004908571104100202.
37. Sterling SA, Henderson K, Jones AE. Coordinating emergency care through telemedicine. In: Value and quality innovations in acute and emergency care. 2017. p. 139–147. https://doi.org/10.1017/9781316779965.
38. Murphy KM, Hughes LS, Conway P. A path to sustain rural hospitals. JAMA. 2018;319(12):1193–4. (1538-3598 (Electronic)).
39. Thomas SR, Holmes GM, Pink GH. To what extent do community characteristics explain differences in closure among financially distressed rural hospitals? J Health Care Poor Underserved. 2016;27(4):194–203. https://doi.org/10.1353/hpu.2016.0176.

40. Aaron B. Indigenous men's health: access strategy. Aborig Isl Health Work J. https://doi.org/10.3316/ielapa.207198047604349.
41. Swann JA, Matthews MR, Bay C, Foster KN. Burn injury outcome differences in Native Americans. Burns. 2019;45(2):494–501. https://doi.org/10.1016/j.burns.2018.09.018.
42. Canuto K, Wittert G, Harfield S, Brown A. "I feel more comfortable speaking to a male": aboriginal and Torres Strait Islander men's discourse on utilizing primary health care services. Int J Equity Health. 2018;17(1):185. https://doi.org/10.1186/s12939-018-0902-1.
43. DeWall CN, Van Tongeren DR. No longer religious, but still spending money religiously: religious rituals and community influence consumer behavior among religious dones. Int J Psychol Relig. 2021:1–18. https://doi.org/10.1080/10508619.2020.1871558.
44. Demir E. The evolution of spirituality, religion and health publications: yesterday, today and tomorrow. J Relig Health. 2019;58(1):1–13. https://doi.org/10.1007/s10943-018-00739-w.
45. Ayalew MB, Tegegn HG, Abdela OA. Drug related hospital admissions; a systematic review of the recent literatures. Bull Emerg Trauma. 2019;7(4):339–46. https://doi.org/10.29252/beat-070401.
46. Jonas WB, Eisenberg D, Hufford D, Crawford C. The evolution of complementary and alternative medicine (CAM) in the USA over the last 20 years. Complement Med Res. 2013;20(1):65–72. https://doi.org/10.1159/000348284.
47. Ventola CL. Current issues regarding complementary and alternative medicine (CAM) in the United States: part 1: the widespread use of CAM and the need for better-informed health care professionals to provide patient counseling. P T. 2010;35(8):461–8.
48. Dixit U. Traditional knowledge from and for elderly. Indian J Tradit Knowl. 2011;10(3):429–38.
49. Van Kessel K, Assefi N, Marrazzo J, Eckert L. Common complementary and alternative therapies for yeast vaginitis and bacterial vaginosis: a systematic review. Obstet Gynecol Surv. 2003;58(5):351–8. https://doi.org/10.1097/00006254-200305000-00024.
50. Song LJ, Aryana KJ. Reconstituted yogurt from yogurt cultured milk powder mix has better overall characteristics than reconstituted yogurt from commercial yogurt powder. J Dairy Sci. 2014;97(10):6007–15. https://doi.org/10.3168/jds.2014-8181.
51. Robbins N, Caplan T, Cowen LE. Molecular evolution of antifungal drug resistance. Annu Rev Microbiol. 2017;71(71):753–75. https://doi.org/10.1146/annurev-micro-030117-020345.
52. Kienle GS, Ben-Arye E, Berger B, Cuadrado Nahum C, Falkenberg T, Kapócs G, Kiene H, Martin D, Wolf U, Szöke H. Contributing to global health: development of a consensus-based whole systems research strategy for anthroposophic medicine. Evid Based Complement Alternat Med. 2019;2019:3706143. https://doi.org/10.1155/2019/3706143.
53. Chopra A, Saluja M, Tillu G, Sarmukkaddam S, Venugopalan A, Narsimulu G, Handa R, Sumantran V, Raut A, Bichile L, Joshi K, Patwardhan B. Ayurvedic medicine offers a good alternative to glucosamine and celecoxib in the treatment of symptomatic knee osteoarthritis: a randomized, double-blind, controlled equivalence drug trial. Rheumatology (Oxford). 2013;52(8):1408–17. (1462-0332 (Electronic)).
54. Nair KP. The chemistry of turmeric. In: Turmeric (Curcuma Longa L) and Ginger (Zingiber Officinale Rosc) – world's invaluable medicinal spices: the agronomy and economy of turmeric and ginger. 2019. p. 53–66. https://doi.org/10.1007/978-3-030-29189-1_4.
55. Oviya IR. Integrating bioinformatics in alternative medicine practice: an insight. In: Holistic approaches to infectious diseases. 2017. p. 109–118. https://doi.org/10.1201/b19944-4.
56. Oh M-D, Park WB, Park S-W, Choe PG, Bang JH, Song K-H, Kim ES, Kim HB, Kim NJ. Middle East respiratory syndrome: what we learned from the 2015 outbreak in the Republic of Korea. Korean J Intern Med. 2018;33(2):233–46. https://doi.org/10.3904/kjim.2018.031.
57. Jeong E, Hagose M, Jung H, Ki M, Flahault A. Understanding South Korea's response to the COVID-19 outbreak: a real-time analysis. Int J Environ Res Public Health. 2020;17(24):9571. https://doi.org/10.3390/ijerph17249571.
58. Oh J, Lee J-K, Schwarz D, Ratcliffe HL, Markuns JF, Hirschhorn LR. National response to COVID-19 in the Republic of Korea and lessons learned for other countries. Health Syst Reform. 2020;6(1):e1753464. https://doi.org/10.1080/23288604.2020.1753464.

59. Thomson WA, Ferry PG, King JE, Martinez-Wedig C, Michael LH. Increasing access to medical education for students from medically underserved communities: one program's success. Acad Med. 2003;78(5):454–9.
60. Mohamed MMB, Lukitsch I, Torres-Ortiz AE, Walker JB, Varghese V, Hernandez-Arroyo CF, Alqudsi M, LeDoux JR, Velez JCQ. Acute kidney injury associated with coronavirus disease 2019 in Urban New Orleans. Kidney360. 2020;1(7):614. https://doi.org/10.34067/KID.0002652020.
61. Young A, Chaudhry HJ, Rhyne J, Dugan M. A census of actively licensed physicians in the United States, 2010. J Med Regul. 2010;96(4):10–20. https://doi.org/10.30770/2572-1852-96.4.10.
62. Rowland P, Kumagai AK. Dilemmas of representation: patient engagement in health professions education. Acad Med. 2018;93(6):869–73.
63. Greysen SR, Richards AK, Coupet S, Desai MM, Padela AI. Global health experiences of U.S. Physicians: a mixed methods survey of clinician-researchers and health policy leaders. Glob Health. 2013;9(1):19. https://doi.org/10.1186/1744-8603-9-19.

Chapter 23
Update in Hospital Medicine: Trends in Compensation, COVID-19, Workplace Environment and Malpractice

Kevin Conrad

Hospital medicine is approximately 25 over years old. As a specialty it continues to demonstrate its essential role, especially during the current COVID-19 pandemic. Certainly, the COVID-19 pandemic has given the hospitalist a time to shine. During the current period, few people have seen and valued hospital medicine more than hospital administrators. A period of disruption often provides an opportunity to illuminate issues and facilitates open communication. The COVID-19 pandemic has provided that. Hopefully hospital medicine will take advantage of this period to further define and consolidate their practice.

Flexibility has been the cornerstone of Hospital Medicine's proven value. The ability to quickly adapt has been an essential component of hospital medicine since its inception. Where there is a need or gap, hospital medicine adapts and steps up to the plate. This was essential during the COVID-19 surges and will continue to be needed as once rare events become the new norm.

No specialty has grown as fast and has had a greater impact on the delivery of healthcare than hospital medicine. The scope of hospital medicine continues to evolve but maintains a focus on acute patient care, academic teaching, and research on healthcare delivery. Recent research has focused on value-based care and will continue to do so as the current healthcare practices move toward population health. Readmission reduction and length of stay are two particular research areas where hospital medicine has focused its efforts.

The term hospitalist was first mentioned in a 1996 New England Journal of Medicine article written by Goldman and Wachter [1]. Prior to that several terms were utilized such as acute care physicians and house physicians. No one, including hospitalists themselves, knew exactly what they were, so it took some time to develop an identity. Several other specialized designations have evolved since then

---

K. Conrad (✉)
Ochsner Health, New Orleans, LA, USA
e-mail: kconrad@ochsner.org

such as nocturnists, Skilled Nursing Facilities (SNF)-ists, and transitional care physicians.

Prior to 1996, there were limited physician practices in the United States based solely in the hospital. Several forces, primarily academic and financial, aligned in the 1990s to account for the birth and rapid growth of the specialty. Those primarily were a decrease in fee for service model and a transition to capitated care. Suddenly, a hospital admission became an expense rather than an income generator. Efficient models were needed to provide in-patient care.

Clinic-based physicians were finding it increasingly difficult to manage the complexities of clinical care, documentation, and throughput of a hospital patient which required nearly 24 hours attention per day. The initial success of hospitalist programs led to their rapid expansion. Large healthcare systems were the first to embrace the hospital medicine concept, followed by more regional systems.

Currently, there are more than 60,000 practicing hospitalists in the United States. This represents a steady and slight exponential growth over the past 25 years [2]. This expansion is predicted to continue for the next few years as remaining hospitals develop and expand new hospitalist's programs, and the scope of practice continues to expand. Hospital Medicine is larger than any other sub specialty of Internal Medicine.

Compensation

One trend remains constant in this time of uncertainty – hospitalists have undisputed value. This is reflected in recent compensation reports. Both salaries and institutional support continue to rise.

According to the Society of Hospital Medicines 2020 (SHM 2020) report, the median salary for all hospitalists serving adult patients was $307,000. The median salary of pediatric hospitalist was $224,000. Among all adult academic hospitalists, the mean salary was $237,00. This represents a continued overall increase in salaries over the past 15 years and a 10% increase from 2016 and a 6% increase form 2018. Since 2010, there has been on average a 9% increase in salary each year [2]. This is despite relatively flat trends in work relative value units (wRVU) production over the same time period. There continues to be significant geographical variability, with hospitalists in the South earning the most. Compensation growth is expected to continue to be similar in the near future as hospitalists positions continue to outnumber the available workforce and competition remains in filling positions. Within the last year, nearly 73% of all Hospital Medicine programs report having unfilled positions. It is expected that the majority of the positions will be filled by new residents [2].

Nocturnist receive, on average, 14.7% more pay than those doing only daytime shifts. Hospitalists working in physician-owned practices have had larger compensation increases than those in hospital-owned groups, according to the MGMA

Provider Compensation report [3]. Over that past several years, this pay difference between nocturnist and traditional providers has remained relatively stable.

Other trends among high earners have also emerged from a survey taken in 2016 in Today's Hospitalist magazine. More than 8% earn over $400,000. This is usualy accomplished by working night shifts or additional moonlighting shifts. High compensation is also seen in some geographically isolated regions [4].

The COVID-19 pandemic has had an undetermined finacial impact on hospital medicine, with many groups reporting transient salary reductions. Despite an influx of pateints at many hospitals due to COVID-19, many experienced decreased volumes. This neccesitated temporary staff reductions. The exact pay reduction has not been quantified in any reports. Although most hospitals were under financial strain, a minority of groups were offered hazard pay during the COVID-19 pandemic. However, roughly 40% reported a reduction in pay. The majority of groups reported that this has been a temporary measure and the expectation is that salaries will eventually stabilize to pre-COVID-19 levels [2]. It is uncertain how the pandemic will affect recruitment, retention, and work patterns.

Institutional support of hospitalists remains significant. The average financial support of a single hospitalist according to the SHM 2020 report was $201,761. This was defined as direct costs not covered by professional fees. This does not take into account any shared savings, which continues to increase, through at-risk and value-based contracts [2].

Performance Metrics

The amount of hospitalist compensation tied to performance metrics continues to be steady, with currently 80% being base pay and approximately 15% being production and 5% performance metrics [2]. The three most commonly used metrics are patient satisfaction, core measure performance, and readmission rates.

Since 2014, core measures and documentation are declining as a metric. It is anticipated that the use of performance metrics tied to compensation will continue to increase as the transition to value-based purchasing continues. There continues to be discussions on the efficacy and implementation of performance metrics and their impact on morale. Some have argued that incentivizing expected activities with little ability to modify them does little to improve outcomes and increases burnout. Often what is easy to measure and is included in a performance metric provides little in terms of improved outcomes for the patient or increased revenues. Value-based medicine, with an increased percentage of patients being at financial risk to healthcare institutions, will continue to drive performance metrics as percentage of compensation for hospitalists. These metrics tend to be more complicated, spread across multiple disciplines, and difficult to assign solely to hospital medicine performance. Despite these challenges, it will be essential for hospital medicine to define their role in improving value-based metrics.

COVID-19 Experience: Insight into Career Satisfaction

Hospitalists' experience with COVID-19 continues to evolve. With its roots in disrupting typical healthcare treatment paradigms, hospital medicine was and is well suited to meet the needs of this rapidly changing pandemic. During the pandemic, this was manifested by speed in which hospital medicine programs adapted to clinical, staffing, and supply challenges. The data provided in this chapter is primarily from the year 2020. As programs venture into the second year of the pandemic, sustainable solutions are being developed, many of which will be permanent. It will be some time before the true impact of the COVID-19 pandemic on the practice of hospital medicine is known. As with all disruptions in healthcare, permanent change can be expected.

Volume fluctuation was a major challenge for most programs. Surge planning became an essential component, with daily reallocation of patients being the norm. Communication of both clinical and operational issues became essential with many programs adopting daily huddles. Most hospitalist's programs, approximately 70% across the country, instituted dedicated COVID and non-COVID teams. This allowed for adjusted patient allocation, personal protective equipment (PPE) conservation, and streamlined provider workflows. More than 60% of pediatric units housed adult COVID-19 patients and almost 40% of pediatric hospitalists provided direct care for adult COVID-19 patients [2, 5].

Hospitalists employed clinicians from other hospital service lines including primary care specialists in both medicine and surgical fields to cover shifts or provide other forms of clinical support [5]. Nearly, 39.6% of hospital medicine groups utilized non-hospital medicine group clinicians to help cover service needs. Many specialties had decreased volumes during the COVID-19 pandemic. Providers in these specialties provided both back up and primary care to COVID-19 patients in the hospital [2, 5].

As discussed in a previous chapter, wellness among hospitalists has come to the forefront during the COVID-19 pandemic. Many issues that were previously known gained increased awareness. Burnout, which is a growing factor among all specialties, is an important topic in many if not most hospitalist groups. As previously stated in order to have burnout, you need to be burning. In response to this, many groups have developed formal wellness efforts and office champions. The issue of wellness will continue to rapidly evolve over the next few years and formal efforts as part of most programs.

Turnover has always been a significant and costly part of hospital medicine due to several factors, including the portability of the practice. The onging efforts of recruitment continue to be costly and at times disruptive to many groups. This is both a positive and negative component of the specialty. One struggle will continue to be differentiating turnover due to burnout versus natural career progression. The impact of COVID-19 on turnover is yet to be determined, with various factors promoting and reducing turnover. Disruptive events often reveal hidden issues. Certainly the COVID-19 pandemic has demonstrated the value of hospital medicine and what is needed to make Hospital Medicine a sustainable career.

Regardless, hospital medicine, still a relatively new specialty, will continue to examine what defines the components of career satisfaction. As exponential expansion of the specialty declines, it will make financial sense to place an increased emphasis on retention and career satisfaction.

There will continue to be turnover with positions being filled by new graduating house staff, but possibly a new paradigm needs to be developed and has been suggested that rewards career hospitalists with professional opportunities at a predefined pace. This would ensure some degree of stability within programs. One factor often cited in burnout is stagnation. Many programs have developed career pathways that ensure professional growth among their ranks.

One contributing component to diminished career satisfaction may be the relative lack of research opportunities in the field of hospital medicine. As compared to other specialties, hospital medicine has a relative lack of clinical investigators and academic output [6]. The cause of this is multifactorial, including the broad nature of the specialty and the recent focus on rapid expansion. Defining the expertise of hospital medicine and translating that into research opportunities is not an easy task. The COVID-19 pandemic will certainly make that task a much easier proposition.

Specific reasons cited for the lack of research initiatives include the lack of funding, few mentors, few dedicated fellowships, and lack of financial incentives. To address this, the Society of Hospital Medicine has placed an emphasis expanding fellowships and mentorships within hospital medicine groups [6].

Research opportunities exist for hospital medicine, particularly with the expansion of value-based medicine as discussed in a previous chapter. The COVID-19 pandemic has certainly been a catalyst in defining the expertise of hospital medicine both in the public and in the academic world. It will be incumbent for hospital medicine to take advantage of the current opportunities.

Hospital Medicine and Occupational Risk Related to COVID-19 Infection

Hospitalists were at the center of healthcare delivery during the COVID-19 pandemic. This included significant occupational risk. At the time of the publication, 48.2% of groups reported having lost provider time due to staff contracting COVID-19 [5].

All healthcare workers (HCW) have a high occupational risk related to COVID-19 infection. This was especially evident early in the pandemic among those on the frontlines. China, Italy, and other countries early in the pandemic reported significant risk to providers. This includes primary care, emergency room, and hospital-based physicians. The correct use and limited availability of PPE was a significant factor early on, as well as adopting correct infection control methods.

As the pandemic progressed, this risk to HCW was less evident. Morbidity and mortality among hospitalists from COVID-19 have not been specifically reported on, but as with many specialties, there have been anecdotal reports. Several studies with somewhat conflicting results have examined mortality among physician specialties as the pandemic has progressed. This has varied by region and time frame studied. The full toll that the pandemic has taken on HCW is significant but has not yet been defined, especially in comparison to the general public.

Physicians across the spectrum adopted early vaccinations. As of June 2021, more than 96% are fully vaccinated against COVID-19, with no significant difference in vaccination rates across regions, according to a survey from the American Medical Association [7].

In addition to the risk of COVID-19 infection, psychological stress became a significant side effect of the COVID-19 pandemic. Wellness became formalized in many programs. Retention of employees became major concern not only for physicians but among all clinical staff. Daily destressing rounds were instituted in many locations, as well as peer-driven mental health checkups. Several programs report that this will be a permanent part of their structure going forward [3].

COVID-19 and Telemedicine

In response to the COVID-19 pandemic, the Centers for Medicare & Medicaid Services (CMS), through its emergency authority, granted radical changes to its longstanding telehealth policies in 2019. Prior to COVID-19, telemedicine was slowly entering clinical medicine and to a lesser degree hospital medicine. These efforts were limited by infrastructure, billing limitations, and public acceptance. CMS previously limited telehealth to specific remote geographical locations and limited billable services. Many of the lifted restrictions remain in place at the time of this publication. Billing is comparable to in-patient services. As previously reviewed in a prior chapter in this text, this flexibility enabled groups to create new or expand existing virtual and telemedicine programs. Initially this enabled PPE to be preserved, capacity expanded, and allowed for more efficient workflows. As the pandemic has lessened in some areas, telehealth continued to be employed because it is cost saving and flexible.

After the first year of the pandemic, virtual appointments accounted for approximately 20% of all clinic and hospital-based appointments. Some, still under emergency practices, reported as high as 30%. The perecenatge of virtual appointments is expected to decline, but remain a significant component of clinical practice [6].

Telemedicine and digital health technology are becoming established parts of medical practice and are very likely to persist after the COVID-19 pandemic. Between mid-March and mid-October 2020, over 24.5 million patients (approximately 40% of all Medicare patients) had received a telemedicine service. As of June 2021, CMS is currently debating and requesting public input on the structure of future telehealth services. New guidelines are expected to continue to broadly support the use of telemedicine.

There are still obstacles for further growth including access to broadband, patient familiarity with technology, and future trends in reimbursement. The role of telemedicine in hospital medicine is even less certain as practice patterns normalize. This may seem as an attractive career choice for many providers. As with many innovations seen during the pandemic, some groups may permanently keep the service line while others may only enact it in emergent situations.

Malpractice

Overall, medical malpractice claims have been trending down among all medical specialties. Previous studies have shown that hospitalists had lower claim rates than office-based internal medicine physicians. However, these trends may be changing among hospitalists and heading in the wrong direction.

Hospitalists malpractice claims have remained roughly stable, as compared to other specialties which as noted have seen a decline. They are generally equal to office-based primary care physicians but statistically higher than medical specialties. Claims against hospitalists tend to be on the higher side due to severity of injuries, with a median indemnity payout of $231,000 [7]. Approximately one-third of claims against hospitalists resulted in a payout, a rate similar to other specialties. However, this was significantly lower than the payout rate for emergency physicians.

One possible explanation for the worsening picture may be the broadening scope of a hospitalist practice. Among other specialties, most commonly named as codefendants in hospitalist claims, are general surgery and orthopedics. To a lesser degree, nursing, emergency medicine, and cardiology were also reported. Co-management services among hospitalists have rapidly expanded in the past 10 years. Possibly too fast, without proper evaluation of where value is truly added.

The rapid expansion of hospital medicine as a whole may also play a role, with inexperienced physicians accepting new roles that they are not trained for. Often the newly hired physician is placed in a novel service. A potential solution may be to continue to define the collaborative agreement and roles among services as well as to provide formal onboarding. Further thought must be given to the scope of practice of hospitalists. The recent trend of unabridged expansion seems to have subsided, but it must be examined where hospitalist add true value and what can be done to limit liability exposure. It can be expected that co-management services will continue to be an area of increased liability and must be closely tracked and supported.

Two specific areas most often cited in claims are clinical judgment and communication errors. Improving clinical judgment of clinicians is a challenge. There is limited data supporting the use of electronic medical record support systems, but some have shown promise. A specific success story is the implementation of standardized sepsis protocols and alarm systems. Certainly this area will continue to evolve and will be an integral part of risk reduction moving forward.

Communication support systems, especially at crucial junctures such as hand-offs, are essential and have been reported to significantly reduce adverse events. Despite criticisms, the 7 day on, 7 day off shift model continues to be the norm. Variable models of staffing continue to put stress on communication systems. Hospital medicine will continue to have communication challenges that are among the most difficult among all medical fields.

Patient satisfaction of the physician was also reported to be a key component in those patients who ultimately filed a claim. Much of this is from retrospective studies. To be definitively determined is the impact of patient communication educational activities on reducing law suits.

Workplace Environment and Safety

There is the perception that workplace tension and violence are increasing in hospitals. This may mirror the increase in violence seen on airplanes, school bar meetings, and sports arenas. Possibly, the violence seen within the hospital is reflection of the mounting tensions outside them. National political anger is being manifested locally and is often incited by local regulations such as mask wearing and visitor restrictions. At the same time, patients with illicit narcotic use continue to pose a threat. In an industry already struggling with staffing issues, a fundamental issue in retention has become safety. Many healthcare employees have a fundamental question, "Will you keep me safe?" For many, already debating career choices, this has become the tipping point in deciding to exit the healthcare field.

Federal data reveals that 73% of all nonfatal injuries reported occurred in healthcare in 2018 [8]. It is yet to be seen if the COVID-19 pandemic has worsened this, but antidotal reports certainly suggest that it has. Many studies show that healthcare workers are more susceptible to aggravated assault than any other industry [9]. For frontline workers already exhausted by 18 months of disruption, workplace violence is often too much to bear. An additional pressure is decreased staffing levels. On typical shifts by provders, little time is available to deescalate patient issues.

Hospitalists are obviously at direct risk of workplace violence and must advocate not only for themselves but also for allied health staff and their patients. In the hospital, they are in a unique position of authority, physical presence, and responsibility. In addition to patient care, hospitalists have a unique understanding of the functioning of the hospital.

Hospitalists should recognize that they must be actively engaged in the safe functioning of the hospital at all levels, including a robust working relationship with security teams. It is important for the hospitalist to be actively engaged in these efforts and provide leadership when needed.

Ensuring hospital safety is a multifactorial task that requires input and solutions from a variety of viewpoints. The expertise of the hospitalist should be included in devleoping system wide safety protocols. No one group can provide all the services needed to ensure a safe working environment in the hospital. Mental health, clinical care, housekeeping, and physical plant services all play a part. In the past, much of this was left solely to security teams to manage. Current best practices suggest that all members of the care team should be engaged and successful initiatives have incorporated various members of the healthcare team.

References

1. Wachter RM, Goldman L. The emerging role of "hospitalists" in the American health care system. N Engl J Med. 1996;335(7):514–7. https://doi.org/10.1056/NEJM199608153350713. PMID: 8672160.
2. 2020 State of Hospital Medicine Report, Society of Hospital Medicine.
3. 2016 Medical Group Management Report, https://www.amga.org/amga/media/store/products/660342.pdf. Retrieved 15 July 2021.
4. Todays Hospitalist 2016 Hospital medicine Compensation Report, https://www.todayshospitalist.com/past-issues-7/. Retrieved 20 Aug 2021.
5. 2020 State of Hospital Medicine Report, Society of Hospital Medicine. COVID-19, Addendum.
6. Shannon EM, Chopra V, Greysen SR, Herzig SJ, Kripalani S, O'Leary KJ, Vasilevskis EE, Williams MV, Mueller SK, Auerbach AD, Schnipper JL. Dearth of hospitalist investigators in academic medicine: a call to action. J Hosp Med. 2021;3:189–91. https://doi.org/10.12788/jhm.3536. Published Online First February 17, 2021.
7. https://www.upi.com/Health_News/2021/06/15/coronavirus-vaccine-doctors-most-received-poll/9601623764459/. Retrieved 20 Oct 2021.
8. Schaffer AC, et al. Rates and characteristics of medical malpractice claims against hospitalists. J Hosp Med. 2021;16(7):390–6. https://doi.org/10.12788/jhm.3557.
9. https://www.osha.gov/healthcare/workplace-violence. Retrieved Aug 2021.

Index

A

Academic medicine
    AAMC, 280, 281
    black physicians, 277–279
    burnout, 286, 287
    diversity, equity, and inclusion, 277
    ethnic and racial minorities, 275, 276
    gender, 276, 277
        gender pay gap, 285, 286
        promotion rates, 283–285
    minority identities, 287, 288
    racial disparity, 276, 277
    underrepresented minorities, 282, 283
    women physicians, 279, 280
    women representation, 275, 276
    workforce diversity, 288, 289
Accountable Care Organizations (ACOs), 234, 235
Acetaminophen, 168
ACO investment model (AIM), 235
Acute ischemic stroke, 300
Acute kidney injury, 42–45
Acute pain management, 165
Acute respiratory distress syndrome (ARDS), 9, 81
Acute symptomatic psychosis, 144
Adenosine triphosphate (ATP) depletion, 24
Advance care planning (ACP)
    in America, 214
    barriers to, 215–216, 221–222
    benefits and purpose of, 213–214
    definition, 213
    hospital medicine, 215
    identified barriers, 218–220
    Ochsner Health, 216, 217
Affordable Care Act (ACA), 230, 231
Agency for Healthcare Research and Quality (AHRQ) guidelines, 232, 250–251
Allopathic medicine, 331
Alpha variant, 3
American Board of Medical Specialties (ABMS), 119
Aminoglycosides, 183
Amphotericin, 183
Angiotensin converting enzyme inhibitors (ACEi), 47
Angiotensin-converting enzyme 2 (ACE2), 3
Antibody therapy, 7
Anticonvulsant agents, 169
Antimicrobial resistance (AMR), 78
Association of American Medical Colleges (AAMC), 280, 281
Atrial natriuretic peptide (ANP), 50
Autism, 142

B

Bamlanivimab, 7
Baricitinib, 7, 8
Behavioral management, 163
Beta variant, 3
BiliTool™, 124
Bioelectrical impedance analysis (BIA), 50
Blood urea nitrogen (BUN), 42
Bowman's capsule, 52
Brain disease model of addiction, 154–156

Brain natriuretic peptide (BNP), 50
Breast cancer, 266, 267
Bronchiolitis, 120, 121
Bundled payment systems, 235, 236
Buprenorphine, 174, 175
Burnout, 286, 287

C
Campylobacteri jejuni, 25
Canagliflozin (Invokana®), 52, 53
Canagliflozin cardiovascular assessment study (CANVAS), 53
Canagliflozin/metformin (Invokamet®), 52
Carbon footprint, 317
Cardiovascular disease (CVD), 66, 266
Cefoxitin, 31
Central pain syndromes, 160
Cerebral endotheliopathy, 92
Cerebral vascular accident (CVA), 162
Chest X-ray, 64
Chief wellness officer (CWO), 251
Chloroquine, 6
Chronic kidney disease (CKD), 41
Chronic obstructive pulmonary disease (COPD), 182
Chronic opioids, 153
Chronic pain, 165
Climate change, 312
Cognitive behavioral therapy (CBT), 12
Commonwealth Fund, 317
Community health, 326
Complex regional pain syndrome, 160
Computed tomography enterography (CTE), 29
Coping mechanisms, 248, 249
Coronary artery disease (CAD), 181
Coronavirus disease 2019 (COVID-19), 1, 80, 179, 243, 270, 271, 288, 298, 321, 324, 332, 333
    admission criteria, 4–5
    antenatal care, 13–17
    career satisfaction, 342, 343
    clinic-based physician, 340
    compensation, 340, 341
    delta variant, 3
    epidemiology, 2
    hospital safety, 346, 347
    length of stay, 339
    malpractice, 345, 346
    management
        antibody therapy, 7
        baricitinib, 7, 8
        complications, 9–10
        dexamethasone, 6
        discharge from hospital, 10
        general therapy guidelines, 5–6
        remdesivir, 6
        systemic glucocorticoids, 6
        treatment of coinfections, 8–9
        vaccination, 10
    occupational risk, 343, 344
    performance metrics, 341
    pregnancy issues, 13–17
    psychiatric complications, 11–13
    readmission reduction, 339
    symptoms, 4
    telemedicine, 344, 345
    value based care, 339
    virology, 3
    workplace environment, 346
COVID-19-associated nephropathy (COVAN), 46
COX-2 inhibitors (COXIBs), 168
C-reactive protein (CRP), 28
Crohn's disease (CD), 23
Crohn's disease activity index (CDAI), 27
Cultural competence, 329, 330
Cytomegalovirus (CMV), 29

D
Dapagliflozin (Farxiga®), 52
Dapagliflozin/metformin (Xigduo XR®), 52
Deep vein thrombosis (DVT) prophylaxis, 100–101
Delirium, 131, 184
Delta variant, 3
Delusions, 141
Dexamethasone, 6, 45
Diabetes mellitus (DM), 186, 266
Diabetic ketoacidosis, 9
Diabetic kidney disease (DKD), 51
Digital health technology, 344
Direct oral anticoagulants (DOACs), 185
Diversity, equity, and inclusion (DEI), 283
Doctors without borders, 323

E
Echocardiography, 64
Electrocardiogram (EKG), 137
Electroencephalogram (EEG), 144
Electrolyte abnormalities, 46–48
Empagliflozin (Jardiance®), 52
Empagliflozin/linagliptin (Glyxambi®), 52
Empagliflozin/metformin (Synjardy®), 52
Endocrine, 186–187
End-stage renal disease (ESRD), 41

Enhanced recovery after surgery (ERAS) protocols, 189
Epstein-Barr virus (EBV), 29
Ertapenem, 31
Escherichia coli, 122
Estimated GFR (eGFR), 53
Euglycemic diabetic ketoacidosis (DKA), 53
Evidence-based medicine, 331
    black-box warning, 298–300
    clinical practice, 294
    clot retrieval protocols
        composition prediction, 303
        history, 301, 302
        management, 302
        secondary embolism, 303
        standard of care, 301
    domains, 294
    pulmonary embolism, 295–297
    robotic surgery
        applications, 305, 306
        evolution, 304
        peri-operative care, 304, 305

F
Focal segmental glomerulosclerosis (FSGS), 46

G
Gamma variant, 3
Gender, 256
Global health
    access to healthcare, 328, 329
    alternative medicine and religion, 330–332
    COVID-19, 332, 333
    cultural competence, 329, 330
    economies, 327, 328
    evolution, 322–325
    healthcare, 327, 328
    life expectancy, 321, 326, 327
    models of care, 321
    mortality, 326, 327
    reverse innovation, 328, 329
    social determinants of health, 325, 326
Group B *Streptococcus* (GBS), 122
Guideline directed medical therapy (GDMT), 65
Gulf Cooperation Council (GCC), 327

H
Hallucinations, 141
Harvey-Bradshaw Index (HBI), 27
Health care organizations (HCOs), 251
Health Maintenance Organization (HMO) Act, 229
Healthcare Without Harm, 318
Healthcare workers (HCW), 343
Heart failure (HF)
    advancements in management, 66–67
    barriers to health care, 67
    biomarkers, 64
    blood tests, 64–65
    chest X-ray, 64
    clinical presentation, 62
    echocardiography, 64
    epidemiology, 59–60
    GDMT, 65
    history, 62, 63
    pathophysiology, 60–62
    physical exam, 63
Hemorrhagic strokes, 86
Hepatojugular reflex, 63
High quality health systems (HQSS), 325
Hospital Readmissions Reductions Program (HRRP), 231, 237
Hospital shopping, 163
Hospital value based purchasing (VBP) program, 236, 237
Hydroxychloroquine, 6
Hyperkalemia, 46
Hypofrontality, 155
Hyponatremia, 48–51

I
Implicit bias, 280, 281
Inferior vena cava (IVC) collapse index, 51
Inflammatory bowel disease (IBD)
    causing factors, 24–25
    Crohn's disease
        cardinal symptoms, 26
        enteritis, 26
        evaluation of, 28–29
        fistulas, 26
        intrabdominal abscesses, 31
        management for, 29–31
        percutaneous *vs.* surgical drainage, 31–32
        severity of, 27–28
        structural issues, 32–33
    flare/worsen existing symptoms, 24
    ulcerative colitis
        evaluation of, 34–35
        management of, 35–37
        severity of, 34
Internal carotid artery (ICA), 86
Intrabdominal abscesses (IAA), 31

Intracerebral hemorrhage (ICH), 86
Ischemic strokes, 86
IV methylprednisolone (IVMP), 35
IV of hydrocortisone (IVHC), 35

K
Kaiser permanente, 313, 314
Kawasaki disease, 4
Kawasaki-like symptoms, 4
Kayexalate, 47
Kidney disease improving global outcome (KDIGO), 42

L
Lancet commissions, 325
Lesbian, gay, and bisexual (LGB) care, 262
LGBTQ+
    anti-androgens, 260, 261
    definitions, 255, 256
    environment, 257, 258
    epidemiology, 255–257
    estrogen, 260
    forms and documentation, 258
    gender-affirming care, 259
    health care, 255–257
    hormone therapy, 259
    introduction, 258
    LGB care, 262
    medical education, 262, 263
    medical history, 259
    testosterone, 261
    vocabulary use, 259
Liposomal bupivacaine, 169
Lokelma, 48
Low molecular weight heparin (LMWH), 185

M
Magnesium, 89
Magnetic resonance enterography (MRE), 29
Médecins Sans Frontières (MSF), 323
Medicaid, 229
Medical missions, 322, 323
Medicare, 229
Medication assisted therapy (MAT), 163, 172–175
Metabolic abnormalities, 142
Metabolic syndrome, 145
Methadone, 174
Microaggressions, 282, 283

Middle cerebral artery (MCA), 86
Middle East respiratory syndrome (MERS), 11
Minority tax, 283
Morphinism, 151
Moxifloxacin, 31
mRNA vaccines, 10, 11
Multimodal analgesic (MMA) model, 110
Multiple organ dysfunction score (MODS), 81
Multisystem inflammatory syndrome in children (MIS-C), 124–127
Musculoskeletal system, 102
Music therapy, 209

N
National Institute of Health (NIH), 5
Neonatal hyperbilirubinemia, 123–124
Neonatal sepsis, 121–123
Nephrology
    acute kidney injury, 42–45
    COVID-19, 45
    dapagliflozin (Farxiga), 52
    electrolyte abnormalities, 46–48
    hyponatremia, 48–51
    SGLT2 inhibitors, 51–53
    urine output, 42
Nerinetide, 89
Neuraxial anesthesia, 16
Neuroprotection, 89
Nicotine replacement therapy (NRT), 188
N-methyl-D-aspartate receptor (NMDA) antagonists, 89, 169
Non-invasive positive pressure ventilation (NIPPV), 9
Nonopioid analgesic therapies, 166
Non-pharmacologic approaches, 171
Non-steroidal anti-inflammatory drugs (NSAIDs), 110, 111, 168, 183

O
Obsessive compulsive disorder (OCD), 142
Ochsner health system, 196–198, 216, 217
Ochsner's protocol, 126
Opioid epidemic
    brain disease model of addiction, 154–156
    cardinal features of, 154
    central pain syndromes, 160
    chronic pain, 160
    complex regional pain syndrome, 160
    fear and anxiety, 161
    MAT, 173–175

Index 353

multimodal therapy
  class of, 168, 169
  compassionate withdrawal, 170–173
  DSM-5 opioid use disorder, 173
  opioid dependence, 172
  timeline of withdrawal, 171–172
non-addictive, 153
opioid stewardship, 161–168
opioid withdrawal, 161
pain matrix, 156–158
shared neural networks, 158–160
Opioid-induced hyperalgesia, 160
Opioid maintenance therapy, 152
Opioid stewardship, 161–168
Opioid-withdrawal hypersensitivity, 168
Orthopedic co-management
  blending, 114–115
  chronic medical comorbidities, 100
  co-management program, 102
  consulting, 113
  daily acute post-operative complications, 100
  discharge disposition, 105–106
  hospital length of stay, 104
  hospital medications, 112
  ICU admissions, 111–112
  mortality rate, 105
  orthopedic patients, 102–103
  pain management, 108–111
  readmission rate, 106
  roles, 100–102
  satisfaction, 107–108
  surgical complications, 113, 114
  total cost of care, 107
  value-based healthcare setting, 100
Orthopedic-geriatric service, 99
Orthostatic hypotension, 145
OxyContin, 153

P

Pain catastrophizing behavior, 157
Pain matrix, 156–158
Palliative care
  communication, 203–207
  interdisciplinary approach, 201
  music therapy, 209
  pain and symptom management, 202
  telemedicine in, 204–208
  virtual reality, 208
Patient centered medical home (PCMH) model, 233
Patiromer, 48
Pediatric hospital medicine (PHM)
  bronchiolitis, 120, 121
  evidence-based tools and protocols, 119
  MIS-C, 124–127
  neonatal hyperbilirubinemia, 123–124
  neonatal sepsis, 121–123
Perioperative care
  advanced care planning, 189
  anticoagulation, 185–186
  assessment and plan, 180–181
  CAD, 181
  clinic medical evaluation, 180–181
  connective tissue disease, 187
  COPD, 182
  COVID-19 pandemic, 189
  definition, 180
  delirium, 184
  endocrine, 186–187
  ERAS protocols, 189
  frailty, 185
  hematological conditions, 185–186
  informed consent, 189
  laboratory investigations, 188
  liver disease, 184
  medication history, 188
  postoperative complications, 182
  renal disease, 183–184
  risk assessment process, 180
  surgical site infections, 187
Perioperative surgical home (PSH), 189
Personal protective equipment (PPE), 246
Physicians wellness
  AHRQ guidelines, 250
  burnout, 245–246
  coping mechanisms, 248, 249
  COVID-19 infections, 244
  first year of pandemic, 244–245
  historical perspective, 247–248
  mental health, 244
  system level promotion, 249
  system-level interventions, 251
Polymerase chain reaction (PCR), 80
Post traumatic stress disorder (PTSD), 142
Post-stroke depression (PSD), 93
Post-traumatic stress disorder (PTSD), 12
Potassium sparing diuretics, 47
Poverty, 269
Preferred Provider Organizations (PPOs), 230
Primary health center (PHCs), 328

Pro-brain natriuretic peptide (pro-BNP), 50
Psychiatric disorders
   delirium
      assessment, 136–137
      diagnostic criteria, 134–135
      epidemiology of, 132, 133
      etiology, 132
      management, 137–138
      prevention, 139
      risk factors, 133–134
      select medications, 134
      subtypes, 135–136
   psychosis
      bipolar personality disorder, 139
      clinical manifestations, 141–142
      differential diagnosis, 142–143
      epidemiology, 140–141
      management, 144–146
      preliminary medical workup, 143, 144
Psychosis, 131
Pulmonary capillary wedge pressure (PCWP), 63
Pulmonary embolism, 295–297
Pulmonary embolism rule-out criteria (PERC), 296, 297
Pulsus alternans, 63

Q
QT prolongation, 145

R
Racial disparities
   analgesia, 267
   breast cancer, 266, 267
   cardiovascular disease, 266
   COVID-19, 270, 271
   cultural exposure, 271
   diabetes mellitus, 266
   health insurance coverage, 268, 269
   healthcare providers, 268
   HIV/AIDS, 267
   income and life expectancy, 269
   maternal health and pregnancy, 270
   minority groups, 265
   poverty, 269
   Veteran's Health Administration, 266
Radio contrast agents, 183
Regional anesthesia, 169
Rehabilitation therapy, 94
Remdesivir, 6, 45
Respiratory depression, 162
Robotic surgery
   applications, 305, 306
   evolution, 304
   peri-operative care, 304, 305

S
Schizophrenia, 141
Selective serotonin reuptake inhibitor (SSRI), 168
Sepsis and shock
   antimicrobial stewardship, 78–80
   and COVID 19, 80–81
   definition, 71, 72
   1-hour bundle, 77
   practice statements, 72–76
   recommendations, 72–76
   SOFA score, 72
Serotonin-norepinephrine reuptake inhibitor (SNRI), 168
Severe acute kidney injuries (AKI), 9
Severe acute respiratory syndrome (SARS-CoV-1) virus, 3, 11
Severe acute respiratory syndrome coronavirus 2 (SARS-CoV-2), 1
Sexual orientation, 256
Shigella flexneri, 25
Social determinants of health, 256, 257
Society of Hospital Medicine (SHM), 104, 215
Sodium-glucose cotransporters (SGLTs), 51
Sodium glucose transport inhibitors (SGLTi), 51
Solar energy, 313
Sotrovimab, 7
STEGHs, 323, 324
Stroke management
   COVID-19, 91, 92
   epidemiology of, 85–86
   hemorrhagic strokes, 86
   ischemic stroke management
      collateral blood flow, 88–89
      intravenous thrombolysis, 87
      IV thrombolysis guidelines, 87
      mechanical thrombectomy, 87
      mechanical thrombectomy guidelines, 87–88
      neuroprotection, 89
      non-contrast CT, 86
   ischemic strokes, 86

post-stroke care, 94–95
post-stroke depression, 93
and women, 90
Structural racism, 281
Subarachnoid hemorrhage (SAH), 86
Suboxone, 174
Substance use disorder (SUD), 163
Sustainability
    Boston Green Ribbon Healthcare Working Group, 315, 316
    Cleveland Clinic, 316, 317
    climate change, 311
    healthcare guidelines, 312
    healthcare providers, 312
    Kaiser Permanente, 313, 314
    medical industry, 312
    Practice Greenhealth, 317, 318
    startup costs, 312
Sustainable healthcare, 312
Systemic glucocorticoids, 6
Systemic inflammatory response syndrome (SIRS), 71

T
Telehospitalist, 196
Telemedicine, 195, 344, 345
Tigecycline, 31
Tissue plasminogen activator (tPA), 195
Tofacitinib, 37
Toxic shock syndrome, 4
Tramadol, 168
Transcutaneous electrical stimulation (TENS), 110
Transgender, 256
Transmasculine, 256
Transthoracic echocardiograms (TTE), 9

U
Ulcerative colitis (UC), 23
Urinary tract infection (UTI), 113

V
Vaccination, 10
Value based care
    ACA, 230, 231
    ACOs, 234, 235
    AHRQ, 232
    bundled payment systems, 235, 236
    definition, 225
    economic principle, 231
    education, 237–238
    employer-based commercial health insurance, 228
    health insurance, 227–228
    healthcare quality, 226
    HMO plan, 229
    medicare and medicaid, 228–229
    multi-part process, 226
    national healthcare system, 230
    PCMHs model, 233
    referenced indicators, 226
    socioeconomic factors, 226
    transition healthcare, 232
    in United States, 227
    VBP program, 236, 237
Vedolizumab, 37
Venous thromboembolism (VTE), 10
Veterans health administration (VHA), 196
Virtual hospital medicine
    COVID-19 pandemic, 196
    inpatient telehealth, 195
    Ochsner health system, 196–198
    Ochsner's "telemedicine champions," 198
Virtual hospital medicine (VHM), 195
Virtual reality (VR), 208, 304
VITALtalk communication resource, 202
VOCAL-Penn variables, 184

W
Well's criteria, 295, 296
White fragility, 281

9783030951634